Small Animal Oncology

Small Animal Oncology

Joanna Morris

*Formerly of Department of Clinical Veterinary Medicine,
University of Cambridge Veterinary School*

and

Jane Dobson

*Department of Clinical Veterinary Medicine,
University of Cambridge Veterinary School*

b

Blackwell
Science

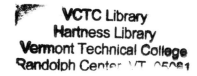

© 2001
Blackwell Science Ltd
Editorial Offices:
Osney Mead, Oxford OX2 0EL
25 John Street, London WC1N 2BS
23 Ainslie Place, Edinburgh EH3 6AJ
350 Main Street, Malden
  MA 02148 5018, USA
54 University Street, Carlton
  Victoria 3053, Australia
10, rue Casimir Delavigne
  75006 Paris, France

Other Editorial Offices:

Blackwell Wissenschafts-Verlag GmbH
Kurfürstendamm 57
10707 Berlin, Germany

Blackwell Science KK
MG Kodenmacho Building
7–10 Kodenmacho Nihombashi
Chuo-ku, Tokyo 104, Japan

Iowa State University Press
A Blackwell Science Company
2121 S. State Avenue
Ames, Iowa 50014-8300, USA

First published 2001

Set in 9.5 on 11.5 pt Times
by Best-set Typesetter Ltd., Hong Kong
Printed and bound in Great Britain at
the Alder Press Ltd, Oxford and Northampton

The Blackwell Science logo is a
trade mark of Blackwell Science Ltd,
registered at the United Kingdom
Trade Marks Registry

DISTRIBUTORS
Marston Book Services Ltd
PO Box 269
Abingdon
Oxon OX14 4YN
(*Orders*: Tel: 01235 465500
            Fax: 01235 465555)

USA and Canada
Iowa State University Press
A Blackwell Science Company
2121 S. State Avenue
Ames, Iowa 50014-8300
(*Orders*: Tel: 800-862-6657
            Fax: 515-292-3348
            Web www.isupress.com
            email:orders@isupress.com)

Australia
Blackwell Science Pty Ltd
54 University Street
Carlton, Victoria 3053
(*Orders*: Tel: 03 9347 0300
            Fax: 03 9347 5001)

A catalogue record for this title
is available from the British Library

ISBN 0-632-05282-1

Library of Congress
Cataloging-in-Publication Data
Morris, Joanna.
   Small animal oncology/Joanna Morris and Jane
   Dobson.
      p. cm.
   Includes bibliographical references (p.).
   ISNB 0-632-05282-1 (pb)
   1. Dogs – Diseases.   2. Cats – Diseases.
   3. Veterinary oncology.   I. Dobson, Jane M.
   II. Title.

SF992.C35 M65 2000
636.089′6992 – dc21   00-058599

For further information on
Blackwell Science, visit our website:
www.blackwell-science.com

Contents

Please note: the plate section falls between pp. 162 and 163

Acknowledgements

The authors gratefully acknowledge the help and support of friends, families and colleagues in the writing and production of this book.

In particular we would like to thank David Bostock, Phil Nicholls, Elizabeth Villiers, Kathleen Tennant, Andy Jefferies, Mike Herrtage, Malcolm Brearley, Ruth Dennis, Dick White and the Radiology Department, Queens Veterinary School Hospital, Cambridge, for contributing many of the pictures used to illustrate the text. We should also acknowledge the artistic skills of John Fuller who was responsible for the original line drawings reproduced in this book.

We are also grateful to Dr Davina Anderson for her help in reading the text and advice on surgical matters, Malcolm Brearley for his help with Chapter 13, Nervous System, Dr David Williams, Chapter 16, on the eye, and Mike Herrtage, Chapter 14, Endocrine System.

DISCLAIMER

The authors have made every effort to ensure that therapeutic recommendations particularly concerning drug selection and dosage set out in the text are in accord with current recommendations and practice. However, in view of ongoing research, changes in government regulations and the constant flow of information relating to drug therapy and drug reactions, the reader is urged to check the drug manufacturer's instructions for any added warnings and precautions.

The cytotoxic drugs detailed in this book are not licensed for veterinary use. All of these agents are potentially hazardous to the patient and to persons handling or administering them. Veterinary surgeons who prescribe such drugs to patients in their care must assume responsibility for their use and safe handling. Veterinary surgeons who are not familiar with the use of cytotoxic agents should seek further information and advice from a veterinary oncologist.

Introduction

Neoplasia is a common problem in small animal veterinary practice. As facilities in general practices improve and more investigations are conducted into the cause of dog and cat illnesses, it is being increasingly diagnosed. Although accurate figures on the incidence of tumours in cats and dogs are lacking, conservative estimates suggest that one in ten cats or dogs will develop a tumour during their natural life. A few epidemiological studies on small animal cancer do exist but most of these refer to dogs. In the USA, a post mortem study on 2000 dogs revealed that cancer was the most common cause of death, with 23% of animals dying from the disease (Bronson 1982). In a more recent study based on questionnaire responses in the UK, 16% of dogs died from cancer (Michell 1999). Cancer was the most frequently recognised cause of death in both male and female dogs, but in neutered males heart disease was of equal importance.

Another recently conducted study on the incidence of tumours in a population of insured dogs in the UK has provided up-to-date information on the distribution of tumour types (Samuel *et al.* 1999). The skin and soft tissues were found to be the most common sites for tumour development, followed by mammary gland, haematopoietic tissues (including lymphoid), urogenital system, endocrine organs, alimentary system and oropharynx (Fig. I.1). These results are similar to those reported by Dorn and others (Dorn *et al.* 1968a, b) in California who used diagnosis of neoplasia in veterinary practices in specified areas of the country combined with histological examination in a central laboratory and a probability survey to calculate the population at risk. The skin, mammary gland and haematopoietic tissues were the three most common sites for cancer in this study. In the UK study, the three most common tumour types were benign. Canine cutaneous histiocytoma predominated, followed by lipoma and adenoma. Mast cell tumour and lymphoma were the next most common tumour types (Fig. I.2).

Comparable up-to-date epidemiological figures are not available for cats in the UK. In other surveys, lymphoma and other haematopoietic tumours are the most common tumour types and are much more frequent than in the dog. Although skin and soft tissue tumours are important in the cat, malignant neoplasms such as squamous cell carcinoma and soft tissue sarcoma are probably more frequent than benign lesions. Mammary tumours are less frequent in the cat, but a greater proportion are malignant.

The demand for treatment of pets with cancer is increasing and seems likely to do so for the foreseeable future as more animals become insured and their treatment costs are covered. Conventional methods for cancer therapy in animals, as in humans, are surgery, radiotherapy and chemotherapy. These techniques, however, need not be used in isolation. Indeed, as our understanding of the biology of cancer has increased, it has become clear that combining surgical management of a primary mass with chemotherapy directed at systemic disease, is the most logical and potentially effective way of managing malignant tumours. Fears of the side-effects associated with cancer treatment in pet animals are not well founded since most are drawn from comparisons with human cancer therapy where the aim of treatment is to prolong life at all costs. The management of animal cancer also seeks to prolong lifespan but aims to

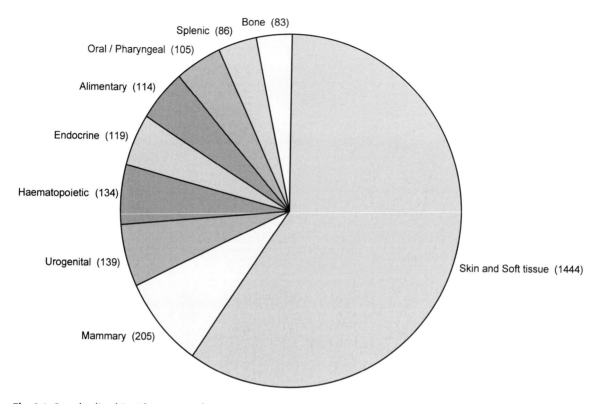

Fig. I.1 Standardised incidence rates for main tumour sites (per 100 000 dogs/year).

achieve a good quality of life as well. All treatment modalities are adjusted to achieve this aim and if any patient is deemed to be suffering, treatment can be stopped or the animal euthanased.

The purpose of this book is to provide a basic clinical approach to the diagnosis and treatment of the more common tumours in cats and dogs for the practising veterinary surgeon, undergraduate student and veterinary nurse. It is not intended to be a comprehensive reference textbook, covering all aspects of veterinary oncology, since several such texts exist (see general reading list in Appendix I). Rather it seeks to provide a core of basic, easily accessible and clinically relevant information on general aspects of veterinary oncology.

The first three chapters present general background information on pathogenesis, tumour biology, managing the cancer patient and the most frequently used methods of treatment. Surgical approaches and instructions are not given since this information is best sought from specific surgical texts or, if particularly specialised, should be carried out by a referral centre. Practical details of chemotherapy and guidance on safety, however, are given, since an increasing number of general practices are using cytotoxic drugs and it is essential that stringent handling practice is adhered to. Again, more detailed texts exist and specialist help is available at a referral centre. Although, at present, Cambridge University has the only radiotherapy unit in the UK dedicated to small animal use, radiotherapy is covered in some detail since it is helpful for general practitioners to be aware of the aims of treatment and the tumour types which are suitable for referral.

The remaining chapters provide specific information on the epidemiology, aetiology, pathology, presentation, staging, management and prognosis for tumours occurring in the different body systems. These specific sub-headings are used in each of the system chapters to enable the reader to find the relevant information more easily. Chapters are minimally referenced using large case series or reviews where possible.

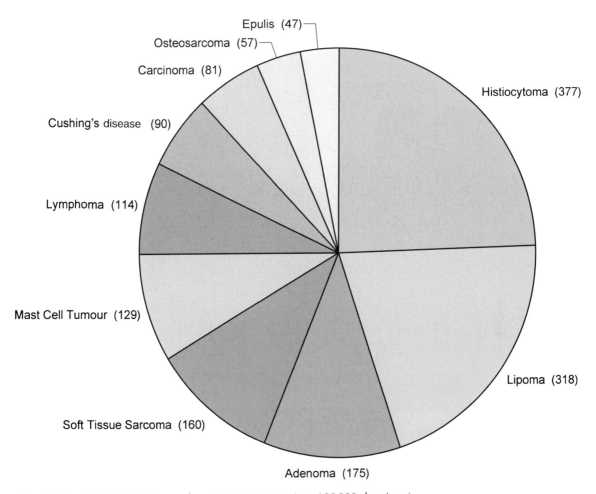

Fig. I.2 Standardised incidence of main tumour types (per 100 000 dogs/year).

References

Bronson, R.T. (1982) Variation in age at death of dogs of different sexes and breeds. *American Journal of Veterinary Research*, (43), 2057–9.

Dorn, C.R., Taylor, D.O.N., Frye, F.L. & Hibbard, H.H. (1968a) Survey of animal neoplasms in Alameda and Contra Costa counties, California. I Methodology and description of cases. *Journal of the National Cancer Institute*, (40), 295–305.

Dorn, C.R., Taylor, D.O.N., Schneider, R., Hibbard, H.H. & Klauber, M.R. (1968b) Survey of animal neoplasms in Alameda and Contra Costa counties, California. II Cancer morbidity in dogs and cats from Alameda County. *Journal of the National Cancer Institute*, (40), 307–18.

Michell, A.R. (1999) Longevity of British breeds of dog and its relationships with sex, size, cardiovascular variables and disease. *Veterinary Record*, (145), 625–9.

Samuel, S., Milstein, H., Dobson, J.M. & Wood, J.L.N. (1999) An epidemiological study into the incidence of neoplasia in a population of insured dogs in the UK. *Proceedings of the British Small Animal Veterinary Association Congress*.

1
Pathogenesis and Tumour Biology

PATHOGENESIS

What is cancer?

Neoplasms are abnormal 'new growths' of tissue which develop faster than adjacent normal tissues and in an uncoordinated, persistent manner. They may be benign or malignant but the term 'cancer' is generally restricted to the malignant growths. Neoplastic cells differ from normal cells in that they show:

• Uncontrolled proliferation which is independent of the requirement for new cells
• Impaired cellular differentiation
• Altered cell communication and adhesion.

What causes cancer?

Cancer development is a multistep process which involves an accumulation of changes or 'errors' in cellular DNA. The steps that lead to neoplastic transformation of a cell are not fully understood but the fundamental change involves disruption of the genes which control cell growth and differentiation. Specific genes may either:

• Be activated (known as oncogenes); or
• Be inactivated (known as tumour suppressor genes); or
• Have their level of expression altered.

Sometimes oncogenes or tumour suppressor genes may be altered indirectly by genetic changes occurring in DNA repair genes. These fail to carry out their normal repair function, causing abnormal sections of DNA to accumulate, some of which may be in important for cell growth.

The transition from a normal growth-controlled cell to a malignant cancer cell requires several mutations. Research on human colon cancer shows that the progression of the disease from benign adenoma (polyp) to invasive carcinoma is paralleled by an increase in the number of genes, predominantly tumour suppressor genes, which are mutated. At least four or five mutated genes are needed for carcinoma development but fewer changes are required for adenomas. Similarly, as human gliomas increase in histopathological grade and become more aggressive, the number of mutated genes increases from 2 to 3 (grade II) to 6 to 8 (grade IV). In both examples, it is the total number of accumulated mutated genes that is paramount and not the order in which they occur.

Genetic changes may occur in germ line cells and therefore be present in all cells of the body at birth, or much more commonly, they may occur spontaneously in somatic cells as part of the ageing process. The accumulation of spontaneous mutations occurs quite slowly but often external risk factors speed up the rate of accumulation. Cancer development can therefore be discussed under the following headings:

- Spontaneous genetic events
- External stimuli
  - biological (viruses, parasites, hormones)
  - physical (UV light, radiation, trauma)
  - chemical
- Inherited genetic events (familial cancers).

Spontaneous genetic events

The majority of cancers result from spontaneous genetic events and these can occur at either the chromosomal or molecular level. Although spontaneous cancer is usually associated with older animals because of the time needed to accumulate genetic changes, there are some exceptions which affect young animals, for example canine cutaneous histiocytoma, some types of feline lymphoma and some anaplastic sarcomas.

Molecular changes

As cells divide and their DNA replicates, errors which alter the DNA may occur. Usually, DNA repair mechanisms act very effectively to correct the errors, but as an individual ages, more events escape the repair mechanisms and permanent DNA changes accumulate. The multistep accumulation of these changes leads to cell transformation and the development of a cancer cell. Although the key changes occur within the DNA sequence, additional changes may also occur in the conversion of DNA to mRNA (transcription) or the synthesis of proteins (translation).

Changes which affect gene function include:

- Point mutation – loss or substitution of one base for another in the DNA helix, thus coding for a different amino acid or none at all.
- Small or large deletion – loss of a few or several

hundred base pairs, thus altering the gene product or stopping its production.
- Amplification – repetition of sections of DNA, perhaps increasing the number of copies of part or all of a gene, although not necessarily increasing its level of expression.

The protein product coded from the DNA may be altered by one amino acid, truncated, overexpressed or not expressed at all. Only isolated reports of mutations in dog and cat genes have appeared in the literature in the last decade (Table 1.1). However, this area of research in pet animals is expanding rapidly and knowledge of the molecular changes in animal cancers will probably increase very quickly in the next five or ten years. There is often conservation of genes between species allowing some of the probes which have been developed for human or other animal reasearch to be used for canine and feline work (Miyoshi *et al.* 1991a, b; Momoi *et al.* 1993). Recently, there has been much interest in the tumour suppressor gene p53 which codes for a protein of molecular mass 53 kilodaltons, and which plays a key role in the carcinogenesis of many human tumours. It has been shown to be mutated in a number of canine and feline tumours (Table 1.1).

Chromosomal changes

Changes in cellular DNA can also be brought about by gross chromosomal changes which may be either numerical or structural. Losses or gains of whole chromosomes alter the total DNA content of a cell and the number of copies of the genes present on those chromosomes. This may either reduce or amplify the level of expression of a particular gene within the cell. Alterations to chromosome structure such as deletions, insertions, inversions, translocations or local amplifications may also occur, affecting the function of genes located at the altered regions of the chromosome. Many such changes are well documented in human cancers. Specific reciprocal translocations have been identified in several types of human leukaemia and non-Hodgkin's lymphoma and more recently in some types of human sarcoma (Rabbitts 1994; Look 1995). The translocations bring together genes from different chromosomes, resulting in a new fusion gene(s) and therefore a new fusion protein(s).

Table 1.1 Molecular changes in dog and cat tumours.

Altered gene	Species	Tumour types	Reference
p53	Dog	Osteosarcoma Squamous cell carcinoma Nasal adenocarcinoma Peri-anal gland adenocarcinoma Mammary adenoma/carcinoma Lymphoma	Sagartz *et al.* 1996 Gamblin *et al.* 1997 Mayr *et al.* 1998a, 1999 Veldhoen *et al.* 1999 Nasir & Argyle 1999
p53	Cat	Mammary carcinoma Osteosarcoma Fibrosarcoma Spindle cell sarcoma Pleomorphic sarcoma	Mayr *et al.* 1998b, c
K-ras	Dog	Lung carcinoma	Kraegel *et al.* 1992
N-ras	Dog	Acute non-lymphocytic leukaemia	Gumerlock *et al.* 1989
yes-1	Dog	Mammary and other tumours	Miyoshi *et al.* 1991b Rungsipipat *et al.* 1999
myc	Dog Cat	Plasma cell tumours Lymphoma	Frazier *et al.* 1993 Neil *et al.* 1984

Table 1.2 Chromosome translocations in human tumours.

Tumour/disease	Translocation	Genes affected
Acute T cell leukaemia	t(8;14)	TCRα and MYC
Acute promyelocytic leukaemia	t(15;17)	RAR and PML
Chronic myeloid leukaemia	t(9;22)	BCR and ABL
Burkitt's lymphoma	t(8;14)	IgH and MYC
	t(2;8)	IgL kappa and MYC
	t(8;22)	IgL lambda and MYC
Follicular lymphoma	t(14;18)	IgH and BCL1
	t(11;14)	IgH and BCL2
Alveolar rhabdomyosarcoma	t(1;13)	FKHR and PAX7
	t(2;13)	FKHR and PAX3
Synovial sarcoma	t(X;18)	SYT and SSX
Ewing's sarcoma	t(11;22)	EWS and FLI-1,
	t(21;22)	EWS and ERG
	t(7;22)	EWS and ETV-1
Liposarcoma	t(12;16)	FUS and CHOP

Alternatively, they may bring genes at the breakpoints close to different regulatory elements which result in altered gene expression. Examples of such translocations are given in Table 1.2. In contrast to the situation with haematopoietic tumours, few translocations have yet been identified for the majority of human solid tumours since they usually have very complex chromosome rearrangements which are difficult to interpret using conventional Giemsa-banding techniques.

Structural and numerical chromosome changes have been reported in dog and cat tumours but the literature is still relatively sparse (Grindem & Bouen 1986; Hahn *et al.* 1994; Mayr *et al.* 1994; Mayr *et al.* 1998a,d; Reimann *et al.* 1998). A common observation in dog tumours is a reduction in the total number of chromosomes due to the formation of large metacentric chromosomes, probably generated by centric or telomeric fusion (Reimann *et al.* 1994). Although the cat has 36 chromosomes which are reasonably easy to identify using conventional banding techniques, the dog has 78 chromosomes, most of which are very similar in appearance and there is still no agreed Giemsa-banding standard for chromosomes 22–36 with which to refer (Switonski *et al.* 1996). A banded karyotype using the fluorescent dye DAPI has recently been published, however, and this will facilitate the identification of canine chromosomes viewed under a fluorescence microscope (Breen *et al.* 1999). Whole chromosome-specific fluorescence *in situ* (FISH) probes known as 'chromosome paints' (Fig. 1.1) have also been developed for the

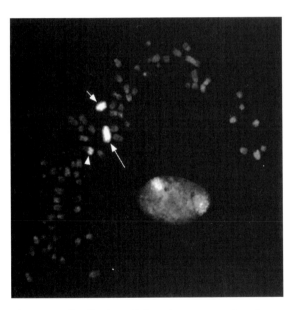

Fig. 1.1 Hybridisation of dog chromosome 1 paint to a metaphase from a canine sarcoma. Chromosome 1 paint is labelled with the fluorescent dye Cy3 (pink) and the other chromosomes are counterstained with DAPI (blue). One normal copy of chromosome 1 (large arrow) is present in the metaphase, but the other copy (small arrow) has split and translocated to a third chromosome (arrow head). This shows that there is a translocation involving chromosome 1 and another as yet unidentified chromosome in this sarcoma. (Chromosome paint as from Yang *et al.* 1999) (Colour plate 1, facing p. 162.)

dog (Langford *et al.* 1996; Yang *et al.* 1999) and these will help future cytogenetic studies of canine tumours enormously (Tap *et al.* 1998).

External stimuli

A variety of external factors may produce genetic changes within the cell.

Biological factors

Viruses

Viruses may influence tumour development either by affecting the cellular DNA directly or by increasing the rate of cell division so that spontaneous changes occur more rapidly within the cell and may not be repaired effectively.

Several animal viruses (both DNA and RNA-containing viruses) are responsible for tumour formation (Table 1.3). DNA-containing viruses normally propagate within host cells without causing cancer. More rarely, they integrate all or part of their genome into the host genome and do not replicate themselves. Stable integration may lead to cell transformation when viral genes which control the host's replicative machinery are transcribed and act as oncogenes. Occasionally, expression of several viral oncogenes or cellular oncogenes is needed for full transformation. Few DNA-containing viruses cause tumours in dogs and cats, although papilloma viruses may be responsible for a recently described type of squamous cell carcinoma in the cat (Bowen's disease) and transformation of papilloma to squamous cell carcinoma has also been rarely reported in the dog.

Retroviruses, a group of RNA-containing viruses, play a much more important role in cancer formation in the cat and probably some types of cancer in the dog too, although direct evidence for the latter is not yet available. Feline leukaemia virus (FeLV) causes lymphoma and leukaemia in cats although not all cases of these cancers are virus positive (Chapter 15). The virus is prevalent in young cats, particularly in breeding colonies or catteries. Multiple strains of a related virus, feline sarcoma virus (FeSV), cause sarcoma formation, also in young cats (Chapter 5) but affected animals are also FeLV positive. There is no evidence that FeSV can be transmitted between cats or to other species.

Table 1.3 Tumour-causing viruses.

Virus	Tumour	Species
DNA viruses		
Hepadnavirus family (hepatitis B virus)	Hepatocellular carcinoma	Man
Herpesvirus family (Epstein-Barr virus)	Burkitt's lymphoma in Africa, Nasopharyngeal carcinoma in China	Man
HHV-8	Kaposi's sarcoma	Man
Mareks disease virus	Mareks disease/lymphoma	Chicken
Papovavirus family	Papillomas/warts	Man and animals
(papilloma viruses)	Carcinomas of cervix	Man
	?Bowen's disease/squamous cell carcinoma	Cat
Adenovirus family	Adenomas	Sheep
RNA viruses		
Retrovirus family		
HTLV-1	Adult T cell leukaemia/lymphoma	Man
FeLV	Leukaemia/lymphoma	Cat
BLV	Bovine leukosis/lymphoma	Cow
ALV	Avian leukosis/lymphoma	Chicken

The mRNA within a retrovirus is reverse transcribed to a double-stranded DNA provirus which can insert into the host genome. The DNA polymerase enzyme 'reverse transcriptase' is coded for in the viral genome to allow this process. Some retroviruses also contain 'oncogenes' which replace one of the virus genes and which have been incorporated from the host genome by a process called transduction. These viruses are unable to replicate without a related helper virus because the oncogene replaces part of the necessary replication machinery. They are known as acutely transforming retroviruses because when inserted into the host genome they act rapidly to transform the cell. The various strains of FeSV belong to this group, each containing an oncogene such as *fms*, *kit*, or *fgr* from the feline genome. Helper FeLV virus is needed for replication. Other retroviruses such as FeLV or bovine leukosis virus (BLV) do not contain oncogenes. The insertion of the viral genome into the host DNA causes the activation of cellular oncogenes instead. These retroviruses have a long latency and are replication competent. FeLV often inserts adjacent to the myc oncogene, affecting the regulatory elements which control the transcription of this gene and resulting in an increased level of gene expression (Neil *et al.* 1984).

Parasites

Few parasites are responsible for cancer formation in animals. The most frequently quoted example is that of *Spirocerca lupi* which causes oesophageal tumours in the dog, fox, wolf and jaguar in Africa and south-east USA, where the helminth is endemic (see Chapter 8). Worm eggs develop to form encysted third stage larvae when eaten by intermediate host dung beetles. Beetles may be ingested by another intermediate host such as chicken, small mammal or reptile or eaten directly by the host carnivore. Ingested larvae migrate via the aorta to the oesophagus, mature into adult worms and produce loose inflammatory nodules around themselves. The lesions are highly vascular with fibroblastic proliferation and central areas containing worm eggs. As the lesion progresses, the blood vessels decrease and fibroblasts become more numerous and active. With continued proliferation, the fibroblasts transform into neoplastic foci that eventually combine to form a fibrosarcoma. Secretion of a carcinogen may help the progression to fibrosarcoma or, if bone and osteoid are produced, osteosarcoma.

Hormones

Certain hormones can influence cancer development by increasing cell replication and the progression of cells which have already accumulated other initiating events. Oestrogen and to a lesser extent progesterone influence the development of mammary cancer in humans, dogs and cats (see Chapter 12). Early ovariohysterectomy to remove hormonal fluctuations significantly reduces the risk of developing mammary cancer. Anti-oestrogen therapy (tamoxifen) is widely used in post-menopausal women to prevent breast cancer recurrence and metastasis, but has not been successful in animals because of the different way in which it is metabolised. Oestrogen also influences the development of benign vaginal fibromas in dogs, and ovariohysterectomy is usually necessary to prevent recurrence (see Chapter 11).

In male dogs, testosterone is responsible for the development of perianal adenoma, and castration is therefore advisable to prevent the risk of further tumours. Other male dog tumours, such as prostatic cancer, however, are unaffected by testosterone secretion.

Physical factors

A range of physical or environmental factors may also influence cancer development.

UV light

In recent years the climate has subtly changed, and the harmful effects of UV light which lead to the development of skin cancer have been increasingly acknowledged, along with a change in behaviour of many individuals with respect to holidays abroad and sunbathing. A depletion of the ozone layer, particularly over Antarctica has produced an 8% increase in UVB at ground level in the southern hemisphere since 1980, leading to an increase in non-melanoma skin cancer in man. Ozone depletion has occurred to a lesser extent in the northern hemisphere but is masked to a degree in industrial coun-

tries by the production of ozone at ground level in a photochemical reaction with exhaust fumes.

UVB and to a lesser extent UVA induce specific DNA changes in the skin, leading to the production of cyclobutane dimers and (6–4) photoproducts. Characteristic mutations which are never seen in internal tumours take place, such as the conversion of cytosine to thymine, and the dimerisation of two adjacent thymines, which disrupts base-pairing. In addition, suppression of the immune response by UV light may play a role in allowing tumours to develop.

Long-term exposure to UV light allows skin tumours such as squamous cell carcinoma to develop in animals, particularly in areas that lack protective pigment. Any patches of white skin or non-pigmented mucous membranes can be affected, for example the nasal planum, lips, periocuar skin or ventral abdomen. Early sun-induced changes such as erythema, hair loss or scaling may be mistaken for inflammatory lesions, but if left untreated these will progress to squamous cell carcinoma (Chapter 4, Figs 4.6–4.8).

Other irradiation

Animals may be exposed to radiation in various ways. An increasing number of dogs and cats may be exposed to X-rays as part of a routine diagnostic investigation and a smaller number to either X-rays or γ-rays if they receive radiotherapy for a tumour. The doses received from diagnostic X-rays are relatively small and carry a low risk and those from radiotherapy are only given if there is a malignant cancer already present, making the development of a further cancer at the site of treatment less likely within the animal's already shortened life span.

Environmental exposure to radon gas or radioactive ores may occur more in some parts of the UK than others, but generally carries a low risk of cancer development in animals. Similarly, experimental exposure of animals to radioactive substances is now rare, although past experimental work has shown that exposure to strontium 90 causes osteosarcoma and lymphoid tumours, and to radium or plutonium, osteosarcoma and bronchoalveolar carcinoma.

At the cellular level, particulate radiation acts directly on the DNA to break chemical bonds whereas electromagnetic radiation causes indirect

DNA damage by the production of free radicals. Although the main effect is probably on DNA, damage to other cell components such as RNA and proteins may also be important.

Trauma/chronic inflammation

There is evidence to suggest that squamous cell carcinoma and sarcomas can develop at the site of thermal or chemical burns or chronic inflammation, suggesting that these conditions predispose in some way to cancer formation. Repeated microtrauma to the metaphyses of long bones produced by weight bearing stresses may play a role in the development of osteosarcoma in large and giant breeds, as may the insertion of metal implants at the site of long bone fractures. These may cause subclinical osteomyelitis at the implant site and stimulate a chronic inflammatory response which predisposes to tumour formation, often after a latent period of several years. In cats, intra-ocular sarcoma has been associated with the chronic inflammatory reaction caused by lens trauma.

In the last decade, increasing numbers of feline soft tissue fibrosarcomas have developed in animals given rabies and FeLV vaccines, with tumours arising at classical injection sites, especially in the interscapular space (Hendrick *et al*. 1992; Esplin *et al*. 1993; Doddy *et al*. 1996). Histologically, most tumours appear pleomorphic and aggressive, with a chronic inflammatory cell infiltrate. In many, the peripheral macrophages contain adjuvant, suggesting a foreign body type reaction to the vaccine. Despite the strong association of vaccine site, inflammatory reaction and sarcoma formation, the precise relationship between the act of vaccination and tumour development is unknown.

Chemical factors

Much of the information about carcinogenic chemicals such as food additives, PVC packaging and environmental contaminants is derived from the human literature, although many chemical carcinogens have been tested on laboratory animals, and other specific examples for domestic animals do exist. Many chemicals are inactive until converted to the active form in the body and so species differences are frequent.

Long-term administration of chemotherapeutic agents to treat a malignant cancer may lead to a secondary cancer if the animal survives for long enough, and use of cyclophosphamide in particular has been associated with the development of bladder cancer in dogs. Chronic ingestion of bracken can produce cancers of the gastro-intestinal and urinary tract in ruminants but is not a problem for small animals.

The extent to which air pollution affects cancer development in animals is not known although tonsillar squamous cell carcinoma in dogs and lingual squamous cell carcinoma were reportedly higher in industrial cities when smoke pollution was a major problem. Inhalation of asbestos dust produces mesothelioma in pet animals and often occurs in the owner at the same time due to a common source of exposure.

Inherited genetic events

A number of familial cancers have been identified in man and these usually develop because of changes to tumour suppressor genes such as Rb which causes the childhood cancer, retinoblastoma, or p53 which is affected in a number of different cancers. Tumour suppressor genes act in a recessive fashion, requiring both alleles to be inactivated to inhibit the gene's activity. One copy of an abnormal gene is inherited and therefore present at birth, and the second copy of the gene becomes abnormal or is lost at some stage in the lifetime of the individual. This usually happens more quickly than if the individual had to lose both copies of the gene by spontaneous events and thus familial cancers usually arise in children or young adults rather than at the age at which most spontaneous cancers occur in the general population. Some inherited human cancers and the genes responsible for them are listed in Table 1.4.

No specific hereditary genes have been identified in domestic animals but a number of tumour types, particularly sarcomas, seem to show breed predispositions and these are listed in Table 1.5. A familial incidence of some cancers has been demonstrated within certain breeds, for example malignant histiocytosis in the Bernese mountain dog and lymphoma in the bullmastiff (Onions 1984; Padgett *et al*. 1995).

Table 1.4 Familial cancers occurring in humans.

Disease/tumour	Gene	Chromosome location
Retinoblastoma	RB1	13q
Wilms tumour	WT1	11p
von Hippel Lindau	VPL	3p
Multiple endocrine neoplasia	MEN1	11q
	MEN2	10q
Neurofibromatosis	NF1	17q
	NF2	22q
Li-Fraumeni syndrome	p53	17p
Familial adenomatous polyposis	APC/FAP	5q
Hereditary non-polyposis colon cancer	MLH1	3p
	MSH2	2p
Malignant melanoma	MLM	9p
Breast cancer	BRCA1	17q
	BRCA2	13q

Table 1.5 Breed predispositions for cancers occurring in dogs.

Disease/tumour	Breed
Systemic/malignant histiocytosis	Bernese mountain dog
Soft tissue sarcoma	Flat-coated retriever
Fibrosarcoma	Golden retriever
Haemangiosarcoma	German shepherd dog
Osteosarcoma	Irish wolfhound, Great Dane, St Bernard
Mast cell tumour	Boxer, golden/Labrador retriever
Chemoreceptor tumours	Boxer, Boston terrier
Gastric carcinoma	Belgian shepherd dog

TUMOUR BIOLOGY

Neoplasms are classified according to their growth and behavioural characteristics as being benign or malignant (Table 1.6). Malignant neoplasms are characterised by a locally invasive and destructive manner of growth and the ability to metastasise to other sites in the body. These will cause death unless radical clinical action is taken. Benign tumours tend to grow by expansion rather than invasion and do not metastasise. They have a more predictable clinical course and are not usually life threatening. Although this division is useful for descriptive purposes, neoplasms in fact display a spectrum of behaviour. Some canine tumours, for example oral acanthomatous epulis (basal cell carcinoma) and haemangiopericytoma, have local characteristics of malignancy but metastasis is rare. Other tumours,

for example mast cell tumours, can display a wide range of behaviour with some being benign or low grade, and others highly malignant. The morphological features of a tumour, for example its cellular and nuclear characteristics and mitotic rate, can be used to predict its likely behaviour. The histological grade or appearance of the tumour is therefore important in prognosis (see Chapter 2).

The ability of malignant tumours to spread and grow in distant organs is their most serious and life-threatening characteristic. Tumours may metastasise via the lymphatic route to local and regional lymph nodes or via the haematogenous route allowing secondary tumours to develop in any body organ. These two systems are widely interconnected and many tumours use these connections to spread

Table 1.6 Features of benign and malignant tumours.

	Benign	Malignant
Rate of growth	Relatively slow Growth may cease in some cases	Often rapid Rarely ceases growing
Manner of growth	Expansive Usually well defined boundary between neoplastic and normal tissues. May become encapsulated.	Invasive Poorly defined borders, tumour cells extend into and may be scattered throughout adjacent normal tissues.
Effects on adjacent tissues	Often minimal May cause pressure necrosis and anatomical deformity	Often serious Tumour growth and invasion results in destruction of adjacent normal tissues, manifest as ulceration of superficial tissues, lysis of bone
Metastasis	Does not occur	Occurs by lymphatic and haematogenous routes and transcoelomic spread
Effect on host	Often minimal (can be life threatening if tumour develops in a vital organ, e.g. brain)	Often life-threatening by virtue of destructive nature of growth and metastatic dissemination to other, vital organs.

through the body. In humans, different types of cancer show different target organ specificity for metastasis. For example:

- Prostatic carcinoma – bone
- Breast carcinoma – bone, brain, adrenal, lung, liver
- Cutaneous melanoma – liver, brain, bowel.

In small animals, the lungs are the most common site for the development of haematogenous secondary tumours but other sites including liver, spleen, kidneys, skin and bone should not be overlooked. Carcinomas and mast cell tumours usually metastasise by the lymphatic route and sarcomas and melanomas by the haematogenous route but tumours do not always follow expected patterns of behaviour and some tumours may spread by both lymphatic and haematogenous routes.

The mechanisms involved in the process of metastasis are not fully understood. In order to form a metastasic growth, a cancer cell must detach from the primary tumour, move into the vasculature to travel to a new location, aggregate with platelets and fibrin to arrest at the new site, extravasate into surrounding parenchyma and establish growth. During this process the cell must evade host defence mechanisms and survive in the circulation. Current theories suggest that only certain clones of cells within a tumour develop all the abilities required for metastasis but that these clones probably arise and disseminate in the early stages of that tumour's growth, often prior to the detection of the primary tumour.

References

Breen, M., Bullerdiek, J. & Langford, C. (1999) The DAPI banded karyotype of the domestic dog (*Canis familiaris*) generated using chromosome-specific paint probes. *Chromosome Research*, (7), 401–6.

Doddy, F.D., Glickman, L.T., Glickman, N.W. & Janovitz, F.B. (1996) Feline fibrosarcomas at vaccination sites and non-vaccination sites. *Journal of Comparative Pathology*, (114), 165–74.

Esplin, D.G., McGill, L.D., Meininger, A.C. & Wilson, S.R. (1993) Postvaccination sarcomas in cats. *Journal of the American Veterinary Medical Association*, (11), 1440–44.

Frazier, K.S., Hines, M.E., Hurvitz, A.I., Robinson, P.G. & Herron, A.J. (1993) Analysis of DNA aneuploidy and c-*myc* oncoprotein content of canine plasma cell tumours using flow cytometry. *Veterinary Pathology*, (30), 505–11.

Gamblin, R.M., Sagartz, J.E. & Couto, C.G. (1997) Overexpression of p53 tumour suppressor protein in spontaneously arising neoplasms of dogs. *American Journal of Veterinary Research*, (58), 857–63.

Grindem, C.B. & Buoen, L.C. (1986) Cytogenetic analysis of leukaemic cells in the dog. A report of ten cases and a review of the literature. *Journal of Comparative Pathology*, (96), 623–35.

Gumerlock, P.H., Meyers, F.J., Foster, B.A., Kawakami, T.G. & deVere White, R.W. (1989) Activated c-N-ras in radiation induced acute nonlymphocytic leukaemia: twelfth codon aspartic acid. *Radiation Research*, (117), 198–206.

Hahn, K.A., Richardson, R.C., Hahn, E.A. & Chrisman, C.L. (1994) Diagnostic and prognostic importance of chromosomal aberrations identified in 61 dogs with lymphosarcoma. *Veterinary Pathology*, (31), 528–40.

Hendrick, M.J., Goldschmidt, M.H., Shofer, F.S. *et al.* (1992) Postvaccinal sarcomas in the cat: epidemiology and electron probe microanalytical identification of aluminium. *Cancer Research*, (52), 5391–4.

Kraegal, S.A., Gumerlock, P.H., Dungworth, D.L., Oreffo, V.I., & Madewell, B.R. (1992) K-ras activation in nonsmall cell lung cancer in the dog. *Cancer Research*, (52), 4724–7.

Langford, C.F., Fischer, P.E., Binns, M.M., Holmes, N.G. & Carter, N.P. (1996) Chromosome-specific paints from a high-resolution flow karyotype of the dog. *Chromosome Research*, (4), 115–23.

Look, A.T. (1995) Oncogenic role of 'master' transcription factors in human leukemias and sarcomas: a developmental model. *Advances in Cancer Research*, (67), 25–57.

Mayr, B., Reifinger, M., Weissenbock, H. *et al.* (1994) Cytogenetic analyses of four solid tumours in dogs. *Research in Veterinary Science*, (57), 88–95.

Mayr, B., Dressler, A., Reifinger, M. & Feil, C. (1998a) Cytogenetic alterations in eight mammary tumours and tumour suppressor gene p53 mutation in one mammary tumour from dogs. *American Journal of Veterinary Research*, (59), 69–78.

Mayr, B., Reifinger, M. & Loupal, G. (1998b) Polymorphisms in feline tumour suppressor gene p53. Mutations in an osteosarcoma and a mammary carcinoma. *Veterinary Journal*, (155), 103–106.

Mayr, B., Reifinger, M, Alton, K. & Schaffner, G. (1998c) Novel p53 tumour suppressor mutations in cases of spindle cell sarcoma, pleomorphic sarcoma and fibrosarcoma in cats. *Veterinary Research Communications*, (22), 249–55.

Mayr, B., Wegscheider, H., Reifinger, M. & Jugl, T. (1998d) Cytogenetic alterations in four feline soft-tissue tumours. *Veterinary Research Communications*, (22), 21–9.

Mayr, B., Reifinger, M. & Alton, K. (1999) Novel canine tumour suppressor gene mutations in cases of skin and mammary neoplasms. *Veterinary Research Communications*, (23), 285–91.

Miyoshi, N., Tateyama, S., Ogawa, K.L. *et al.* (1991a) Proto-oncogenes of genomic DNA in clinically normal animals of various species. *American Journal of Veterinary Research*, (52), 940–43.

Miyoshi, N., Tateyama, S., Ogawa, K.L. *et al.* (1991b) Abnormal structure of the canine oncogene, related to the human c-*yes*-1 oncogene, in canine mammary tumour tissue. *American Journal of Veterinary Research*, (52), 2046–9.

Momoi, Y., Nagase, M., Okamoto, Y. *et al.* (1993) Rearrangements of immunoglobulin and T-cell receptor genes in canine lymphoma/leukaemia cells. *Journal of Veterinary Medicine and Science*, (55), 775–80.

Nasir, L. & Argyle, D.J. (1999) Mutational analysis of the tumour suppressor gene p53 in lymphosarcoma in two bull mastiffs. *Veterinary Record*, (145), 23–4.

Neil, J.C., Hughes, D., McFarlane, R. *et al.* (1984) Transduction and rearrangement of the myc gene by feline leukaemia virus in naturally occurring T-cell leukaemias. *Nature*, (308), 814–20.

Onions, D.E. (1984) A prospective study of familial canine lymphosarcoma. *Journal of the National Cancer Institute*, (72), 909–12.

Padgett, G.A., Madewell, B.R., Keller, E.T., Jodar, L. & Packard, M. (1995) Inheritance of histiocytosis in Bernese mountain dogs. *Journal of Small Animal Practice*, (36), 93–8.

Rabbitts, T.H. (1994) Chromosomal translocations in human cancer. *Nature*, (372), 143–9.

Reimann, N., Rogalla, P., Kazmierczak, B. *et al.* (1994) Evidence that metacentric and submetacentric chromosomes in canine tumours can result from telomeric fusions. *Cytogenetics and Cell Genetics*, (67), 81–5.

Reimann, N., Bartnitzke, S., Bullerdiek, J. *et al.* (1998) Trisomy 1 in a canine acute leukemia indicating importance of polysomy 1 in leukemias of the dog. *Cancer Genetics and Cytogenetics*, (101), 49–52.

Rungsipipat, A., Tateyama, S., Yamaguchi, R., Uchida, K. & Miyoshi, N. (1999) Expression of c-yes oncogene product in various animal tissues and spontaneous canine tumours. *Research in Veterinary Science*, (66), 205–10.

Sagartz, J.E., Bodley, W.L., Gamblin, R.M., Couto, C.G., Tierney, L.A. & Capen, C.C. (1996) p53 tumour suppressor protein overexpression in osteogenic tumours of dogs. *Veterinary Pathology*, (33), 213–21.

Switonski, M., Reimann, N., Bosma, A.A. *et al.* (1996) Report on the progress of standardization of the G-banded canine (Canis familiaris) karyotype. *Chromosome Research*, (4), 306–09.

Tap, O.T., Rutteman, G.R., Zijlstra, C., de Haan, N.A. & Bosma, A.A. (1998) Analysis of chromosome aberrations in a mammary carcinoma cell line from a dog by using canine painting probes. *Cytogenetics and Cell Genetics*, (82), 75–9.

Veldhoen, N., Watterson, J., Brash, M. & Milner, J. (1999) Identification of tumour-associated and germ line p53 mutations in canine mammary cancer. *British Journal of Cancer*, (81), 409–15.

Yang, F., O'Brien, P.C.M., Milne, B.S. *et al.* (1999) A com-

plete comparative chromosome map for the dog, red
fox and human and its integration with canine genetic
maps. *Genomics*, (62), 189–202.

Further reading

Alberts, B., Bray, D., Lewis, J., Raff, M., Roberts, K. &
    Watson, J.D. (1994) *The Molecular Biology of the Cell*,
    3rd edn. Garland Publishing Inc, New York.
Hardy, W.D. (1981) The feline leukemia virus. *Journal of
    the American Animal Hospital Association*, (17), 951–80.
Hardy, W.D. (1981) The feline sarcoma viruses. *Journal of
    the American Animal Hospital Association*, (17), 981–97.

Jarrett, O. (1985) Feline leukaemia virus. *In Practice*, (7),
    125–6.
Jarrett, O. (1994) Feline leukaemia virus. In: *Feline Medi-
    cine and Therapeutics*, (eds E.A. Chandler, C.J. Gaskell
    & R.M. Gaskell), 2nd edn, pp. 473–87. Blackwells,
    Oxford.
Miller, W.H., Affolter, V., Scott, D.W. & Suter, M.M. (1992)
    Multicentric squamous cell carcinomas in situ resem-
    bling Bowen's disease in five cats. *Veterinary Derma-
    tology*, (3), 177–82.
Rosenkrantz, W.S. (1993) Solar dermatitis. In: *Current Vet-
    erinary Dermatology, The Science and Art of Therapy*.
    (eds C.E. Griffin, K.W. Kwochka & J.M. MacDonald),
    pp. 309–15. Mosby Year Book, St Louis.

2
Diagnosis and Staging

The treatment and prognosis for an individual with cancer will depend on the nature and the extent of their disease. Thus for treatment to succeed, the histological type (and grade) of the tumour and its size and anatomical extent must be defined prior to treatment. It is also important to detect possible haematological or metabolic complications related to the disease and to investigate concurrent illness, since all of these factors may influence the method of treatment and prognosis or whether the patient is treated at all.

The objectives of the initial evaluation of the cancer patient may thus be summarised:

- Diagnosis of the histological type and grade of the disease
- Determination of the extent or stage of the disease
- Investigation of tumour-related complications
- Investigation of any concurrent disorder.

TUMOUR DIAGNOSIS

Neoplastic tissues have certain features which distinguish them from hyperplastic or inflammatory conditions and further features which distinguish benign from malignant growths, as shown in Table 2.1. Although an experienced clinician can sometimes make an informed guess as to the likely nature of a tumour according to its site, gross appearance and history, a definitive diagnosis can only be made by microscopic examination of representative tissue or cells from the tumour. This may be achieved by either:

- Collection of tissue from the tumour – histological diagnosis; *or*
- Collection of cells from the tumour – cytological diagnosis.

Histology

Histological examination of representative tissue from a tumour is the most accurate method of cancer diagnosis. A biopsy provides the pathologist with the opportunity to examine the cellular components of the tumour, its architecture and its relationship to adjacent normal tissues.

A variety of biopsy techniques may be used to collect tumour samples:

- Needle biopsy – e.g. 'tru-cut' for soft tissue tumours, 'Jamshidi' for bone
- Skin punch biopsy – for skin and superficial soft tissue tumours
- Crocodile action 'grab' biopsy forceps – may be used with endoscopic techniques for tumours

Table 2.1 Cytological and histological features of malignancy.

Cytological features	
Cell population	Pleomorphism
	Presence of mitoses, especially abnormal or bizarre forms
Cellular features	Large cell size/giant cells (anisocytosis)
	Poorly differentiated, anaplastic cells
	High nuclear to cytoplasmic ratio
Nuclear features	Large nuclear size, nuclear pleomorphism (anisokaryosis)
	Multiple nuclei (often of variable size)
	Hyperchromatic nuclei with clumping or stippling of chromatin
	Prominent and often multiple nucleoli of variable size and shape
Histological features	
Cellular features	As outlined for 'cytology'
Tumour architecture	Lack of structural organisation of cells into recognisable form
Relationship with adjacent tissues	Invasion of cells into adjacent normal tissues
Evidence of metastatic behaviour	Tumour cells invading or present within lymphatics or venules

sited in the respiratory, gastro-intestinal and urogenital tracts
• Incisional biopsy
• Excisional biopsy.

In most circumstances it is preferable to make the tumour diagnosis prior to treatment, even when the treatment will be surgical, because only when the nature of the disease is known can an appropriate treatment be planned. The margins of surgical resection required to remove a canine cutaneous histiocytoma are considerably less than those required to remove a cutaneous mast cell tumour. Thus in order to prevent an inadequate surgery, leading to local tumour recurrence, a needle, grab or incisional biopsy is preferable to an excisional biopsy (cytology can also be useful in this respect).

The exception to this general rule is when prior knowledge of the histological type of tumour will not influence the surgical approach; for example, tumours involving internal organs (such as kidney or spleen) where removal of that entire organ is the most feasible surgical approach, or in the case of canine mammary tumours, where, irrespective of whether the tumour is a benign mixed mammary tumour or a carcinoma, the only surgical approach is to remove the entire mass, often with the affected gland. Providing all the tumour is removed, the post-surgical prognosis for canine mammary tumours is not dependent on the degree of surgery.

On occasions it may be difficult to procure representative tumour tissue, particularly where there is surface ulceration or extensive necrosis in a tumour. Factors that should be taken into consideration in order to obtain a representative biopsy sample with minimum risk to the patient are summarised in Table 2.2. In addition to giving a definitive diagnosis, by providing information regarding cell type, mitotic rate and tissue architecture, histology can also provide an indication of the 'grade' of a tumour, i.e. its likely clinical behaviour in terms of local invasion and distant metastasis. Increasingly it is appreciated that the histological grade of a tumour is of equal importance to histological type in treatment selection and prognosis (see soft tissue sarcoma and mast cell tumours). The following features may all be used to help predict tumour behaviour:

• Degree of cellular differentiation
• Degree of cellular and nuclear pleomorphism
• Mitotic rate (number of mitotic figures per high power field)
• Presence and amount of necrosis
• Presence of an inflammatory infiltrate
• Stromal reaction
• Degree of invasion, i.e. the relationship between the tumour and adjacent normal tissues.

Other ways to assess tumour prognosis include measuring DNA content or ploidy by flow cytometry, cell proliferation or abnormal expression of oncogenes (e.g. ErbB2) or tumour suppressor genes

Table 2.2 Factors to consider when planning a tumour biopsy.	
Objective	Considerations
Procure a representative sample of the tumour	Avoid superfical ulceration, areas of inflammation or necrosis Ensure adequate depth of biopsy, particularly for oral tumours Try to include tumour – normal tissue boundary in the biopsy sample
Avoid local tumour recurrence or local spread	Minimise handling of tumour by adequate surgical exposure Ensure adequate haemostasis Minimise trauma to tumour and normal tissues Avoid contamination of normal tissue by surgical instruments
Do not compromise subsequent therapy	Site any biopsy procedure well within the margins of future excision

(e.g. p53). Cell proliferation may be quantified by using monoclonal antibodies to nuclear antigens which are present in the nuclear matrix of proliferating cells but not in non-proliferating cells. These include Ki-67, DNA polymerase alpha, PCNA. Alternatively, silver staining to detect agrophillic nucleolar organiser regions (AgNORs) can also be helpful in assessing proliferation. For poorly differentiated tumours, haematoxylin and eosin stains may not be sufficient to reach a definitive diagnosis and special staining techniques can be applied to help differentiate possible tumour types.

Cytology

Cells may be collected from tumours by a variety of techniques:

- Fine needle aspirate
- Exfoliation – tissue imprint, scrape or exudate smears
- Cytospins of body fluids.

Microscopic examination of such samples provides information regarding the cell population and the morphology of individual cells. Fine needle aspi-

rates or impression smears from solid tumours and the cellular content of fluids collected from organs or body cavities can provide a great deal of information about the lesion and will often differentiate between inflammatory and neoplastic processes. The morphology of neoplastic cells will also often provide an indication of the likely nature of a tumour and its degree of malignancy. Fine needle aspiration is a quick and simple technique requiring a minimum of equipment that can easily be performed in practice. The technique is summarised in Figs 2.1–2.4. Many commercial clinical pathology laboratories will report on cytological samples and with practice most veterinarians should be able to use cytology to discriminate between reactive and neoplastic lesions and even to diagnose some particularly characteristic tumours, for example mast cell tumours.

Obtaining aspirates for cytology is often quicker, cheaper and easier to perform than obtaining biopsies for histopathology but the latter has the advantage that tissue architecture can be assessed, along with the degree of invasiveness, haemorrhage and necrosis, and thus not only provide a definitive tumour diagnosis but also information about the grade of malignancy.

TUMOUR STAGING

The 'stage', that is the extent of a tumour, is of equal importance to its histological type in determining prognosis and the feasibility of therapy. Successful treatment depends on eradication of all tumour stem cells and this can only be achieved if the extent of the disease is fully appreciated. It is there-

fore important to determine the local extent of a tumour and investigate the possibility of metastasis as part of the initial evaluation of the cancer patient, and a logical system for such evaluation should be followed.

Anatomical classification or clinical staging of

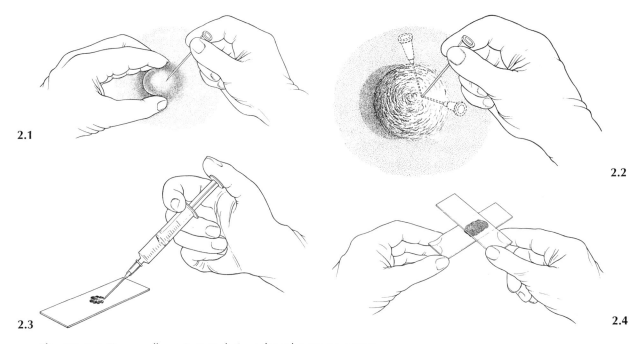

2.1

2.2

2.3

2.4

Figs 2.1–2.4 Fine needle aspirate technique for subcutaneous mass.
Fig. 2.1. The lesion is located and fixed with one hand. Fig. 2.2. The fine needle (usually 23 guage, 1 in.) is inserted into the mass and redirected several times in a stabbing motion. Fig. 2.3. The needle is withdrawn and connected to an air filled syringe to expel the needle contents onto a clean glass slide. Fig. 2.4. The sample is smeared by laying a second slide perpendicular to the first and carefully drawing the two apart. (Reprinted from Dobson (1999) with permission.)

tumours is based on an objective approach to (Fig. 2.5):

- The primary tumour (T)
- The local and regional lymph nodes (N)
- Distant metastases (M).

Primary tumour (T)

Malignant neoplasms are characterised by an invasive, infiltrating pattern of growth. The tendency for local recurrence of such tumours following excisional surgery is a result of a failure to remove or eradicate all tumour (i.e. a failure of the surgery) rather than a preset characteristic of the tumour.

It is essential, therefore, to define the extent of the primary tumour as accurately as possible prior to therapy so that appropriate treatment margins can be applied. A tumour is a three-dimensional entity and all surrounding structures including skin, fascia, muscles, bone and adjacent viscera must be

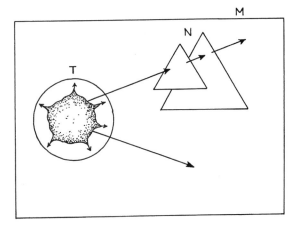

Fig. 2.5 Diagrammatic representation of the TNM tumour staging system. (T = primary tumour, N = local and regional lymph nodes, M = metastases.)

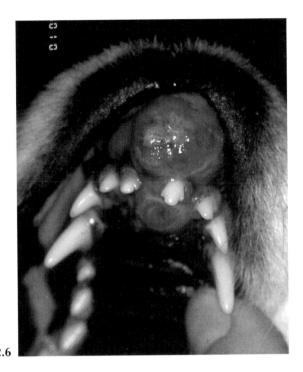

2.6

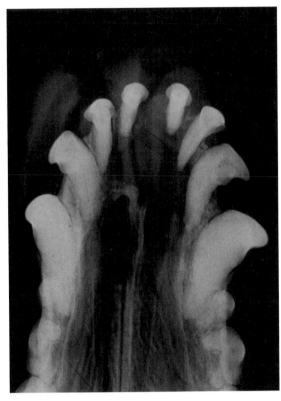

2.7

Fig. 2.6 Basal cell carcinoma of the premaxilla. The dental displacement and extension of the tumour mass on both sides of the dental arcade are indicators of bone invasion by the tumour as is shown in **Fig. 2.7**, an intraoral radiograph of the tumour site.

evaluated for evidence of tumour infiltration. The ease of evaluation of the primary tumour will depend on its location and accessibility. Methods of evaluation include the following.

Physical examination

- Tumour site and relationship to normal anatomic structures
- Size or volume of the primary mass
- Mobility of the tumour with respect to surrounding tissues: fixation usually denotes tumour infiltration of adjacent structures
- Ulceration denotes infiltration and disruption of the epidermis.

For deeper tumours, operative procedures – for instance celiotomy or thoracotomy – may be necessary to provide access to the tumour for both histological and anatomical classification.

Radiography

Radiography is especially useful for:

- Tumours involving or adjacent to bone (e.g. tumours of the oral cavity (Figs 2.6 and 2.7)).
- Tumours sited within body cavities. Contrast studies may be required to assist visualisation of tumours sited within hollow organs.

Ultrasonography

Ultrasonography can provide useful information about lesions affecting soft tissues and internal organs such as the liver, spleen and kidneys.

Endoscopy

Endoscopy allows visual examination of the respiratory, gastro-intestinal and urogenital tracts.

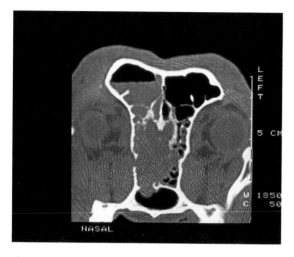

Fig. 2.8 CT scan of dog's nose with nasal tumour. (Courtesy of Animal Medical Centre, Referral Services, Manchester.)

Biopsy

In addition to providing a histological diagnosis, well-orientated biopsies may be used to determine the extent of tumour invasion.

Specialist imaging techniques

Computed tomography (CT) and magnetic resonance imaging (MRI) are increasing in use. These techniques allow detailed, three dimensional imaging of soft tissues and bone (see Fig. 2.8).

Lymph nodes (N)

Lymph node metastasis is most common in:

- Carcinomas
- Melanomas
- Mast cell tumours.

But soft tissue sarcomas may also metastasise by this route. Methods of evaluation of local and regional lymph nodes include the following.

Physical examination

The size, shape, texture and mobility of local and regional lymph nodes should be assessed. Gross enlargement, irregularity, firmness and fixation are all features indicative of neoplastic involvement. A more subtle lymphadenopathy may indicate a small metastatic deposit or may arise as a result of reactive hyperplasia.

Aspirate/biopsy

Aspirate/biopsy of lymph node(s) may be required to distinguish between reactive and neoplastic enlargement.

Imaging techniques

Internal lymph nodes may be evaluated by radiography, ultrasonography, CT or MRI.

Internal lymph nodes may also be evaluated at the time of surgery.

Distant metastasis (M)

Haematogenous dissemination of malignant tumours gives rise to metastases in distant organs. Soft tissue and osteosarcomas and malignant melanoma characteristically metastasise in this way but some carcinomas and mast cell tumours also spread via the blood to distant sites. Although the lungs are the most common site for the development of metastases in small animals, other potential sites for metastatic spread should not be overlooked:

- Skin
- Bones
- Brain and spinal cord
- Internal organs, spleen, liver, kidneys, heart.

The detection of metastases is problematic: tumours only become large enough to detect at a relatively late stage in their development and micro-metastases are below the threshold of currently available detection methods (Fig. 2.9). Nevertheless a range of investigative methods for screening the patient with suspected metastatic disease can be considered:

- History and physical examination
- Radiography – especially thorax, right and left lateral and dorsoventral views; skeletal survey if bone metastases suspected
- Ultrasonography – liver, spleen, kidneys
- Scintigraphy – sensitive method for detection of bone metastasis

- CT or MRI – internal organs including brain
- Laboratory investigations – of little value in most cases
- Bone marrow aspirate.

Discrete pulmonary tumours can only be detected on thoracic radiographs once they have reached

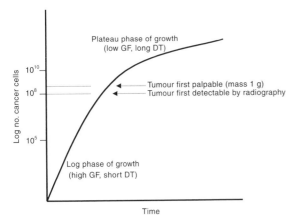

Fig. 2.9 Graph of tumour growth versus clinical detection. A tumour cannot be detected by palpation or radiography until it reaches approximately 1 cm in diameter or 0.5–1 g in weight, by which time it has undergone approximately 30 doublings and contains in the order of 10^8–10^9 cells.

the size of 0.5–1.0 cm in diameter. Right and left lateral thoracic radiographs should be included as a routine part of the initial 'work-up' of any animal with a malignant tumour because the finding of pulmonary metastases usually leads to a poor prognosis (Figs 2.10 and 2.11). The finding of a 'clear' thoracic film does not however exclude the possibility of micro-metastases. Metastatic tumour in the liver, spleen or kidneys may be diffuse or nodular in distribution and may not significantly alter the shape or outline of those organs until the tumour reaches advanced stages. Ultrasonography is more useful than radiography in screening these organs but metastatic disease may also be below the threshold of ultrasonic detection (Figs 2.12 and 2.13).

Clinical tumour staging systems

The TNM anatomical classification of tumours can be used to provide a precise means of recording the apparent extent of the disease at the time of assessment. Coupled with a knowledge of the clinical

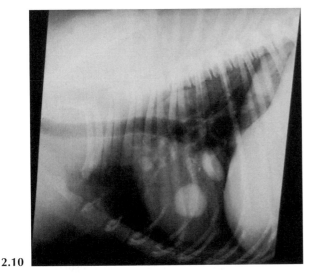

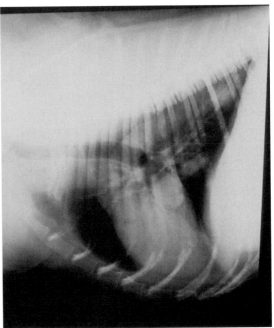

2.10

2.11

Figs 2.10 and 2.11 Left and right lateral views of the thorax of a dog. The secondary pulmonary tumours are only clearly visible on the left view which indicates that they are in the right lung. Visualisation of pulmonary metastases depends on the contrast between the air filled lung and the soft tissue of the tumour. Thus tumours are more likely to be detected in the upper, inflated lung as opposed to the lower lung which is compressed.

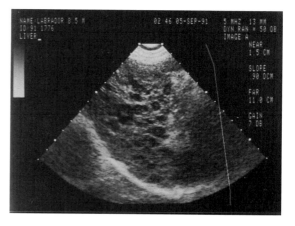

Fig. 2.13 Ultrasonogram of the liver showing multiple hypoechogenic areas correlating with hepatic metastases. (Courtesy of Mr M. E. Herrtage, Department of Clinical Veterinary Medicine, Cambridge.)

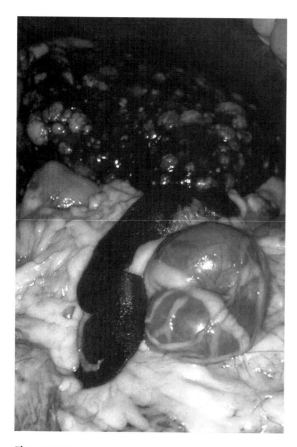

Fig. 2.12 Extensive nodular metastases from a cutaneous mast cell tumour in the liver of a dog.

behaviour of individual tumours at specific sites, this information can be used to group tumours according to their prognosis: clinical staging. Where relevant, clinical staging systems are included under individual tumour types in later sections of this book.

Clinical staging does not necessarily imply a regular and predictable progression of the disease. Some cancers do proceed in a typical course, advancing from primary to nodal to metastatic disease, but many variations exist and it is not unknown for metastasis to be the first sign of the disease.

When relating clinical stage to prognosis, two important points must be taken into consideration:

- There is a difference between the clinical stage and the true pathological stage of a disease because it is not possible to detect microscopic tumour extensions or deposits.
- Other factors, apart from clinical stage, are of prognostic significance including the location of the tumour, its histological type and grade.

In practice, cancer therapy must be directed at least towards the clinically-defined stage of the tumour. Local treatment may be selected for tumours of low grade or tumours with a low metastatic potential (e.g. basal cell carcinoma of the skin). However, local treatment will not be adequate for more aggressive tumours with a high potential for metastasis (e.g. malignant melanoma, osteosarcoma) and ideally these tumours should be treated as being potentially stage IV (i.e. as if they had occult disseminated metastasis) even if they present clinically as stage I.

TUMOUR-RELATED COMPLICATIONS

An animal with a tumour may be presented as a result of an obvious mass but often the clinical presentation of cancer patients relates to the direct or indirect effects of the tumour, rather than the tumour mass itself. Tumours may cause clinical signs due to:

- Direct effects of tumour growth on adjacent organs/body systems
- Haematological complications
- Metabolic/endocrine complications ('paraneoplastic' syndromes).

Table 2.3 Direct effects of tumour growth on selected organ systems.

Neurologic	
CNS	Increased intracranial pressure, depression, altered mental state, seizures, disorientation, neurological deficits, endocrine disorders
Spinal cord	Spinal cord compression or invasion – pain, paresis, paralysis
Cardiopulmonary	
Nasopharyngeal	Upper airway obstruction
Anterior mediastinum	Superior vena cava syndrome – facial swelling
	Pleural/mediastinal effusion – dyspnoea
Heart	Arrhythmias
	Pericardial effusion and cardiac tamponade
Gastrointestinal	
Stomach	Gastrointestinal obstruction or perforation,
Small intestine	intra-abdominal haemorrhage, peritonitis,
Large intestine	intra-lumenal haemorrhage, vomiting, diarrhoea, dyschezia
Urogenital	
Renal	Haematuria, dysuria, post renal obstruction
Bladder	with azotemia
Urethra	
Prostate	

Direct effects of tumour growth

Local growth of neoplasms invariably causes destruction of adjacent normal tissues which may result in dysfunction of vital organs. Any organ system can be affected in this way either by primary or secondary tumour growth. Some of the more commonly affected or more important organ systems are summarised in Table 2.3.

Haematological complications

Tumours may cause a number of haematological complications through a variety of mechanisms, the more common of which are summarised in Table 2.4. The haematological problem may be the presenting clinical sign but anaemia and thrombocytopenia are quite common findings in cancer patients and may be detected on routine haematological investigations. In addition to affecting the production of blood cells, tumours can also affect the dynamics of blood flow. The viscosity of the blood may be increased in neoplastic conditions such as polycythaemia, and some forms of leukaemia by high cell numbers, or due to high protein content from immunoglobulin secreting tumours such as multiple myeloma.

Supportive treatment may be required to stabilise and maintain the patient until the underlying problem can be identified and treated:

• Whole blood transfusion may be indicated in cases of severe anaemia or for animals in disseminated intravascular coagulation (DIC).
• Heparin therapy (mini-dose: 5 to 10 IU/kg sc q 8h) is indicated to halt the intravascular coagulation in DIC but must be given with whole blood or fresh frozen plasma to provide anti-thrombin III.
• Phlebotomy may also be used for management of polycythaemia. Up to 20 ml whole blood/kg body weight may be removed and replaced with plasma or crystalloid fluids.
• Plasmapheresis may be indicated for treatment

Table 2.4 Haematological complications of tumours.

Tumour directly affects production of blood cells Neoplastic invasion of the bone marrow (myelophthisis) seen with lymphoproliferative and myeloproliferative conditions.	Usually manifest as reduction in cell numbers (cytopenia): Non-regenerative anaemia Thrombocytopenia Leucopenia May be elevated numbers of abnormal cells in the blood in leukaemia (see below)
Tumour indirectly affects production of blood cells Oestrogen producing tumours (Sertoli cell and granulosa cell tumours) lead to oestrogen-induced myelotoxicity Myelofibrosis may be tumour induced	Usually manifest as: Non-regenerative anaemia Thrombocytopenia Granulocytopenia
Hyperviscosity syndromes Lymphoproliferative and myeloproliferative diseases, forms of leukaemia and primary polycythaemia Renal tumours, also reported with testicular tumours and haemangiosarcoma. Secretory multiple myeloma	Lethargy, disorientation, ataxia, tremors, episodic weakness, seizures, thrombo-embolic disease, bleeding diathesis, retinal detachment Excessive numbers of circulating (neoplastic) blood cells cause sludging of blood and poor circulation Excessive production of erythropoietin leading to secondary polycythaemia Excessive production of gammaglobulins may also lead to hyperviscosity syndrome
Other tumour-mediated abnormalities	Regenerative anaemia/thrombocytopenia may be associated with auto-immune haemolytic anaemia, or immune-mediated thrombocytopenia secondary to lymphoid neoplasia Microangiopathic anaemia, associated with fragmentation of red blood cells in haemangiosarcoma Thrombocytopenia due to sequestration of platelets in large abnormal tumour blood vessels, e.g. haemangiosarcoma Disseminated intravascular coagulopathy (DIC) – triggered by many disseminated malignant tumours, results in thrombocytopenia and bleeding diathesis
Blood loss	Regenerative anaemia/thrombocytopenia may be due to: Haemorrhage from a tumour Bleeding from gastroduodenal ulceration due to hypergastrinaemia or hyperhistaminaemia Secondary to a bleeding disorder

of severe hyperviscosity due to hypergammaglobulinaemia. This is achieved by collecting 20 ml blood/kg body weight and replacing this with centrifuged blood cells from the patient, which have been resuspended in crystalloid fluid.

Haematological assessment of the cancer patient is also very important to provide a base-line from which to monitor the response and toxicity of future treatment.

Metabolic and endocrine complications – paraneoplastic syndromes

Tumours can produce profound systemic or metabolic disturbances through the production of hormones or hormone-like substances that act on organs at sites distant to the primary tumour. The resulting clinical syndromes are termed 'paraneoplastic syndromes' and it is often this metabolic/endocrine disorder which alerts the owner to a problem. Some paraneoplastic conditions are specific to certain tumours or certain metabolic abnormalities (see later); others are more general, for example cancer cachexia is a well recognised syndrome where tumour induced metabolic alterations in carbohydrate, protein and lipid metabolism lead to a net loss of energy to the patient despite adequate energy intake. In many cases the problem is compounded by tumour or treatment induced anorexia, impaired digestion and absorption and protein loss through effusions or haemorrhage. Cancer cachexia is a major cause of morbidity and death in human cancer patients and is of significance in veterinary cancer medicine (Vail *et al.* 1990) (Fig. 2.14). Fever is another syndrome which accompanies many types of tumour usually associated with the production of cytokines, such as tumour necrosis factor and interferon.

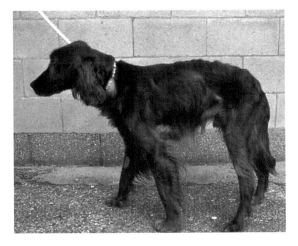

Fig. 2.14 Cachectic patient. Severe cachexia is not common in canine cancer patients.

Paraneoplastic syndromes can arise as a result of autonomous secretion of normal hormones by functional tumours of endocrine origin, as listed in Table 2.5 and discussed in Chapter 14. Various non-endocrine tumours can also produce and release hormones or hormone-like substances. Several commonly recognised syndromes are listed in Table 2.6. Tumours may also cause cutaneous, neurological and skeletal manifestations, some of which are summarised in Table 2.7.

Table 2.5 Endocrine disorders resulting from tumours of endocrine origin.

Syndrome	Tumour(s)	Clinical signs*
Hyperadrenocorticism (Cushing's syndrome)	Adrenal adenoma Adrenal adenocarcinoma Pituitary adenoma	Polydipsia/polyuria Polyphagia Coat changes: alopecia, calcinosis cutis Muscle weakness Hepatomegaly Pendulous abdomen

Hyperthyroidism	Thyroid adenoma (cats)
	Thyroid adenocarcinoma
	  (dogs and occasionally cats)
		Polyphagia, polydipsia
		Weight loss, diarrhoea
		Tachycardia associated with hypertrophic
		  cardiomyopathy
		Hyperexcitability

Primary hyperparathyroidism	Parathyroid adenoma	Due to hypercalcaemia: Polydipsia/polyuria Anorexia, vomiting Muscle weakness Bradycardia/arrhythmias

Hypoglycaemia	Pancreatic islet (beta) cell
	  tumour (insulinoma)
		Episodic weakness, collapse, disorientation
		  and seizures

Hypergastrinaemia (Zollinger-Ellison syndrome)	Pancreatic gastrin producing neoplasm	Gastric and duodenal ulceration Vomiting (haematemesis)

* See Chapter 14 for more detailed information on these conditions.

Table 2.6 Common paraneoplastic syndromes in small animals.

Syndrome	Tumour(s)	Clinical signs
Hypercalcaemia	Lymphoid tumours, myeloid tumours Anal gland adenocarcinoma Solid tumours with skeletal metastases Other solid tumours	Polyuria/polydipsia Anorexia, vomiting Dehydration Muscular weakness, tremor Bradycardia
Hypoglycaemia	Hepatic tumours, especially hepatocelluar carcinoma Other tumours, especially large intra-abdominal tumours	Episodic weakness, collapse, disorientation and seizures
Hyperhistaminaemia	Mast cell tumours	Gastroduodenal ulceration Anorexia, vomiting Haematemesis, melaena, Anaemia

Hypercalcaemia

Neoplasia is the most common cause of hypercalcaemia in the dog and cat, although other, non-neoplastic causes are recognised (e.g. hypoadrenocorticism). Cancer associated hypercalcaemia results from the production of substances by haematopoietic and solid neoplasms which stimulate bone resorption. Several hypercalcaemic mediators produced by tumours have been identified, including parathyroid hormone (PTH), a parathyroid hormone-related protein (PTHrP), and a lymphokine osteoclast activating factor (OAF). In many cases, however, the active substance is not known. In the dog, hypercalcaemia is most commonly associated with:

- Lymphoproliferative disorders, e.g. lymphoma
- Adenocarcinoma of the apocrine glands of the anal sac
- Other solid tumours with or without bone metastases
- Functional adenoma of the parathyroid gland (primary hyperparathyroidism).

Clinical signs of hypercalcaemia
The predominant clinical signs are:

- Polydipsia/polyuria – due to the renal effects of hypercalcaemia
- Anorexia, vomiting – due to gastro-intestinal effects
- Lethargy, depression and muscular weakness – due to neuromuscular effects.

Hypercalcaemia can also affect the heart, resulting in bradycardia and arrhythmias.

The renal effects of hypercalcaemia are of greatest importance. In the early stages hypercalcaemia affects the renal tubules causing an inability to concentrate urine which leads to hyposthenuria and polyuria with secondary polydipsia. The renal nephropathy is initially reversible but if the hypercalcaemia persists, the renal damage becomes irreversible and eventually metastatic calcification of the renal tubular epithelium and basement membranes occurs. The renal effects of hypercalcaemia cause the animal to become dehydrated and hypovolaemic and further fluid loss may occur from vomiting. Renal failure caused by the hypercalcaemia is therefore exacerbated by pre-renal failure due to hypovolaemia, and the animal becomes azotemic.

Diagnosis
In most cases hypercalcaemia is detected on biochemical analysis. Most laboratories routinely measure the total plasma calcium which comprises:

- Ionised, biologically active calcium; *and*
- Calcium that is complexed or bound to protein.

An equilibrium exists between the two states such that in normal circumstances the total plasma calcium is a good indicator of the biologically active, ionised calcium. This equilibrium can be disturbed in cases of hypoalbuminaemia, where ionised calcium will make a proportionately greater contribution to the total value. It may also be influenced by the acid:base balance.

Table 2.7 Paraneoplastic syndromes affecting skin, bone and neuromuscular system.

System affected	Syndrome	Associated tumours/ references
Bone	*Hypertrophic (pulmonary) osteopathy (Marie's disease)* Painful, proliferative periosteal new bone growth on distal limbs associated with rapid increase in peripheral blood flow to the distal extremities. Exact aetiology unknown	Primary or secondary lung tumours Oesophageal tumours Rhabdomyosarcoma of bladder, Nephroblastoma Carcinoma of the liver Other non-neoplastic causes
Skin	*Hepatocutaneous syndrome/epidermal necrosis* Ulcerative dermatosis resembling human necrolytic migratory erythema Hyperkeratosis and fissuring of the foot pads with symmetrical erythema, ulceration and crusting of the face, feet and external genitalia	Glucagon producing pancreatic carcinoma (Gross *et al.* 1990), also reported with hepatic disease, often concurrent with diabetes mellitus (Bond *et al.* 1995)
	Exfoliative dermatitis Generalised scale and erythema	Thymoma in cats (Scott *et al.* 1995)
	Alopecia Progressive alopecia involving limbs and ventrum	Cats with pancreatic carcinoma, metastatic to liver and other distant sites. (Brooks *et al.* 1994; Tasker *et al.* 1999)
	Sterile nodular panniculitis	Bile duct carcinoma leading to pancreatic necrosis (Paterson 1994)
	Nodular dermatofibrosis Cutaneous nodules usually affecting the extremities associated with bilateral renal tumours. Autosomal inheritance in German shepherd dog. Cutaneous lesions may be due to growth factors secreted by the tumour	Renal cystadenocarcinoma (Moe & Lium 1997)
Neuromuscular	*Peripheral nerve syndromes* A variety of neuropathies, including demyelination and axonal degeneration in peripheral nerves have been reported in dogs with tumours	Bronchogenic carcinoma, insulinoma, leiomyosarcoma, haemangiosarcoma, undifferentiated sarcoma, synovial sarcoma and adrenal adenocarcinoma. (Braund 1990, 1996) Multiple myeloma (Villiers & Dobson 1998)
	Myasthenia gravis Failure of neuromuscular transmission, in cancer patients probably immune-mediated due to autoantibodies directed against nicotinic acetylcholine receptors	Thymoma and other tumours, cholangiocellular carcinoma, osteogenic sarcoma

Determining the cause of the hypercalcaemia can be straightforward, if for example the dog is presented with generalised lymphadenopathy. In some cases, however, the cause of the hypercal- caemia is not immediately obvious and a series of investigations (as summarised in Table 2.8) may be carried out based on the known causes of hypercalcaemia.

Table 2.8 Investigation of hypercalcaemia.

(1) *Look for lymphoma/leukaemia* – lymphoproliferative disease is the most common cause of hypercalcaemia in the dog
Check all peripheral lymph nodes and aspirate/biopsy any that are slightly enlarged or firmer than usual
Radiograph the thorax – anterior mediastinal and thymic forms of lymphoma are often associated with hypercalcaemia
Check haematology – is there any abnormality which might indicate lymphoproliferative or myeloproliferative disease?
Evaluate bone marrow

(2) *Check the anal glands* – Apocrine gland adenocarcinoma tends to be most common in middle aged bitch. Tumours can be quite small and only appear as a slight thickening of the anal sac

(3) *Check for hypoadrenocorticism* – sodium and potassium values, ACTH stimulation test

(4) *Consider a parathyroid tumour*
Palpate/examine by ultrasound the neck – looking for enlargement of one parathyroid gland
Parathyroid hormone (PTH) assay

Note:
Hypercalcaemia has been associated with assorted generalised inflammatory/skeletal problems
Calcium is normally elevated in young animals
Always check for laboratory error

Table 2.9 Treatment of hypercalcaemia.

Objective	Action
Restore circulating volume	Intravenous fluid therapy: 0.9% sodium chloride over 24 + hours
Reduce plasma calcium concentration	Saline diuresis: 0.9% NaCl at 2–3 × maintenance rate Frusemide 2 mg/kg bid or tid Glucocorticoids for lymphoid tumours, e.g. prednisolone 2 mg/kg daily
Identify and treat inciting cause	Specific chemotherapy, surgery or radiation as appropriate

Treatment of hypercalcaemia (Table 2.9)
Immediate management of hypercalcaemia is aimed at rehydration of the patient. Normal saline (0.9%) is the fluid of choice. Restoration of circulating volume will aid the lowering of the serum calcium by improving the glomerular filtration rate and thereby assisting renal excretion of calcium. Once the animal is rehydrated, calcium excretion can be further promoted by saline diuresis (0.9% saline at two to three times maintenance rate) and assisted by frusemide.

In hypercalcaemia associated with lymphoproliferative neoplasms, lowering of serum calcium can be assisted by the use of glucocorticoids (prednisolone 1–2 mg/kg daily). These agents are cytotoxic to lymphoid cells and also reduce serum calcium by limiting bone resorption, reducing intestinal calcium absorption and enhancing renal excretion of calcium. The value of glucocorticoids in the treatment of hypercalcaemia associated with non-lymphoid neoplasms is debatable. Once the animal's condition is stabilised, treatment of the primary cause of the hypercalcaemia is essential for long-term control.

There are a number of drugs which have been developed for the symptomatic treatment of human cancer patients where hypercalcaemia may be associated with refractory tumours, including:

Table 2.10 Check-list for diagnostic evaluation of the cancer patient.

Technique	Apply to
Aspirate/biopsy	Primary tumour
	Enlarged lymph nodes
	Any other suspicious lesions
	Bone marrow, if relevant
Radiography	Primary site, if relevant
	Thorax (right and left lateral chest views)
	(abdomen)
Ultrasound	Primary site, if relevant
	Internal organs, liver, spleen, kidneys
Routine haematology	Haematological complications
Routine biochemistry	Metabolic/endocrine complications
FeLV/FIV serology	In cats

- Bisphosphonates – currently treatment of choice in human medicine, e.g. alendronate, etidronate, pamidronate, clodronate
- Mithramycin ($25\,\mu g/kg$ single dose) – used less since development of bisphosphonates
- (Calcitonin)
- (iv infusion of phosphate solutions, phosphate enemas, sodium EDTA and peritoneal dialysis – all largely outdated).

It is unusual for these agents to be required in veterinary medicine as most cases of hypercalcaemia in animals can be managed effectively by fluid therapy and treatment of the primary cause.

Mast cell tumours and hyper-histaminaemia

Mast cells are characterised by intra-cytoplasmic granules that contain vaso-active amines and proteases including histamine and heparin. Degranulation may occur spontaneously in some mast cell tumours or may be precipitated by manipulation of the tumour or therapeutic intervention. The inflammatory mediators thus released may have both local and systemic effects.

Local effects
Local effects include oedematous swelling of the tumour and surrounding area, erythema and sometimes pruritis. If significant amounts of heparin are present there may be a tendency for local bleeding.

Proteases may also cause delayed wound healing or wound breakdown following surgery.

Systemic effects
Massive and sudden histamine release may precipitate an anaphylactic reaction which requires emergency treatment with fluids, corticosteroids and anti-histamines. Although this is extremely unusual, premedication of animals with antihistamine (e.g. chlorpheniramine) prior to surgical manipulation of such tumours is often recommended.

A more common yet less obvious effect of hyperhistaminaemia occurs in the gastro-intestinal tract, where overstimulation of the gastric H_2 receptors results in excessive gastric acid production and changes in the vascular supply and motility of the gastric mucosa leading to gastro-duodenal ulceration. Clinical signs vary according to the severity and duration of the problem and range from mild anorexia to vomiting, haematemesis, melaena and anaemia resulting from intra-luminal bleeding. Ultimately the ulcers may perforate leading to peritonitis, collapse and death. Cimetidine $5–10\,mg/kg$ two to four times daily, or ranitidine $2\,mg/kg$ twice daily, block H_2 receptors and reduce the secretion of gastric acid.

Summary

In summary, tumours can behave and manifest themselves in many different ways. An animal with cancer may present with an obvious mass or as a result of a tumour-related complication. In every case it is important to adopt a methodical approach to the patient in order to define the nature and extent of the problem. Only when this is achieved can an appropriate treatment be devised. A checklist for the 'work-up' of a cancer patient is provided in Table 2.10.

References

Bond, R., McNeil, P.E., Evans, H. & Srebernik, N. (1995) Metabolic epidermal necrosis in two dogs with different underlying diseases. *Veterinary Record*, (136), 466–71.

Braund, K.G. (1990) Remote effects of cancer on the nervous system. *Seminars in Veterinary Medicine and Surgery (Small Animal)*, (5), 262–70.

Braund, K.G. (1996) Endogenous causes of neuropathies in dogs and cats. *Veterinary Medicine*, (91), 740–54.

Brooks, D.G., Campbell, K.L., Dennis, J.S. *et al.* (1994) Pancreatic paraneoplastic alopecia in three cats. *Journal of the American Animal Hospital Association*, (30), 557–63.

Dobson, J.M. (1999) Principles of cancer therapy. In: *Texbook of Small Animal Medicine*, (ed. J.K. Dunn), pp. 985–1028. W. B. Saunders, London.

Gross, T.L., O'Brien, T.D., Davies, A.P. & Long, R.E. (1990) Glucagon producing pancreatic endocrine tumours in two dogs with superficial necrolytic dermatitis. *Journal of the American Veterinary Medical Association*, (197), 1619–22.

Moe, L. & Lium, B. (1997) Hereditary multifocal renal cystadenocarcinomas and nodular dermatofibrosis in 51 German shepherd dogs. *Journal of Small Animal Practice*, (38), 498–505.

Paterson, S. (1994) Panniculitis associated with pancreatic necrosis in a dog. *Journal of Small Animal Practice*, (35), 116–18.

Scott, D.W., Yager, J.A. & Johnson, K.M. (1995) Exfoliative dermatitis in association with thymoma in three cats. *Feline Practice*, (23), 8–13.

Tasker, S., Griffon, D.J., Nuttall, T.J. & Hill, P.B. (1999) Resolution of paraneoplastic alopecia following surgical removal of a pancreatic carcinoma in a cat. *Journal of Small Animal Practice*, (40), 16–19.

Vail, D.M., Ogilvie, G.K. & Wheeler, S.L. (1990) Metabolic alterations in patients with cancer cachexia. *Compendium of Continuing Education for the Practising Veterinarian*, (12), 381–7.

Villiers, E. & Dobson, J.M. (1998) Multiple myeloma with associated polyneuropathy in a German shepherd dog. *Journal of Small Animal Practice*, (39), 249–51.

3
Treatment Options

The three main methods of cancer treatment in animals, as in humans, are:

• Surgery
• Radiotherapy
• Anti-cancer/cytotoxic chemotherapy.

Cancer therapy must always be tailored to suit the individual case, taking account of the biology, histology, grade and extent of that tumour (see Chapter 2). Clearly a cure, i.e. total eradication of all tumour stem cells, is the desirable outcome of treatment, but even the most effective methods of treatment currently available cannot achieve this aim in every case. The decision to treat an animal with cancer is one which must be made jointly by the veterinarian and the owner. Owners must be counselled thoroughly in the nature of the disease, the prognosis, the options for treatment and the expectations of such treatment and should be given time to consider the options and reach a decision. The methods of cancer therapy which will be described are generally tolerated very well by animal patients provided that there are no pre-existing complications which make the patient more susceptible to toxicity.

SURGERY

Surgery is the most effective means of treatment for the majority of solid neoplasms in animals and usually offers the best chance of cure for such tumours.

Indications

Surgery may play a number of roles in the diagnosis and treatment of cancer:

• Diagnosis – biopsy, needle, incisional or excisional (see Chapter 2)
• Definitive treatment for solid, solitary, low grade tumours (see below)
• Cytoreduction of tumour mass prior to radiotherapy (see later)
• Pain management – for example amputation of a limb in the case of a painful tumour or pathological fracture
• Prophylaxis – for example, spaying a bitch before her first or second oestrus significantly reduces the risk of later development of mammary tumours.

The primary objective of surgical treatment of any tumour, be it benign or malignant, is to physically remove all the tumour cells. In most cases it will be necessary to include a margin of normal tissue in the surgical excision in order to achieve this aim. Failure of surgical treatment may result from:

- The tumour being incompletely resected at the first attempt, in which case the tumour will regrow at or adjacent to the primary site
- Contamination of normal tissue with tumour cells at the time of surgery through haemorrhage, from surgical instruments or via surgical drains
- The tumour having metastasised to distant organs prior to surgical treatment, in which case the animal will subsequently develop problems relating to metastatic tumour elsewhere.

Surgery is rarely an effective or feasible means of managing disseminated disease and chemotherapy is more appropriate in such cases. Local tumour recurrence is strongly influenced by the surgical approach and the main advances in surgical oncology have been in defining the margins of excision which are necessary to achieve eradication of different tumours and in developing techniques whereby such margins can be achieved. It is not within the remit of this chapter to cover the surgical and reconstructive techniques used in oncology in detail but a brief description of surgical techniques which have proved efficacious in the management of certain tumours is appropriate.

Surgical principles

- Plan the surgical approach based on the biopsy result and the anatomy of the affected area.
- Try not to change the surgical plan mid treatment. If a tumour seems unexpectedly aggressive, collection of further biopsy material to review the original diagnosis may be the best immediate course of action.
- Aim not to touch tumour tissue or invade the tumour capsule with instruments (or hands).
- If tumour tissue does contaminate instruments, then gloves and instruments should be changed before dissecting into normal tissue.
- Take advantage of clean fascial planes and tissue compartments.
- Submit excised tissue to confirm the biopsy diagnosis.

- Ask the pathologist to examine the margins of the excision. These can be marked with ink or coloured sutures to identify the orientation and sites of concern.

Surgical approaches

Local excision

Truly benign tumours, e.g. fibroma, lipoma and mammary adenoma, can be cured by local surgical resection with a minimal margin of normal tissue (Fig. 3.1). Local surgical resection is a simple and straightforward procedure when lesions are small. A tumour which is left to enlarge will eventually require a more extensive procedure which is less likely to be curative.

Wide local excision

Locally invasive tumours, e.g. basal cell carcinoma and squamous cell carcinoma are characterised by local extension of the tumour into surrounding normal tissues. In such cases local surgical excision is unlikely to remove all tumour cells and local recurrence will ensue unless a more aggressive surgical approach is adopted. Thus wider margins of

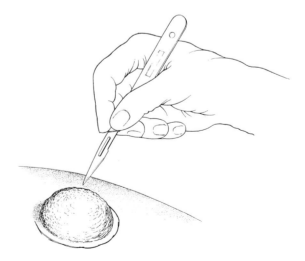

Fig. 3.1 Diagram depicting local surgical excision (excisional biopsy). The tumour is excised through its immediate boundaries with a minimal border of surrounding normal tissue. (Reprinted from Dobson (1999) with permission.)

excision, including at least 1–2 cm of apparently normal tissues lateral and deep to the tumour, are often required to achieve a successful outcome. Some tumours, e.g. mast cell tumours, may require more generous margins than this to effect a complete excision. Such a procedure is termed a 'wide local excision' (Fig. 3.2).

For tumours sited on the chest or abdominal walls, achieving excisional margins of this magnitude is usually possible. Problems may arise, however, in the case of tumours sited on limbs or in the head region, particularly in the oral cavity. For tumours on limbs and the head, excisional margins can usually be achieved but, because of the lack of mobile skin and soft tissues, reconstructive techniques may be necessary to close the resulting deficit. Tumours in the oral cavity present a particular problem because of their proximity to bone. Locally invasive tumours arising at this site frequently extend into the underlying bone such that successful surgery requires removal of portions of bone. Various techniques for mandibulectomy, premaxillectomy and maxillectomy have been well documented (White 1991; Salisbury 1993). These procedures are tolerated very well in dogs and the results for low grade oral tumours are very good (Fig. 3.3) (see Chapter 7).

Compartmental excision

Certain solid tumours such as soft tissue sarcoma (e.g. fibrosarcoma, haemangiopericytoma), infiltrate adjacent tissues so widely that even 1–2 cm margins of excision are not adequate to ensure complete removal of all tumour cells. Surgical removal of tumours such as these requires resection of every tissue compartment which the tumour involves, termed a 'compartmental' or 'en bloc' resection (Fig. 3.4). To achieve such a resection in tumours arising on the trunk invariably requires full thickness resection of either the abdominal or chest wall. The resulting deficits must be reconstructed using prostheses and skin flaps (Pavletic 1999). In tumours arising in the proximal limb, it is sometimes possible to achieve an 'en bloc' resection by removal of a muscle mass and overlying skin, leaving the animal with a functional limb. In other cases amputation may have to be considered.

All the surgical techniques described require

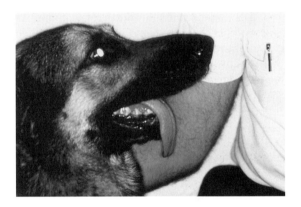

Fig. 3.3 Appearance of dog following a bilateral mandibulectomy. (Courtesy of Dr R.A.S. White, Department of Clinical Veterinary Medicine, Cambridge.)

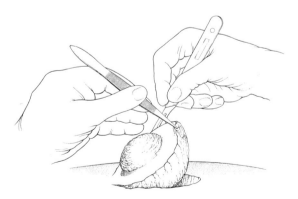

Fig. 3.2 Diagram depicting wide local excision. The tumour is excised with a predetermined margin of surrounding tissue both lateral and deep to the tumour mass. (Reprinted from Dobson (1999) with permission.)

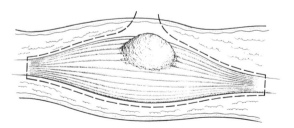

Fig. 3.4 Compartmental or 'en bloc' resection. The tumour is resected together with the contents of the anatomic compartment in which is it contained. Fascial planes which are undisturbed by tumour invasion form the outer margins of the resection. (Reprinted from Dobson (1999) with permission.)

careful planning, particularly when reconstructive techniques are involved. The treatment and the expected cosmetic and functional results should be fully discussed with the owner. It is therefore essential that the nature of the tumour is identified, preferably by biopsy (or cytology), and that regional lymph nodes are carefully assessed prior to embarking on the definitive treatment. It is increasingly appreciated that the best chance of eradication of locally aggressive tumours is at the first surgical attempt. Subsequent surgical procedures are fraught with difficulties due to loss of normal anatomical relationships through scarring and fibrosis, and local dissemination of the tumour at the previous surgery through haemorrhage or on instruments.

RADIOTHERAPY

Radiotherapy (RT) is widely used in the treatment of human cancer patients and is equally applicable to the treatment of the disease in small animals. Radiotherapy requires specialised equipment and facilities which are expensive to install and maintain (Fig. 3.5). Consequently, the use of radiation therapy in animals is restricted to larger referral establishments. Although most veterinarians in practice will not have direct access to such facilities, it is useful to review the principles and practice of radiation therapy, in order that suitable cases might be identified and referred at an appropriate stage.

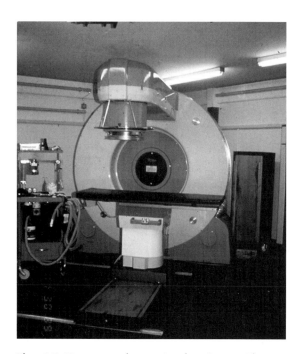

Fig. 3.5 Linear accelerator in the Cancer Therapy Unit, Department of Clinical Veterinary Medicine, Cambridge.

Principles of radiotherapy

The mode of action of radiation

Radiation is a form of energy which, when absorbed by living tissues, causes excitation and ionisation of component atoms or molecules in the path of the beam. Subsequent chemical reactions result in breaking of molecular bonds and can result in apoptotic cell death if molecules critical for cell viability are disrupted. The 'critical target' is generally regarded as being nuclear DNA but other molecules in other parts of the cell (e.g. proteins and lipids) may also be damaged and contribute to radiation-induced cellular injury.

Types of radiation used for therapy

Different types of ionising radiation may be used for therapeutic purposes, including:

- X-rays
- Gamma rays
- Electrons.

There are essentially two techniques for the application of radiation to tumours:

- *Teletherapy* – radiation is applied in the form of an external beam of X-rays, gamma rays or electrons which are directed into the tumour (Fig. 3.6).
- *Brachytherapy* – radioactive substances which emit gamma or beta rays, may be applied to the surface of a tumour, implanted within the tumour (Fig. 3.7) or administered systemically to the patient, for example iodine[131] therapy for thyroid tumours in cats (see Chapter 14, Endocrine system).

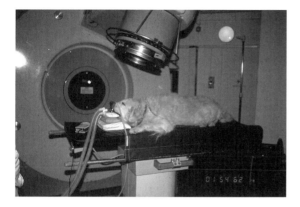

Fig. 3.6 External beam therapy. The patient and machine are positioned to direct the radiation beam into and through the treatment field, in this case a tumour of the nasal cavity.

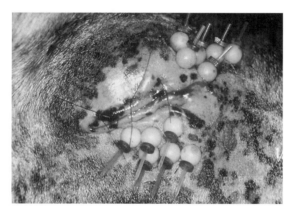

Fig. 3.7 Brachytherapy – irridium wires in afterloading catheters implanted following cytoreductive surgery for a periocular squamous cell carcinoma in a horse.

Each technique has advantages and disadvantages. Whilst external beam therapy is relatively safe for the operator, the equipment is expensive and multiple doses of radiation are required over a four to six week course of treatment. Brachytherapy often offers better localisation of the radiation and permits the delivery of high doses of radiation to the tumour with minimal normal tissue toxicity. However, the implant and the implanted patient present a radiation hazard for the operator and any staff caring for the patient. Radioactive isotopes can only be used on licensed premises and strict local rules for handling the isotope and patient must be applied. Both techniques require careful

planning in consultation with medical physicists to ensure that the required dose of radiation is delivered to the tumour.

Radiation biology

The response of living cells and tissues to radiation depends on the applied dose of radiation and the radiosensitivity of the cell population. Radiosensitivity varies according to a number of factors, one of the most important being the growth fraction of the cell population.

- Dividing cells are generally more sensitive to radiation than non-dividing, differentiated cells. Thus tissues with a high proportion of dividing cells, e.g. bone marrow, gastrointestinal epithelium, are more radiosensitive than non-proliferating tissues, e.g. fibrous tissue and skeletal muscle.
- The same applies to tumours: those with a high growth fraction tend to be more sensitive to radiation than those with low growth fractions.
- Individual cells vary in their radiosensitivity as they pass through the phases of the cell cycle. Cells in the M (mitotic) phase of the cycle are most radiosensitive and those in the S (DNA synthesis) phase are most resistant. The resting (G_o) cells are also radioresistant.
- The oxygenation of cells is also thought to be significant in determining radiosensitivity. Tumour cells which exist at a low oxygen tension, i.e. hypoxic cells, may be two and a half to three times less sensitive to radiation than normally oxygenated cells.

Whilst radiation is a potent means of causing tumour cell death, it is not selective and can be equally damaging to normal tissues; indeed certain normal tissues may be more sensitive to radiation than many tumours. In order to be of therapeutic benefit, radiation must be employed in such a way as to minimise normal tissue injury whilst achieving maximum tumour cell kill. One way in which this may be approached is by attempting to localise the radiation to the tumour. Radioactive implants and radio-labelled substances which are taken up by tumour cells (e.g. radioactive iodine for thyroid tumours) afford a degree of selectivity. With external beam radiation, the beam can be collimated to the area of the tumour and several treatment ports employed in order to reduce the amount of entry and exit beam radiation affecting the surrounding normal tissues.

A further means of reducing normal tissue injury from external beam therapy is to 'fractionate' the treatment, that is to apply the radiation in multiple small doses over a period of time rather than as one large dose. In this way tumour cell kill may be increased whilst normal tissue damage can be limited to some extent by allowing time for repair between doses. At the present time most radiation schedules for human patients employ daily or alternate day treatments over a period of four to six weeks. In animals, where general anaesthesia is required for restraint of the patient during treatment and where radiation facilities are not widely available, larger less frequent fractions tend to be used, although some centres in North America are able to treat animals on a daily basis.

Tumour response and normal tissue toxicity

Whilst the chemical events leading to radiation-induced damage occur almost instantaneously, the biological expression of this injury may take days, weeks or even years to become apparent. Radiation therefore appears to have delayed actions in terms of both tumour response and normal tissue toxicity.

Tumours vary considerably in their response to radiation. In general, small, rapidly growing tumours tend to respond more favourably to radiation than large, slowly growing tumours where radiation treatment is unlikely to achieve more than a partial and temporary remission. The relative radiosensitivity of common animal tumours is summarised in Table 3.1.

Normal tissue toxicity

Radiation has a reputation for causing serious toxicity to the patient; however, radiation sickness and severe morbidity only arise when large areas of the body or vital organs are exposed to high doses. In order to avoid such side effects, radiation is rarely used in this manner in the treatment of animals. Tumours most suitable for radiotherapy tend to be superficial or those sited on the extremities of the body. The skin, superficial connective tissues, oral and nasal mucous membranes and bone are therefore the tissues most commonly included in the treatment field and some radiation-induced changes will occur in these tissues.

Radiation toxicity is usually described in terms of 'acute' reactions occurring during and shortly after the radiation treatment and 'late' reactions which are not observed for weeks or even months following treatment. This division is not absolute.

Table 3.1 Relative radiosensitivity of common animal tumours.

Relative radiosensitivity	Tumour
High	Lymphoproliferative disorders Myeloproliferative disorders Transmissible venereal tumour
Sensitive	Squamous cell carcinoma Basal cell carcinoma Adenocarcinoma (various)
Moderate	Mast cell tumours (variable) Malignant melanoma of the oral cavity
Low	Fibrosarcoma Osteosarcoma Chondrosarcoma Haemangiopericytoma

Factors such as tumour site and tumour extent also influence the suitability of a particular tumour for radiotherapy.

Acute reactions

- Result from the death of actively dividing cell populations, e.g. epithelium of the skin and mucous membranes
- Range from a mild reddening or erythema of the skin/mucosa to desquamation and severe exfoliative dermatitis/necrosis (the latter is rare) (Fig. 3.8)
- Usually resolve spontaneously as the normal cell population regenerates.

Localised hair loss is a common result of irradiation of the skin in animals (Fig. 3.9). This results from damage to the hair follicle epithelium at the time of treatment but the resulting alopecia does not usually occur until the existing hair is shed and not replaced. Ultimately some hair usually regrows but this may be patchy and lacking pigmentation.

Late toxicity

- Is less predictable and more serious
- Tends to occur in slowly proliferating tissues, e.g. connective tissues and bone
- Is often progressive and irreversible.

Examples of late radiation toxicity:

- *Skin* – Radiation induces fibrosis in the dermal connective tissues resulting in a thickened,

rubbery texture and subsequently contraction of the skin and subcutis can occur. As a result of the fibrosis and vascular changes, irradiated skin and soft tissues can be very slow to heal. Wounds in such tissues are difficult to repair as they are avascular and even the most minor surgical procedure can result in a non-healing, necrotic wound.
- *Bone* – Osteonecrosis is a major concern in fields containing bone, particularly in cases where the bone is already compromised by tumour invasion.
- *Nervous tissue* – Late reactions in nervous tissues can result in neural degeneration and necrosis. Irradiation of the spine should be avoided if at all possible as it can result in paralysis.
- *Eye* – Retinal degeneration and cataract formation may be late consequences of radiation of the eye.

Indications for radiation therapy in small animals

It follows from the above that the main indications for radiotherapy in animals are in the control of malignant solid tumours sited on the extremities, which cannot be controlled by surgical means

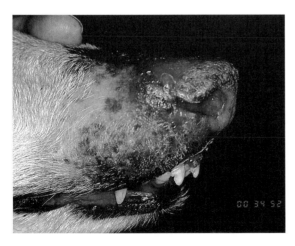

Fig. 3.8 Acute radiation skin reaction – erythema of the skin and moist desquamation of the nasal planum following treatment of a SCC of the nasal planum. (See also Colour plate 2, facing p. 162.)

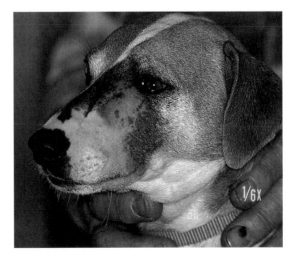

Fig. 3.9 Post radiation alopecia. (See also Colour plate 3, facing p. 162.)

Table 3.2 Tumours commonly treated with radiotherapy in small animals.

Anatomical site	Tumour types
Nasal cavity and paranasal sinuses (Chapter 7)	Adenocarcinoma Squamous cell carcinoma Chondrosarcoma, and other sarcomas (Lymphoma)
Oral cavity (Chapter 7)	(Basal cell carcinoma)** Squamous cell carcinoma Fibrosarcoma and other sarcomas* Malignant melanoma
Skin and soft tissues Head, neck and limbs (Chapters 4, 6, 7 and 14)	Mast cell tumours* Soft tissue sarcomas* Thyroid carcinoma in dogs
Brain (Chapter 13)	Glioma Meningioma

* Post-operative radiotherapy used as an adjunct to cytoreductive surgery in these tumours.
** Surgery is the preferred treatment for such tumours because of the risk of later development of a second malignancy at the same site (White *et al.* 1986).

alone. The types of tumour most commonly treated with radiotherapy in small animals are summarised in Table 3.2. It is desirable that local and/or distant metastases are not present, although local lymph nodes can be included in the treatment fields.

Because of the difficulties in localisation and the risk of toxicity, tumours sited deep in the chest, abdomen or pelvis are not usually treated with radiation in animals. Benign tumours are often not very radiosensitive, and, because radiation is potentially carcinogenic, other means of treatment should always be sought to manage such tumours.

Radiation may be combined with surgery in the management of selected tumours which cannot be treated adequately by surgery alone. Radiation can be used prior to, following or during surgery. Post-operative radiation is the most common method of combining these two modalities. Cytoreductive surgery reduces the tumour burden to microscopic levels leaving small numbers of well oxygenated and rapidly proliferating cells which, in theory, should be sensitive to radiation. Radiation will, however, delay the healing of the surgical wound and must be commenced either immediately following surgery or once the wound has healed. The combination of radiation and surgery in this manner is potentially most beneficial in the management of problematic solid tumours, e.g. soft tissue sarcomas and intermediate grade mast cell tumours. It is preferable that radiation and surgery should be combined as a carefully planned therapeutic strategy. The use of radiation as an afterthought to salvage inadequate surgery is fraught with difficulties in planning the radiation fields and this practice is strongly discouraged.

CHEMOTHERAPY

Anticancer chemotherapy has become an accepted method of cancer treatment in small animal practice and the indications for cytotoxic drugs are ever increasing.

Principles of chemotherapy

What are cytotoxic drugs and how do they work?

Many pharmacologically different drugs have been identified as having anti-cancer activity. These agents can be divided into groups on the basis of their mode of action, anti-tumour activity and toxicity as shown in Table 3.3 and Fig. 3.10.

Alkylating agents, anti-tumour antibiotics and some of the miscellaneous agents interfere with the replication and transcription of DNA. Anti-metabolites interfere with the synthesis of DNA or RNA by enzyme inhibition or by causing the synthesis of non-functional molecules. The vinca alkaloids are anti-mitotic, acting specifically on the mitotic spindle and causing a metaphase arrest.

Thus all these agents act on the processes of cell growth and division and therefore cytotoxic drugs are most effective against growing or dividing cells.

Tumour response

Different tumours are not equally sensitive or responsive to cytotoxic drugs (Table 3.4). The major factors that determine the response of a tumour to drugs are:

- Tumour growth rate, as previously discussed
- Drug resistance.

Table 3.4 Relative tumour sensitivity to cytotoxic drugs.

Chemosensitivity	Tumour type
High	Lymphoma Myeloma Forms of leukaemia (Transmissible venereal tumour)
Moderate	High grade sarcomas (E.g. osteosarcoma, haemangiosarcoma) Mast cell tumours
Low	Slowly growing sarcomas Carcinomas Melanoma

Table 3.3 Classes of cytotoxic drugs.

Alkylating agents	Cyclophosphamide Melphalan Chlorambucil
Anti-metabolites	Cytarabine 5-Fluorouracil Methotrexate (Azathioprine)
Anti-tumour antibiotics	Doxorubicin Epirubicin Mitoxantrone Bleomycin
Vinca alkaloids	Vincristine Vinblastine
Miscellaneous agents	Cisplatin Carboplatin L-Asparaginase

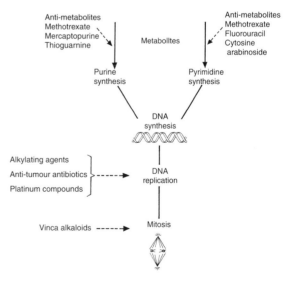

Fig. 3.10 Diagrammatic representation of the mode of action of cytotoxic drugs. (Reprinted from Dobson & Gorman (1993) with permission.)

The growth fraction (GF) is the single most important factor governing tumour response to chemotherapy because most cytotoxic drugs are only active against dividing cells.

Drug resistance describes the ability of a tumour cell to survive the actions of an anti-cancer drug when administered at a dose which would normally be expected to cause cell damage and death. Certain tumours or tumour cells are intrinsically resistant and can circumvent the actions of cytotoxic drugs through various biochemical/metabolic mechanisms. Tumour cells may also acquire drug resistance, as exemplified by the clinical situation in which a previously drug-responsive tumour regrows or relapses and is no longer sensitive to further treatment with the same agent. Tumour cells can acquire resistance to drugs which are unrelated to the drug groups used to treat the tumour initially, through a process known as multi-drug resistance (MDR). MDR is associated with a transmembrane P-glycoprotein pump which can transport cytotoxic drugs directly from the cell membrane before such drugs enter the cytoplasm, or from the cytoplasm, thus limiting the concentration of the drug reaching the target.

Cytotoxic drug administration

Cytotoxic drugs kill tumour cells according to first order kinetics, i.e. a given dose of a cytotoxic drug kills a fixed percentage of the total tumour population as opposed to a set number of tumour cells. Thus:

- Cytotoxic drugs should always be used at the highest possible dose to effect the highest possible fractional kill
- Even a highly effective drug acting on a highly sensitive tumour cell population is unlikely to eradicate the tumour cell population in a single dose
- Chemotherapy should be instituted when the tumour burden is at its lowest
- Chemotherapy is unlikely to be effective if used as a last resort for the treatment of extensive and advanced disease.

Stages of therapy

Chemotherapy usually involves courses of treatment in which different phases are described

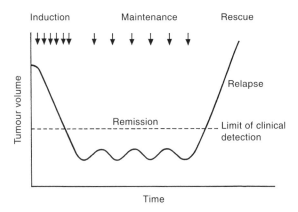

Fig. 3.11 Diagrammatic representation of the phases of chemotherapy. (Reprinted from Dobson & Gorman (1993) with permission.)

according to the intended result, as depicted in Fig. 3.11. (This does not apply when chemotherapy is used as an adjuvant to surgery in the treatment of solid tumours.)

Induction therapy
The aim of induction therapy is to reduce the tumour burden to a minimal level below the limits of detection, i.e. remission. Induction usually involves an intensive course of treatment administered over a defined period of time. A clinical remission is not synonymous with cure and unless treatment is continued a rapid expansion of the residual tumour mass will result in a 'relapse' or recurrence of the disease.

Maintenance therapy
Where clinical remission can be achieved by induction treatment, a less intensive treatment regime may be adopted to maintain this remission.

Rescue therapy
In some cases the tumour may not respond to the initial therapy; in others, the initial response appears to be good but the tumour recurs or relapses despite continued treatment (usually as a result of drug resistance). The aim of rescue therapy is to establish a further remission of the tumour and this usually involves recourse to more aggressive therapy, preferably with agents to which the tumour has not been exposed.

Single agent versus combination therapy

In general, combinations of cytotoxic agents have proved to be more effective in cancer therapy than a single agent. By treating a tumour with a combination of agents which employ different mechanisms of action and have different spectra of normal tissue toxicity, the overall response can be enhanced without an increase in toxicity. A typical example of combination chemotherapy in veterinary practice is the COP protocol for treatment of lymphoma which employs:

• C cyclophosphamide – alkylating agent
• O vincristine – vinca alkaloid
• P prednisolone – glucocorticoid.

Dosage and timing of treatments

Cytotoxic drugs are usually administered at repeated intervals (or in 'pulses'), allowing time for the normal tissues to recover between treatments. The interval between treatments has to be carefully timed to allow for recovery of the normal tissues without expansion of the residual tumour population. For most myelosuppressive cytotoxic agents (e.g. doxorubicin) maximum bone marrow suppression occurs at about day 7–10 following treatment, with recovery by day 21. Hence three week cycles of treatment are used in clinical practice. For other agents or combinations of agents, weekly treatment regimes or semi-continuous protocols may also be used (see Chapter 15).

Dosage
As a general rule the dosages of cytotoxics used in human therapy are not appropriate in the dog and cat because the severe toxicity resulting from such treatment cannot be managed on a routine basis in veterinary medicine. Dosages recommended for animals are invariably a compromise between efficacy and toxicity.

Dose rate calculation
Doses of cytotoxic drugs are usually calculated as a function of body surface area (in square metres: m^2) rather than body weight (in kg) because the blood supply to the organs responsible for detoxification and excretion (liver and kidneys) is more closely

related to surface area than body weight. Conversion charts are provided in Appendix III at the end of this book.

Indications for chemotherapy

The main indication for chemotherapy as a first line treatment is in lymphoproliferative and myeloproliferative disorders, for example:

• Lymphoma
• Myeloma
• Types of leukaemia.

These diseases are systemic in their nature and usually respond favourably to cytotoxic drugs. Details of treatment protocols for these conditions can be found in Chapter 15. Chemotherapy is rarely of value as the sole treatment for solid, i.e. non-lymphoid, tumours, for example carcinomas, sarcomas and melanomas. Such tumours are best treated by surgical resection and/or radiotherapy.

Adjunctive chemotherapy

It is increasingly appreciated that cytotoxic drugs may have a role as an adjunct to surgical (or radiotherapeutic) management of some solid tumours, for example:

• Osteosarcoma – cisplatin or carboplatin
• Haemangiosarcoma – doxorubicin (± cyclophosphamide and vincristine),

where they may be used to prevent or delay development of metastases. In such circumstances, where there is no measurable tumour from the outset of chemotherapy, a set number of treatments (usually four to six) are prescribed as the total course.

Complications of chemotherapy

Normal tissue toxicity (side effects)

Complications of chemotherapy can arise at any time during therapy. Some cytotoxic agents can induce immediate hypersensitivity reactions; some agents are highly irritant and can cause severe local tissue reactions if perivascular leakage occurs. The actions of cytotoxic drugs are not selective for tumour cells and their effects on normal tissues result in toxicity or side effects. Organs containing

---

a high proportion of dividing cells are most susceptible to drug-induced toxicity. Hence the most common side effects of chemotherapy are:

- *Bone marrow* toxicity – myelosuppression, neutropenia and thrombocytopenia
- *Gastrointestinal* toxicity – anorexia, nausea, vomiting and diarrhoea.

Fortunately, these normal tissues are able to recover from cytotoxic drug damage through recruitment of resting stem cells. Hence, although potentially life threatening, these toxic effects are usually quickly reversible on discontinuation of treatment.

Some cytotoxic agents have other toxic actions that are less reversible. These include:

- Cyclophosphamide – haemorrhagic cystitis
- Doxorubicin – cardiomyopathy
- Cisplatin – nephrotoxicity.

Myelosuppression and infection

Most cytotoxic drugs are myelosuppressive. The most notable exceptions are:

- Vincristine
- L-asparaginase.

Myelosuppression is the main dose-limiting factor in veterinary chemotherapy. The main effects of myelosuppression are:

- *Anaemia* – rarely clinically significant and often indistinguishable from anaemia associated with the neoplasm itself.
- *Neutropenia* (a neutrophil count of less than $2 \times 10^9/l$) – results in a clinically significant risk of overwhelming infection and sepsis.
- *Thrombocytopenia* (a platelet count of less than $70 \times 10^9/l$) – rarely severe enough to cause spontaneous bleeding but may require care with biopsies/surgery.

Haematological monitoring is vital in all cases receiving potentially myelosuppressive drugs and these drugs should never be administered until baseline haematological values have been established for that patient.

Neutropenia predisposes the cancer patient to infection and sepsis. Absorption of enteric bacteria e.g. *E. coli* and *Klebsiella* spp., through damaged intestinal mucosa is the most common source of infection in animal cancer patients. Identification or detection of sepsis can be difficult in the neutropenic patient because the inflammatory response is altered by the neutropenia. Pyrexia is the most consistent sign of sepsis.

Treatment
Management of neutropenic patients depends on the neutrophil count and clinical presentation, as summarised in Table 3.5. Most animals recover spontaneously from drug induced myelosuppression within 36–72 hours of ceasing administration of the offending agent through stem cell recruitment. Lithium carbonate may be used to assist this recovery and a number of human recombinant granulocyte (G-CSF) and granulocyte-monocyte (GM-CSF) stimulating factors are available to speed recovery from myelosuppression in human cancer patients. Human recombinant cytokines have been shown to be useful for treatment in cats and dogs with chemotherapy-induced neutropenia and although these species may mount a neutralising antibody response to the human recombinant protein, this does not seem to be a problem in these circumstances (Ogilvie 1993a; Henry *et al.* 1998). Their use in veterinary medicine may be limited by cost.

Anorexia, vomiting and gastrointestinal toxicity

Many cytotoxic drugs have adverse effects on the gastro-intestinal tract either as a direct result of the action of the drug on the oral, gastric and intestinal epithelium or as a result of non-specific myelosuppression. Death and desquamation of alimentary epithelium usually occurs 5–10 days following administration of the drug and leads to stomatitis, vomiting and mucoid or haemorrhagic diarrhoea. In most cases such problems are self-limiting and the animal recovers spontaneously as the normal alimentary epithelium regenerates. Some drugs induce nausea and vomiting by direct stimulation of the chemoreceptor trigger zone. These include cisplatin and doxorubicin.

Treatment
Treatment is symptomatic:

- Anorexia in cats may be helped with cyproheptadine.

Table 3.5 Haematological monitoring for chemotherapy.

Neutrophil count (× 10⁹/l)	Status of patient	Recommended action
>3	Normal	Continue chemotherapy Repeat white blood count in 3–4 weeks
2–3	Evidence of myelosuppression	Reduce dosage of myelosuppressive drug(s) by 50% Repeat WBC count in 2 weeks
<2	Moderate myelosuppression	Stop myelosuppressive chemotherapy Monitor patient and WBC carefully
	Patient asymptomatic/afebrile	If patient has existing predisposition to infection e.g. ulcerated tumour, administer potentiated sulphonamide or fluoroquinolone antibiotics
<1	Severe myelosuppression Patient asymptomatic/afebrile	Stop all cytotoxic treament Administer potentiated sulphonamide or fluoroquinolone antibiotics
	Patient pyrexic	Collect samples in attempt to identify infective agent Supportive therapy: intravenous fluids, electrolytes, glucose as indicated Bactericidal antibiotics: cephalosporins plus gentamicin, or fluoroquinolones (can alter later based on sensitivity)

- Anti-emetics, e.g. metoclopramide or ondansetron, are useful in the prevention or control of drug-induced vomiting.
- Antacids and ulcer healing drugs may be used to assist in the control of gastric ulceration.

Products containing bismuth subsalicylate (Pepto Bismol) may assist management of enterocolitis caused by doxorubicin in some dogs.

- Intravenous fluid therapy should be given in cases where the vomiting/diarrhoea is severe or prolonged.
- Mucosal injury can also predispose to systemic infection and parenteral antibiotics may be indicated, as discussed above.

Hypersensitivity/anaphylaxis

Hypersensitivity reactions to cytotoxic drugs are rare but have been reported in dogs following administration of:

- L-asparaginase
- Doxorubicin
- (Cisplatin)
- (Cytarabine).

Some cytotoxic drug hypersensitivities are immune-mediated reactions (e.g. L-asparaginase); some drugs (e.g. doxorubicin) cause degranulation of mast cells and others may activate the alternative complement pathway.

Prevention

- The route of administration can affect the incidence of hypersensitivity reactions. L-asparaginase may produce anaphylaxis in up to 30% of dogs when administered intravenously. For this reason it is recommended that the drug should always be given by the intramuscular route.
- Pre-treatment with antihistamines e.g. chlorpheniramine, can reduce the frequency of some drug reactions and this is usually recommended prior to administration of doxorubicin.

Treatment
In the event of a hypersensitivity reaction:

- Stop administration of the drug immediately
- Treat with intravenous fluids, soluble corticosteroids, adrenaline and antihistamines.

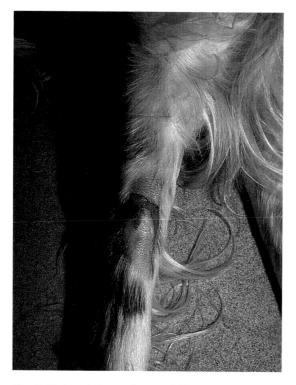

Fig. 3.12 Local tissue damage following perivascular leakage of vincristine. (See also Colour plate 4, facing p. 162.)

Phlebitis and tissue necrosis

Many cytotoxic drugs are irritant or vesicant and may cause severe local tissue necrosis following perivascular injection or extravasation from the intravenous injection site (Fig. 3.12).

- Vesicants include: cisplatin, doxorubicin, epirubicin, vincristine, vinblastine
- Irritants include: carboplatin, mitozantrone.

Prevention
- Adequate restraint of the patient.
- An intravenous catheter must be used for administration of the drug. This should be flushed with saline prior to and following administration of the agent.

Treatment
In the event of perivascular leakage:

- Stop the infusion but do not remove the catheter.
- Aspirate the extravasated drug from the affected area immediately. This may be assisted by subcutaneous injection of 0.9% sodium chloride to dilute any residual drug. Try to draw some blood/fluid back from the catheter.
- Remove catheter.
- Soluble corticosteroids (e.g. hydrocortisone) should be administered systemically, (intravenously), locally as subcutaneous injections and topically (as cream) around the site of extravasation.
- Cold compresses may also help reduce the inflammatory response.
- Specific recommendations for different agents can be found in Appendix IV at the end of the book.

Specific drug associated toxicity

Cyclophosphamide: haemorrhagic cystitis

Metabolites of cyclophosphamide (in particular acrolein) are excreted in the urine and have an irritant action on the bladder mucosa, resulting in an acute inflammation, often accompanied by profuse bleeding. This sterile haemorrhagic cystitis can occur at any time during cyclophosphamide therapy in dogs but is more common following administration of high doses or after long term, continuous low dose therapy. In some cases the cystitis resolves following withdrawal of treatment but, in severe cases, resolution can take considerable time. Haemorrhagic cystitis does not appear to be a problem in cats.

Treatment/prevention
There is no specific treatment for cyclophosphamide-induced haemorrhagic cystitis, although instillation of dimethylsulphoxide (DMSO) into the bladder has been reported to assist in its resolution (Liang *et al.* 1988). Because of the distressing nature of the problem it is preferable to try and minimise the risk of haemorrhagic cystitis in patients receiving cyclophosphamide by:

- Administration of the drug in the early morning
- Ensuring a good fluid intake
- Encouraging frequent emptying of the bladder
- Concurrent glucocorticoid administration will assist diuresis
- The urine of dogs receiving cyclophosphamide

should be checked regularly for blood and protein to help detect the problem in its early stages.

Doxorubicin (and related drugs): cardiotoxicity

Doxorubicin can cause acute and chronic cardiac toxicity through actions on myocardial calcium metabolism. The rate of infusion can influence this cardiac toxicity and it is recommended that the drug is administered as an infusion over at least 15 minutes (see Appendix IV).

- In *acute* cardiac toxicity, tachycardia and arrhythmias may occur on administration of the drug. The pulse rate and character should be monitored throughout administration and immediately afterwards, if tachycardia or other rhythm disturbances occur the infusion should be stopped or slowed.
- *Chronic* changes are due to cumulative, dose-related damage to the myocardium that leads in some cases to an irreversible cardiomyopathy.

Treatment/prevention

- All dogs should have thoracic radiographs, an ECG and ultrasound assessment of ventricular fractional shortening prior to treatment.
- There is no absolute dose at which cardiomyopathy occurs in all dogs, and there is tremendous variation between patients. The total dose of the drug administered should be limited to $240\,mg/m^2$, according to some texts, but cardiomyopathies have been reported at total doses from $180–200\,mg/m^2$.
- Cardioprotectant agents, e.g. dexrazoxane, are used in some parts of the world for human patients, but such agents have not been evaluated in companion animals and dexrazoxane is not licensed for use in the UK.

In cats, doxorubicin can cause nephrotoxicity, especially when used in combined protocols with cyclophosphamide. Renal toxicity has been reported at total doses as low as $80\,mg/m^2$ in this species (Ogilvie 1993b).

Cisplatin (carboplatin) – nephrotoxicity

Platinum co-ordination compounds accumulate in renal tubular epithelial cells where they block oxidative phosphorylation leading to acute proximal tubular necrosis. The drug may also affect renal blood flow. In order to minimise these effects cisplatin must be administered with fluid diuresis, and renal parameters should be monitored carefully throughout the course of treatment. Several different regimes have been described for cisplatin administration (see Appendix IV).

Safety of handling cytotoxic drugs

Many cytotoxic drugs are carcinogenic and mutagenic; some are teratogenic. Some drugs are also extremely irritant and produce harmful local effects after direct contact with the skin or eyes. Persons handling and administering these agents should be aware of the potential dangers and take steps to minimise any risk to themselves, their staff and their clients. Detailed local rules and working practices should be established in practices where cytotoxic drugs are used. The following are general considerations concerning the use of these drugs in veterinary practice.

Cytotoxic drugs are commonly available in two forms:

- Tablets or capsules for oral administration
- Powder or solutions for injection.

Tablets/capsules

- Tablets should never be broken or crushed and capsules should not be opened.
- Disposable latex gloves should be worn when handling any tablet which does not have an inert barrier coat.
- Where tablets are provided in individual wrappers, they should always be dispensed in this form.
- In addition to the statutory requirements for the labelling of medicinal products, all containers used for dispensing cytotoxic drugs must be child-proof and carry a clear warning to keep out of the reach of children. Containers should be clearly labelled with the name of the agent.
- Staff and owners should receive clear instructions on the administration of tablets.
- Disposable latex gloves should be worn when administering these tablets because the protective barrier may break down on contact with saliva.

- Always wash hands following handling of any drug.
- Excess or unwanted drugs should be disposed of by high temperature chemical incineration by a licensed authority.

Injectable solutions

The main risk of exposure arises during the preparation and administration of injectable cytotoxics, many of which are presented as freeze-dried material or powder, requiring reconstitution with a diluent. Potential dangers are:

- The creation of aerosols during preparation/ reconstitution of the solution
- Accidental spillage.

Protective clothing should be worn during reconstitution, administration and disposal of these agents. The level of protection required varies according to the agent. The minimum requirement should be:

- Latex gloves
- Protective arm sleeves *or*
- A gown with long sleeves to protect the skin
- A protective visor or goggles to protect the eyes
- A surgical mask to provide some protection against splashes to the face.

(Specialised chemoprotective clothing is available from several manufacturers, such as the Chemoprotect™ range distributed by Codan Ltd, Wokingham, Berkshire RG11 2PR.)

Reconstitution

- The drug should only be reconstituted by trained personnel.
- Reconstitution of the drug should only be performed in a designated area, free from draughts, and well away from thoroughfares and food.
- If drugs such as doxorubicin are used on a regular basis they should be reconstituted in a protective, biological safety cabinet.
- Careful technique should prevent high pressure being generated within the vials and should minimise the risk of creating aerosols.
- If it is necessary to expel excess air from a filled syringe it should be exhausted into an absorbent pad (disposed of in appropriate manner – see below) and not straight into the atmosphere.

Administration

- Luer lock fittings should be used in preference to push connections on syringes, tubing and giving sets.
- All animal patients must be adequately restrained by trained staff (who should also wear protective clothing). Fractious or lively animals may need to be sedated.

In the event of spillage the following actions should be taken:

- The spilt material should be mopped up with disposable absorbent towels (these should be damp if the spilt material is in powder form). The towels should be disposed of as detailed below.
- Contaminated surfaces should be washed with plenty of water.

Waste disposal

- Adequate care and preparation should be taken for the disposal of items (syringes, needles etc.) used to reconstitute and administer cytotoxic drugs.
- 'Sharps' should be placed in an impenetrable container specified for the purpose, and sent for incineration.
- Solid waste (e.g. contaminated equipment, absorbent paper etc.) should be placed in double sealed polythene bags and disposed of by high temperature chemical incineration by a licensed authority.

NOVEL METHODS OF CANCER THERAPY

There is no doubt that cancer will continue to be a major problem facing veterinary practice. Currently available treatment techniques do not provide a solution for many cancers and carry a high potential for serious patient toxicity. Thus cancer research continues to look for new approaches to cancer therapy. Alongside the conventional methods of surgery, radiation and chemotherapy a number of other techniques, such as hyperthermia and photodynamic therapy, have been used in attempts to selectively kill cancer cells. For the future, developments in immunology and molecular biology may hold the key to a much more targeted approach to cancer therapy.

Hyperthermia

Hyperthermia is a technique for treatment of cancer which is based on the observation that malignant cells can be destroyed selectively by exposure to temperatures of 42–45°C. The mechanisms of this selective cell kill are complex but include direct cellular actions, through inhibition of cellular aerobic metabolism, inhibition of cellular nucleic acid and protein synthesis, increased intracellular lysosomal acitivity and alterations in the permeability of cell membranes. Hyperthermia also acts at a tumour level with direct actions on tumour vasculature, causing stasis, thrombosis and endothelial degeneration.

Hyperthemia is thus of great interest in cancer therapy and as such has been the subject of intensive study over the past 25 years both in laboratory models and in clinical trials. It has been used as a local/regional treatment, often in combination with radiation, and as a whole body treatment, combined with chemotherapy (Dobson 1991). Despite the potential of this technique, it has not become widely used in either human or veterinary clinical practice, largely due to technical difficulties in the local heating of tumours and the complex care and management required for whole body treatment.

Photodynamic therapy

Photodynamic therapy (PDT) is another technique in which there has been considerable interest for many years. PDT is based on the preferential accumulation of a photosensitising agent in malignant cells following systemic or topical application. Stimulation of the tumour (and thus the agent) with light of an appropriate wavelength activates the photosensitiser and causes a photochemical reaction culminating in the production of cytotoxic free radicals and cell death (Fig. 3.13). Porphyrin-based photosensitisers were the first agents used for PDT and argon-pumped dye lasers were used as the light source. Although the technique was shown to be effective in human and veterinary clinical studies, a number of problems were encountered (Peaston *et al.* 1993). Whilst haematoporphyrin-derivatives do accumulate in malignant cells, they

Mechanism for PDT:

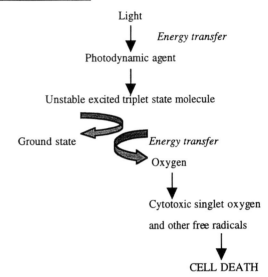

Fig. 3.13 Diagrammatic representation of the mode of action of PDT.

also enter normal cells and result in photosensitisation of the patient. Furthermore, argon-pumped dye lasers were expensive and unwieldy pieces of equipment.

In recent years, new more selective or shorter acting photodynamic agents have been developed, some of which can be applied topically (e.g. ALA cream), laser technology has advanced and it has been recognised that much cheaper sources of red light can be used for treatment of superficial tumours (Stell *et al.* 1999) (Fig. 3.14). As a result PDT has become much more feasible in the clinical setting and whilst it remains an investigational technique in cancer therapy, a number of clinical trials are in progress.

Immunotherapy, gene therapy and new targets

The potential for harnessing the immune system to combat cancer has for a long time been one of the major goals of cancer therapy. A variety of strategies have been devised and applied in veterinary patients with mixed results. Autogenous vaccination of tumour lysates has been used to promote regression of virally induced papilloma in cattle and dogs, but because these tumours often regress spon-

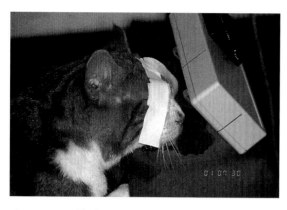

Fig. 3.14 Red light source being used to treat superficial SCC on cat's nose. (See also Colour plate 5, facing p. 162.)

taneously, the true benefit of this approach is unclear (Bell *et al.* 1994). Passive immunotherapy using antibodies directed against tumour cells has not met with much success, but a monoclonal antibody (MAb-231) is available in the USA for the treatment of canine lymphoma (Jeglum 1991). Non-specific immunostimulants have been widely used in veterinary medicine. Bacillus Calmette-Guerin (BCG), an attenuated mycobacterium, was one of the first agents to be used for immunotherapy. BCG has been used to treat dogs with mammary carcinoma but although there was evidence that it delayed onset of metastasis, toxicity proved to be a problem (Bostock & Gorman 1978). Muramyl tripeptide-phosphatidylethanolamine (MTP-PE), a synthetic molecule resembling part of the mycobacterial cell wall, has been shown to be efficacious in prolonging post-amputation survival times in dogs with osteosarcoma (MacEwen *et al.* 1989).

Several other agents have been reported to have non-specific immunostimulatory activity which may be beneficial in treatment of some tumours. Ace-mannan, a complex plant carbohydrate, which is reported to have several effects on immune function is approved for adjunctive treatment of soft tissue sarcomas in the USA (King *et al.* 1995) and the non-steroidal anti-inflammatory agent Piroxicam is used for its 'immunostimulatory' properties in the treatment of transitional cell carcinoma of the bladder in dogs (Knapp *et al.* 1992). The H_2 antagonist cimetidine has also been reported to have immunomodulatory actions, beneficial in the treatment of melanoma, although this has not been substantiated in large scale clinical trials.

Individual cytokines (e.g. interferon, IL-2) and agents such as muramyl tripeptide (MTP) can stimulate cytotoxic activity of effector cells (T lymphocytes, natural killer cells and macrophages) but success in the clinical setting has been limited because, as is now recognised, in addition to being stimulated, these cells need to be directed to their target. Most tumour cells are not easily recognised as 'foreign' by the cells of the immune system as they do not express aberrant cell surface antigens or, if they do, the immune system may either become tolerant to those antigens or suppressed by tumour derived agents. Hence the concept of the 'magic bullet', a monoclonal antibody designed to carry a toxin directly to the tumour cell, has not been realised. However, with improved understanding of the complex mechanisms and interactions of the immune system, strategies are being developed which hold promise for overcoming some such problems, for example the use of dendritic cell vaccination in the treatment of melanoma patients (Nestle *et al.* 1998). The advent of molecular techniques which allow the introduction of new genetic material into cells offers other opportunities and there is no doubt that cytokine technology will play a role with gene therapy in future developments in cancer therapy.

Other developments which hold hope for the future stem from a better understanding of the biology of cancer. Certain growth factor receptors have been identified as having key influence on the growth and development of certain cancers (e.g. epidermal growth factor – breast cancer) and some of these have been targeted. The mechanisms of tumour growth and invasion have been elucidated and strategies are being developed to attack a tumour in a much more specific manner than is currently the case with cytotoxic drugs; for example, through inhibition of enzymes which facilitate tumour invasion and metastasis (e.g. metalloproteinases) and inhibition of tumour driven angiogenesis (e.g. angiostatin, endostatin and interferon-alpha). These strategies look very promising in the laboratory and some are starting to enter human clinical trials.

References

Bell, J.A., Sundberg, J.P., Ghim, S.A. *et al.* (1994) A formalin-inactivated vaccine protects against mucosal papilloma virus infection. A canine model. *Pathobiology*, (62), 194–8.

Bostock, D.E. & Gorman, N.T. (1978) Intravenous BCG therapy of mammary carcinoma in bitches after surgical excision of the primary tumour. *European Journal of Cancer*, (14), 879–83.

Dobson, J.M. (1991) Hyperthermia. *Manual of Small Animal Oncology*, (ed. R.A.S. White), pp. 175–83. British Small Animal Veterinary Association, Cheltenham.

Dobson, J.M. (1999) Principles of Cancer Therapy. In: *Textbook of Small Animal Medicine* (ed. J.K. Dunn), pp. 985–1028. W.B. Saunders, London.

Dobson, J.M. & Gorman, N.T. (1993) *Cancer Chemotherapy in Small Animal Practice*. Blackwell Science Ltd, Oxford.

Henry, C.J., Buss, M.S. & Lothrop, C.D. (1998) Veterinary uses of recombinant human granulocyte colony-stimulating factor. Part I Oncology. *Compendium on Continuing Education, Small Animal*, (20), 728–35.

Jeglum, K.A. (1991) Monoclonal antibody treatment of canine lymphoma. *Proceedings of the Eastern States Veterinary Conference*, (5), 222–3.

King, G.K. *et al.* (1995) The effect of acemannan immunostimulant in combination with surgery and radiation therapy on spontaneous canine and feline fibrosarcomas. *Journal of the American Animal Hospital Association*, (31), 439–47.

Knapp, D.W., Richardson, R.C., Bottoms, G.D., Teclaw, R. & Chan, T.C.K. (1992) Phase I trial of piroxicam in 62 dogs bearing naturally occuring tumours. *Cancer Chemotherapy and Pharmacology*, (29), 214.

Liang, E.J., Muiller, C.W. & Cochrane, S.M. (1988) Treatment of cyclophosphamide-induced haemorrhagic cystitis in five dogs. *Journal of the American Veterinary Medical Association*, (193), 233–6.

MacEwen, E.G. *et al.* (1989) Therapy for osteosarcoma in dogs with liposome-encapsulated muramyl tripeptide. *Journal of the National Cancer Institute*, (81), 935.

Nestle, F.O., Alijagic, S., Gilliet, M., Sun, Y.S. & Grabbe, S. (1998) Vaccination of melanoma patients with peptide or tumour lysate pulsed dendritic cells. *Nature Medicine*, (4), 328–32.

Ogilvie, G.K. (1993a) Haematopoietic growth factors: tools for a revolution in veterinary oncology and haematology. *Compendium on Continuing Education*, (15), 851–4.

Ogilvie, G.K. (1993b) Recent advances in cancer, chemotherapy and medical management of the geriatric cat. *Veterinary International*, (5), 3–12.

Pavletic, M.M. (1999) *Atlas of Small Animal Reconstructive Surgery*, 2nd edn. W.B. Saunders, Philadelphia.

Peaston, A.E., Leach, M.W. & Higgins, R.J. (1993) Photodynamic therapy for nasal and aural squamous cell carcinoma in cats. *Journal of the American Veterinary Medical Association*, (202), 1261–5.

Salisbury, S.K. (1993) Maxillectomy and mandibulectomy. In: *Textbook of Small Animal Surgery*, (ed. D. Slatter, 2nd edition, pp. 521–30.

Stell, A.J., Langmack, K. & Dobson, J.M. (1999) Treatment of superficial squamous cell carcinoma of the nasal planum in cats using photodynamic therapy. *Proceedings of BSAVA Congress*, p. 314.

White, R.A.S. (1991) Mandibulectomy and maxillectomy in the dog: long term survival in 100 cases. *Journal of Small Animal Practice*, (32), 69–74.

White, R.A.S., Jefferies, A.R. & Gorman, N.T. (1986) Sarcoma development following irradiation of acanthomatous epulis in two dogs. *Veterinary Record*, (118), 668.

Further reading

Couto, C.G. (1990) Clinical Management of the Cancer Patient. *Veterinary Clinics of North America, Small Animal Practice*, (20), 4.

Dobson, J.M. & Gorman, N.T. (1993) *Cancer Chemotherapy in Small Animal Practice*. Blackwell Science, Oxford.

Hahn, K.A. & Richardson, R.C. (1995) *Cancer Chemotherapy. A Veterinary Handbook*. Williams & Wilkins, Baltimore.

Safety

COSHH Regulations (1988) *General Approved Code of Practice for the Control of Substances Hazardous to Health and Approved Code of Practice Control of Carcinogenic Substances*. Stationery Office, London. ISBN 0118854682.

Guidance Notes MS21 from the Health and Safety Executive (1983) *Precautions for the safe handling of cytotoxic drugs*. Stationery Office, London. ISBN 0118835718.

Allwood, M. & Wright, P. (eds) (1993) *The Cytotoxics Handbook*, 2nd edn. Radcliffe Medical Press, Oxford.

4
Skin

OVERVIEW

The skin is the largest and most easily observed organ in the body and therefore it is perhaps not surprising that tumours of the skin (and soft tissues) are the most common neoplasms in the dog and cat. By virtue of its complex structure, a large variety of tumours may arise in the skin and it is also a possible site for the development of secondary, metastatic tumours.

This chapter will consider those tumours arising from or within the epidermis, dermis and related structures. Soft tissue tumours, which may arise within dermal connective tissues, are considered in Chapter 5, Soft tissues.

Epidemiology

Cutaneous tumours represent at least one third of all canine tumours. Approximately two thirds of all canine cutaneous tumours are solitary, benign lesions originating from the epithelium or from adnexal structures including sebaceous glands, sweat glands and hair follicles. The age, breed and sex incidence varies from type to type, as discussed in the relevant sections.

The skin is also a common site for tumour devel-opment in the cat, although benign tumours tend to be less frequent than malignant ones in this species.

Aetiology

Several external agents and biological factors are recognised to be important in the development of certain tumours of the skin but for the majority the aetiology is unknown. Long term exposure to ultraviolet light (especially UVB) is implicated in the development of squamous and basal cell tumours in unprotected, non-pigmented and lightly haired skin (see Chapter 1). Cutaneous papillomatosis, induced by host specific DNA papovaviruses, occur infrequently in the dog; virally induced papillomas usually affect the oral cavity in young dogs (solitary cutaneous papilloma in older dogs is not associated with a viral aetiology). In male dogs, testosterone promotes the development of perianal, hepatoid gland adenoma.

Pathology

The skin is a complex organ (Fig. 4.1), essentially comprising two layers:

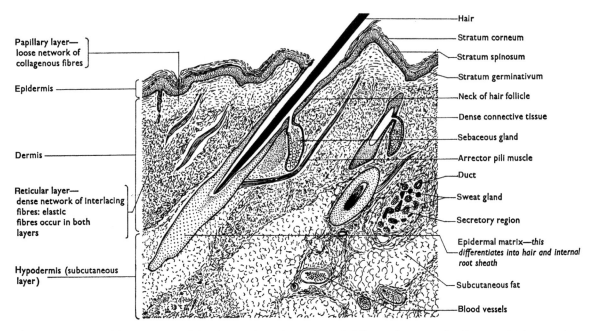

Fig. 4.1 Diagram of the structure of the skin to show the variety of different tissues and cell types which may give rise to tumours affecting the skin. (Reprinted from Freeman & Bracegirdle (1976) with permission.)

- The epidermis, a stratified squamous epithelium
- The dermis, of vascular dense connective tissue.

In addition, there are associated sebaceous and sweat glands and hair follicles, collectively termed the adnexae, plus melanocytes, histiocytes and dermal mast cells. Any of these tissues/cells may give rise to benign or malignant tumours (Table 4.1). In the dog benign tumours are twice as common as malignant tumours of the skin. Canine cutaneous histiocytoma and sebaceous gland adenomas are the most common tumours in this species. Mast cell tumours are the most common 'malignant' tumours, although in reality many canine mast cell tumours follow a relatively benign course (see later). Benign skin tumours are less common in the cat, with the exception of basal cell tumours. Squamous cell carcinoma is the most frequent malignant tumour of the skin in this species.

Tumour behaviour and paraneoplastic syndromes

Because of the diverse nature of tumours affecting the skin, the behaviour, presentation and treatment of the more common tumours will be discussed under separate headings. Paraneoplastic syndromes are only included where relevant.

Investigations

A presumptive diagnosis of a solitary skin tumour may be made on clinical examination, including visual inspection and palpation. Skin tumours which present as multifocal lesions may be harder to distinguish from other dermatological conditions. In both cases skin tumours must be differentiated from:

- Hyperplastic lesions
- Granulomatous lesions
- Inflammatory lesions
- Immune-mediated lesions
- Developmental lesions.

A useful clinical approach to a lesion affecting the skin is to determine the location of the lesion, i.e. whether it is epidermal, dermal or subcutaneous, as this will give some indication of its origin and thus its possible histogenesis. The distinction between solitary and multiple lesions is also of clinical value. However, definitive diagnosis can only be made

Table 4.1 Classification of tumours affecting the skin.

Tissue type	Specific tumours	Sub types
Epithelial tumours	Papilloma Basal cell tumour/carcinoma Squamous cell carcinoma Adnexal tumours Sebaceous gland tumours	
		Sebaceous gland adenoma Sebaceous epithelioma Sebaceous gland adenocarcinoma
	Tumours of perianal glands	Perianal gland adenoma/ adenocarcinoma
	Sweat gland tumours	Adenoma/adenocarcinoma
	Tumours of hair follicles	Pilomatricoma Trichoepithelioma
	Intracutaneous cornifying epithelioma	
Mesenchymal tumours (see Chapter 5)	Fibrous tissue tumours	Fibroma Fibrosarcoma Canine haemangiopericytoma
	Adipose tissue tumours	Lipoma Liposarcoma
	Blood vessel tumours	Haemangioma Haemangiosarcoma
Melanocytic tumours	Benign melanoma Malignant melanoma	
Mast cell tumours	Well differentiated, intermediate and poorly differentiated	
Cutaneous lymphoid neoplasia	Plasmacytoma Primary cutaneous T cell lymphoma Epitheliotrophic lymphoma (mycosis fungoides) 'Histiocytic' lymphoma Lymphomatoid granulomatosis	
Histiocytic and granulomatous skin conditions	Canine cutaneous histiocytoma Cutaneous histiocytosis Sterile pyogranulomatous/granulomas dermatoses Systemic histiocytosis	

upon histopathological examination of representative tissue.

Bloods

Routine haematological/biochemical analyses are not generally very helpful in the diagnosis of skin tumours although some skin tumours may be associated with haematological or paraneoplastic complications (e.g. mast cell tumours – anaemia due to gastric ulceration) and these investigations would be indicated in the general evaluation of such tumours.

Imaging techniques

Radiography of the primary tumour is not usually necessary unless the lesion is invasive and sited close to bone (e.g. squamous cell carcinoma of the digit). Radiography of the thorax is required in the clinical staging of malignant tumours, and ultrasound evaluation of abdominal organs (liver, spleen and kidneys) is important in the clinical staging of mast cell tumours. Both techniques may be used to assess the internal iliac/sublumbar lymph nodes for staging malignant skin tumours sited on the hind limbs and perianal region.

Biopsy/FNA

Cutaneous masses are easily accessible for fine needle aspiration (FNA) and this is a quick, minimally invasive and useful technique for assessing any mass within the skin. In some cases (e.g. mast cell tumours, cutaneous lymphoma) cytology may provide a diagnosis, although histological examination of the tumour is still required to assess the grade of the lesion. Fine needle aspiration of local lymph nodes is also useful to assess metastatic spread.

Skin punch, needle or incisional biopsies are required for a definitve histological diagnosis. Collection of a representative sample of tissue is important. Areas of ulceration and necrosis should be avoided, as should the temptation to collect too superficial a sample of the tumour. Excisional biopsy (i.e. local resection of the whole mass) is not generally recommended, except as a diagnostic procedure in a case with multiple skin lesions.

Staging

Clinical staging of primary tumours of the skin is by clinical examination and radiography. The primary tumour is assessed on the basis of its size, infiltration of the subcutis and involvement of other structures such as fascia, muscle and bone, as shown in Table 4.2.

EPITHELIAL TUMOURS

Papilloma/cutaneous papillomatosis

Cutaneous papillomatosis is a viral disease which is rare in dogs and very rare in cats. Virally-induced oral papillomatosis is seen more frequently in dogs. Lesions usually regress spontaneously as immunity develops, although can persist for as long as nine months. This is distinct from non-virus induced spontaneous

Table 4.2 Clinical stages (TNM) of canine or feline tumours of epidermal or dermal origin (excluding lymphoma and mast cell tumours) (Owen 1980).

T *Primary tumour*
  Tis   Pre-invasive carcinoma (carcinoma *in situ*)
  T0   No evidence of tumour
  T1   Tumour <2 cm maximum diameter, superficial or exophytic
  T2   Tumour 2–5 cm maximum diameter, or with minimal invasion irrespective of size
  T3   Tumour >5 cm maximum diameter, or with invasion of the subcutis, irrespective of size
  T4   Tumour invading other structures such as fascia, muscle, bone or cartilage

(Tumours occurring simultaneously should have the actual number recorded. The tumour with the highest T category is selected and the number of tumours indicated in parenthesis. Successive tumours should be classified independently.)

N *Regional lymph nodes (RLN)*
  N0   No evidence of RLN involvement
  N1   Movable ipsilateral nodes
        N1a nodes not considered to contain growth
        N1b nodes considered to contain growth
  N2   Movable contralateral or bilateral nodes
        N2a nodes not considered to contain growth
        N2b nodes considered to contain growth
  N3   Fixed nodes
        (−) histologically negative, (+) histologically positive

M *Distant metastases*
  M0   No evidence of distant metastasis
  M1   Distant metastasis detected (specify sites)

No stage grouping is at present recommended.

papillomas of skin which occur occasionally in older dogs.

Basal cell tumour/carcinoma

This tumour is relatively common in the dog and cat and usually affects middle-aged to older animals. It is reported to account for 4% of canine and 14% of feline skin tumours (Bostock 1986) or for 11% of canine and 34% of feline epithelial tumours (Goldschmidt & Shofer 1992).

Tumours are usually solitary, discrete, firm, well circumscribed masses, sited in the dermis and sub-cutis of the head and neck. The overlying skin may be ulcerated. Most tumours are small, 0.5–2.0 cm in diameter, although on occasion may reach up to 10 cm. Some basal cell tumours especially in the cat, contain abundant melanin pigment and may therefore be confused on gross inspection with melanoma. Various subtypes have been described based on the histological appearance, e.g. solid, cystic, adenoid and medusoid.

Behaviour/treatment/prognosis

These are usually slow-growing, non-invasive tumours which follow a benign course and rarely metastasise. Occasionally, more invasive tumours may be seen which are similar to the human 'rodent ulcer'. Local/wide local surgical excision is the treatment of choice. The prognosis is good in most cases. Local recurrence can occur following incomplete surgical excision.

Benign adnexal tumours

These are relatively common in the dog but uncommon in the cat.

Tumours of hair follicles

Pilomatricoma and trichoepithelioma are usually solitary lesions sited in the dermis. Both tend to occur in older animals, over 5–6 years of age. No sex or breed predisposition is recognised for tricho-epithelioma, whereas the Kerry blue terrier and possibly the poodle have been reported to be pre-disposed to the development of pilomatricoma (Nielsen & Cole 1960).

Sebaceous gland tumours

These are the most common skin tumour of the older dog with a mean age of affected animals between 9 and 10 years (Nielsen & Cole 1960). The cocker spaniel is predisposed to develop these tumours, and they are also common in poodles. Lesions may be solitary or multiple and arise anywhere on the body but the head and trunk are the most common sites, in particular the eyelid. Various types of benign sebaceous gland tumour are described according to their gross and histological appearance:

- Nodular sebaceous hyperplastic lesions are small, discrete, superficial, lobulated, often pedunclated lesions (Fig. 4.2).
- Sebaceous gland adenomas tend to be larger and less lobulated.
- Sebaceous epitheliomas present as firm, well circumscribed dermal masses with hairless and sometimes ulcerated overlying skin.

Intracutaneous cornifying epithelioma

These are quite common tumours in the dog, accounting for approximately 5% of canine epithelial tumours (Goldschmidt & Shofer 1992). They arise from the outer portion of the hair follicle and present as a dermal or subcutaneous mass, often with a superficial, exophytic component. Many of these tumours contain a dilated pore through which

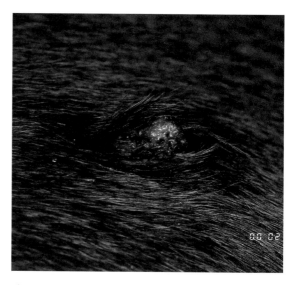

Fig. 4.2 Sebaceous gland tumour. Common skin lesions in older dogs, often referred to as 'a wart'.

grey-brown keratin can be expressed. Sites of predilection are on the back and tail and whilst lesions are usually solitary, some dogs may develop multiple tumours (especially the Norwegian elkhound). Their behaviour is benign and many undergo partial or even complete regression following the initial growth phase.

Behaviour/treatment/prognosis

All these tumours are slowly growing, non-invasive and benign in their behaviour. Treatment is surgical (if required) and the prognosis is good. Sebaceous epithelioma may recur following incomplete surgical excision. In dogs that are prone to developing multiple tumours surgical management may not be appropriate and further lesions are likely. Successful treatment of multiple intracutaneous cornifying epitheliomata using isotretinoin has been reported (Henfrey 1991).

Malignant adnexal tumours

Malignant tumours arising from the adnexal structures of the skin are uncommon in the dog but sebaceous gland and sweat gland adenocarcionomas are occasionally reported. Such tumours are extremely rare in the cat.

Behaviour/treatment/prognosis

These tumours can be very aggressive and locally invasive, often presenting with satellite nodules around the primary mass. They may also result in oedema, ulceration and inflammation of the surrounding skin due to infiltration of dermal lymphatics (Fig. 4.3). The incidence of metastasis is variable but tends to be to local and regional lymph nodes and then to the lungs and other organs.

Surgical excision is the treatment of choice but wide margins of excision are required due to the infiltrative nature of the lesion. Limited experience suggests that these tumours may be reasonably radiosensitive and radiotherapy may offer an alternative for local control in cases where surgery is not possible. The role of chemotherapy in the management of such tumours has not been established.

The prognosis is usually guarded to poor because of the locally invasive and malignant behaviour of these tumours.

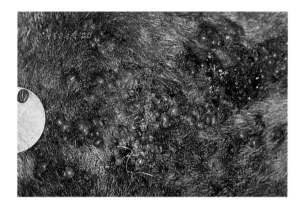

Fig. 4.3 Sweat gland adenocarcinoma, infiltrating widely throughout the skin. (See also Colour plate 6, facing p. 162.)

Perianal/hepatoid gland tumours

Perianal (circumanal, hepatoid) glands are modified sebaceous glands located in the skin of the perianal region. They develop throughout life under the influence of sex hormones and it is often difficult to distinguish hyperplasia of these glands from a benign adenoma.

Perianal gland adenomas

These are common in elderly male dogs and occasionally occur in spayed bitches. No breed predisposition has been reported, although the cocker spaniel, English bulldog, samoyed and beagle had the highest incidence of these tumours in one study (Hayes & Wilson 1977). These tumours do not occur in cats. Tumours usually present as a solitary, discrete, button-like lesion in the perianal skin (Fig. 4.4) but may also occur around the base of the tail, prepuce or midline and can be multiple. As lesions enlarge they tend to ulcerate and whilst most are presented at 1–2 cm diameter they can attain quite large size, up to 10 cm in diameter.

Perianal gland adenocarcinomas

These are far less frequent than their benign counterparts. They arise in similar locations but are characterised by a more rapid and infiltrating growth resulting in large, ulcerated circumanal masses (Fig. 4.5).

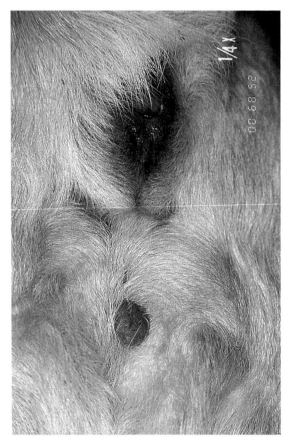

Fig. 4.4 Perianal gland adenoma. (See also Colour plate 7, facing p. 162.)

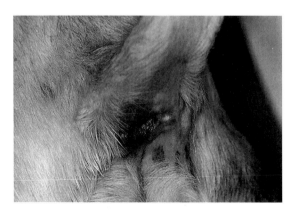

Fig. 4.5 Perianal gland adenocarcinoma. (See also Colour plate 8, facing p. 162) (Courtesy of Dr R. A. S. White, Department of Clinical Veterinary Medicine, Cambridge.)

Behaviour/treatment/prognosis

Most perianal gland tumours follow a benign course. Perianal gland carcinomas metastasise via the lymphatic route to internal iliac lymph nodes and then, via the blood to lung, liver, kidney and bone.

Surgical excision is the treatment of choice for benign adenomas and where possible for carcinomas. Castration will usually prevent the development of benign tumours, and is recommended to prevent recurrence. Carcinomas appear to be less hormonally dependent than adenomas and there is little evidence that castration or hormonal treatment is beneficial in the management of malignant perianal tumours. Perianal gland carcinomas are reasonably radiosensitive and radiotherapy may offer an alternative for local control in cases where surgery is not possible. The role of chemotherapy in the management of such tumours has not been established. The prognosis is favourable for benign tumours but guarded for carcinomas.

Note

Perianal adenoma/adenocarcinoma is distinct from carcinoma of the anus and from adenocarcinoma of the anal sac. These tumours are described in Chapter 8, Gastrointestinal tract.

Squamous cell carcinoma (SCC)

Squamous cell carcinoma (SCC) is one of the more common malignant cutaneous tumours in the dog and the most common in the cat. It usually affects older animals and there is no known breed predisposition in either species. SCC can occur anywhere in the skin. The trunk, legs, scrotum, lips and nail bed are the most frequent sites of occurrence in the dog, whereas lesions are more common on the head of the cat affecting the nasal planum (Fig. 4.6), pinnae, eyelids and lips. SCC may be productive, forming a friable, papillary growth, or it may be erosive, forming an ulcerated lesion. It is not unknown for these tumours to be dismissed as inflammatory or infective lesions on initial presentation.

Aetiology

Prolonged exposure to UV light (especially UVB) is recognised to be an important factor in the development of actinic solar dermatitis, carcinoma *in situ*

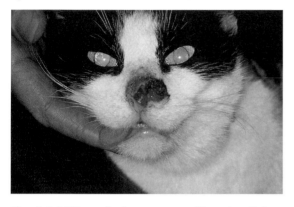

Fig. 4.6 SCC nasal planum – cat. (See also Colour plate 9, facing p. 162.)

and eventually invasive SCC (Figs 4.7. and 4.8) but not all cutaneous SCC are UV induced.

Behaviour/treatment/prognosis

SCC is a locally invasive tumour that infiltrates the underlying dermal and subcutaneous tissue. Metastasis tends to be via the lymphatic route but the incidence of metastasis is variable. SCC of the skin is usually well differentiated and slow to metastasise; at other sites, for example the nail-bed of the digit, behaviour can be much more aggressive.

Wide local surgical excision is the treatment of choice and, in cases where this can be achieved, the prognosis is favourable. SCC is moderately radiosensitive and radiotherapy may be indicated as an alternative or adjunctive treatment in cases where adequate surgical resection is not possible. Photodynamic therapy has been used successfully for treatment of early, superficial lesions of the nasal planum in cats. Chemotherapy is not usually

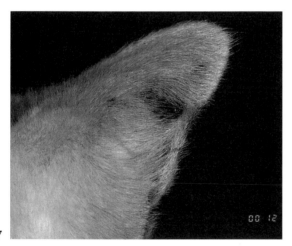

4.7

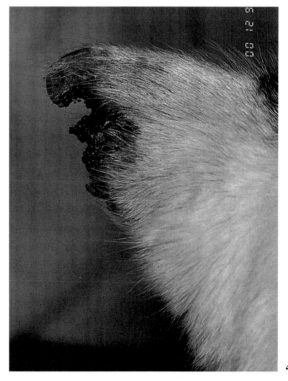

4.8

Figs 4.7 and 4.8 SCC of the pinnae in a cat. (See also Colour plates 10 and 11, facing p. 162) Fig. 4.7 Early stage lesion with erythema and crusting is seen on the right ear. Fig. 4.8 A more advanced, ulcerated and invasive tumour is affecting the left pinna of the same cat.

indicated in the management of localised SCC and the role of chemotherapy in the management of metastatic SCC has not been established.

SCC of the digit

SCC of the nail-bed region of the canine digit is an aggressive tumour and invasion and destruction of the distal phalanx is common (Fig. 4.9). Amputation of the affected digit(s) is the treatment of choice but these tumours may metastasise to the local and regional lymph nodes and the prognosis is guarded.

A phenomenon of SCC affecting several digits has been reported in large breed, black dogs, e.g. standard poodles, giant schnauzers (Paradis *et al.* 1989). These tumours appear to have a lesser tendency for metastasis but over a period of time may affect multiple digits on different feet.

Multiple digital carcinomas have also been reported in cats but here the digital lesions appear to be secondary, metastatic tumours from a primary pulmonary carcinoma (Scott-Moncrieff *et al.* 1989).

MELANOMA

Melanocytic tumours are relatively uncommon tumours of the skin in the dog and cat, representing between 4 and 6% of all canine skin tumours and 1–2% of all feline skin tumours (Bostock 1986; Goldschmidt & Shofer 1992). In dogs, cutaneous melanoma principally affects older animals (7–14 years of age) and is most common in the Scottish terrier, Boston terrier, Airedale and cocker

spaniels (and in other breeds with heavily pigmented skin). Older cats are also affected with a mean age of 8 years; there is no sex or breed predisposition in the cat.

Grossly tumours may appear as flat, plaque-like to domed masses, up to 2 cm in diameter, sited within the dermis. They are usually dark brown to black and quite well defined. Malignant tumours may attain larger size, contain less pigment and frequently ulcerate. In the cat cutaneous melanoma must be distinguished from the more common pigmented basal cell tumour.

Behaviour/treatment/prognosis

Tumour site seems to be an important factor governing the behaviour of cutaneous melanoma. Most melanocytic tumours of the canine skin are solitary, slowly growing lesions which follow a benign course. Tumours arising on the digits and on mucocutaneous junctions, e.g. eyelids and lips, are more aggressive and behave in a similar manner to oral melanoma (see Chapter 7) with a high incidence of metastasis to local lymph nodes and via the blood to the lungs and other organs.

Wide surgical excision is the treatment of choice for benign dermal melanoma and the prognosis following complete surgical excision is good. Tumours may recur locally if excision is incomplete. Surgical excision is also indicated for local control of malignant tumours but the prognosis in such cases is guarded to poor because of the high incidence of metastasis. These tumours are not considered to be chemosensitive.

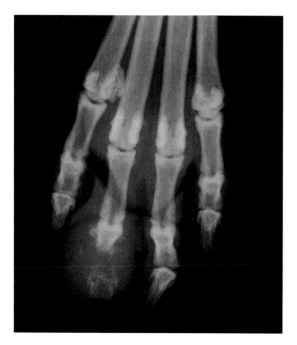

Fig. 4.9 Radiograph of digital SCC with bone destruction.

MAST CELL TUMOURS

Mast cell tumours (MCT) are one of the most common tumours in the skin of the dog, representing up to 20% of all canine skin tumours (Bostock 1986). They tend to affect older animals (mean age 8 years) but may occur at any age, from 4 months to 18 years. There is no sex predilection but several breeds of dog including the boxer, Boston terrier, bull terrier, Staffordshire bull terrier, fox terrier and possibly the Labrador and golden retriever appear to be predisposed to development of this tumour. Cutaneous mast cell tumours occur less frequently in the cat. The presentation and behaviour of mast cell tumours differ between the cat and dog and will be considered as separate entities.

Canine mast cell tumours

Canine mast cell tumours show tremendous diversity in gross appearance, clinical behaviour, rate of metastasis and response to treatment as a result of which they present considerable prognostic and therapeutic problems.

Presentation/clinical signs

There is no typical presentation for a canine mast cell tumour. The gross appearance can mimic any other cutaneous tumour and MCT should be considered in the differential diagnosis of any skin tumour. Low grade, well-differentiated mast cell tumours usually present as a solitary, slowly growing, dermal nodule (Fig. 4.10). Some tumours ulcerate through the skin and in some cases, local release of histamine from tumour cells may cause the lesion to fluctuate in size and become red and 'angry' looking at times. More aggressive mast cell tumours may present as large, ill-defined soft tissue masses and some may be surrounded by satellite nodules as the tumour spreads though surrounding cutaneous lymphatic vessels (Fig. 4.11).

Tumour behaviour

Mast cell tumours can vary in behaviour from slowly growing, low grade tumours which follow a benign course to rapidly growing, invasive, highly malignant tumours, and many stages in-between. Histological grading based on the degree of cellular differentiation, the mitotic index and invasion of

adjacent tissue has been shown to be of prognostic value. Three histological grades of mast cell tumour are described:

- *Well differentiated tumours* are generally of low grade/benign nature and carry a favourable prognosis.
- *Poorly differentiated tumours* are invasive with a high rate of metastasis and therefore a poor prognosis.

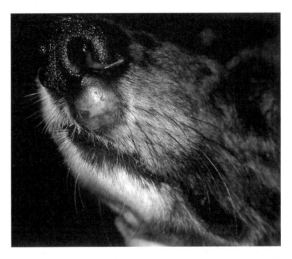

Fig. 4.10 Low grade mast cell tumour – a well circumscribed, erythematous mass on the upper lip adjacent to the nasal planum.

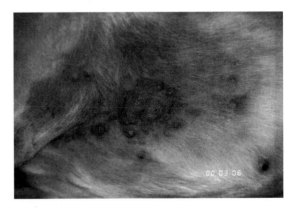

Fig. 4.11 Aggressive mast cell tumour – the main mass is sited in the skin of the axilla; multiple satellite nodules of locally invasive tumour spreading through the dermal lymphatics surround this mass.

• *Moderately differentiated tumours* are intermediate both in their histological appearance and also in behaviour. Unfortunately, many mast cell tumours fall into this intermediate category where the prognosis is difficult to predict.

Malignant mast cell tumours may metastasise either by the lymphatic route or via the blood. In most cases the first sign of metastasis is enlargement of the local lymph node. Discrete pulmonary metastases are rare; disseminated mast cell tumours more commonly metastasise to the spleen, liver and kidneys. The skin is also a common site for development of metastastes.

Paraneoplastic syndromes

Solitary and metastatic mast cell tumours can have local or systemic effects via the release of histamine and other vasoactive amines from the tumour cells. Locally histamine release may be associated with oedema and erythema of the tumour and adjacent tissues. Histamine release may also be associated with gastro-duodenal ulceration leading to anorexia, vomiting, melaena, anaemia and, in some cases, perforation (see Chapter 2).

Investigations

Bloods
Routine haematological assessment is indicated in cases with mast cell tumours. This may indicate anaemia due to blood loss from a bleeding intestinal ulcer. It is rare to see circulating mast cells (mastocytosis), even on buffy coat smears, but eosinophilia may be a feature of widespread, metastatic mast cell tumours.

Biopsy/FNA
Mast cells can be readily identified by FNA cytology (Fig. 4.12), and this simple technique should be performed prior to surgical removal of any cutaneous lesion. MCT cannot be graded accurately on cytology alone, although some indication of the degree of differentiation of the tumour cells may be possible. Thus excisional samples should be submitted for histological grading and assessment of the margins of surgical excision.

Staging
The clinical staging system for canine mast cell tumours is shown in Table 4.3. Local and regional

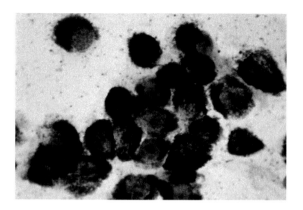

Fig. 4.12 Cytological appearance of a mast cell tumour. Mast cells may be recognised by the characteristic heavily staining cytoplasmic granules. Stained with 'neat-stain'–Haematology and Gram–by Guest Medical (See also Colour plate 12, facing p. 162.)

Table 4.3 The clinical staging of canine mast cell tumours. Owen (1980).

Clinical stage	Description
I	One tumour confined to dermis, no nodal involvement
II	One tumour confined to dermis with local or regional lymph node involvement
III	Large infiltrating tumours with or without regional lymph node involvement
IV	Any tumour with distant metastases

lymph nodes should always be evaluated by palpation, radiography and/or cytology as appropriate. Ultrasound evaluation of liver, spleen and kidneys is valuable in the staging of these tumours; radiography of the chest is less useful. The skin is a common site for mast cell tumour metastasis and skin nodules should be investigated by FNA or biopsy.

Treatment

Surgery
Surgical resection is undoubtedly the treatment of choice for well differentiated mast cell tumours. Even well differentiated tumours can infiltrate into adjacent tissues; hence the minimal requirement to ensure complete resection of the tumour is a wide

Table 4.4 Post-surgical prognosis for canine mast cell tumours.

Histological grade	Number of dogs	Median survival (weeks)	Dead from tumour (%)
Well differentiated	19	40	10
Intermediate	16	36	25
Poorly differentiated	15	13	73

Figures from Bostock *et al.* (1989). This study was based on mast cell tumours excised by veterinary surgeons in general practice. Margins of excision were not examined or specified.

local resection. Surgical resection is also indicated in the management of moderately differentiated or intermediate grade tumours, but in this instance resection of the tumour with generous (3–5 cm) margins around the tumour is required. Deep margins are also important but as mast cell tumours do not usually invade through fascial planes, resection to a clean fascial plane deep to the tumour is usually adequate.

The most common cause of treatment failure for mast cell tumours is inadequate resection of the primary tumour leading to local tumour recurrence. This is often the result of badly planned or executed surgery rather than a feature of a bad tumour! The first surgical attempt stands most chance of success. Cure rates for subsequent surgical excisions or adjunctive therapies are low. For this reason it is vitally important to identify a mast cell tumour prior to any attempt at treatment so that appropriate surgical margins can be planned and achieved at the first attempt. Mast cell tumours are relatively easy to diagnose by cytological examination of fine needle aspirates, as previously described.

Radiotherapy

There is no unequivocal evidence to show that radiotherapy as a sole treatment is particularly beneficial in the management of mast cell tumours of any grade; indeed *in situ* destruction of tumour cells by radiation can precipitate severe local reactions. Radiotherapy may be beneficial as a post-surgical treatment in cases of moderately differentiated tumours where complete surgical resection is not feasible (Al-Sarraf *et al.* 1996) and, on occasions, may be used in conjunction with chemotherapy for the treatment of tumours which cannot be surgically excised due to their site.

Chemotherapy

The use of cytotoxic drugs in the treatment of mast cell tumours remains controversial. Empirical clinical evidence suggests that some mast cell tumours do regress in response to high dose corticosteroid treatment (prednisolone). Whether or not the addition of more potent cytotoxic drugs, e.g. vincristine, vinblastine, cyclophosphamide, doxorubicin, L-asparaginase, or CCNU, improves the response is unknown at this time. Although there have been several publications suggesting that such agents may be beneficial, large scale controlled clinical studies of chemotherapy for canine mast cell tumours are lacking.

Other

Claims that deionised water injected into the tumour bed post-surgery may be beneficial in reducing tumour recurrence rates have not been substantiated in more recent studies (Jaffe *et al.* 2000) and this technique remains the subject of controversy.

Prognosis

The post-surgical prognosis for canine mast cell tumours has been well documented and is summarised in Table 4.4.

A suggested therapeutic approach to canine mast cell tumours based on the histological grade and clinical stage of the tumour is summarised in Table 4.5.

Feline mast cell tumours

Mast cell tumours are less common in the cat than in the dog and are also less of a diagnostic problem.

Table 4.5 Suggested strategies for the clinical management of canine mast cell tumours.

Histological grade	Clinical stage	Therapy
Well differentiated tumour	I	Wide local surgical excision
Intermediate, moderately differentiated tumour	I	As above (Post operative radiation may be required if adequate surgical margins cannot be achieved)
	II	Surgical excision and/or radiation of primary tumour and node. (± chemotherapy)
Poorly differentiated tumour	III	Chemotherapy: Prednisolone $40\,mg/M^2$ daily for 14 days, then gradually reducing to $20\,mg/M^2$ for maintenance
Any tumour with distant metastases	IV	± Cyclophosphamide $50\,mg/M^2$q 48 hours ± Vincristine $0.5\,mg/M^2$ or vinblastine $2\,mg/M^2$ iv weekly

Any animal showing systemic signs should also be treated with either cimetidine or ranitidine (Zantac–Glaxo™).

Two forms of mast cell tumour are recognised in the cat: cutaneous and visceral.

Cutaneous mast cell tumours

The majority of feline cutaneous mast cell tumours are solitary cutaneous/dermal nodules. These tumours are usually histologically well differentiated and have a benign clinical course. On occasion a cat may be affected by multiple skin nodules, or a solitary lesion may be invasive. However, the majority of cutaneous mast cell tumours in the cat are benign, and histological grading of feline cutaneous mast cell tumours has not been shown to be clinically useful.

Treatment and prognosis
Surgical resection is the treatment of choice for feline cutaneous mast cell tumours and the prognosis is usually good (Molander-McCrary et al. 1998). In cats with multiple tumours corticosteroids may be of palliative value. Invasive or incompletely excised tumours may be treated with adjunctive radiotherapy.

Note
A variant of feline mast cell tumour has been reported predominantly affecting Siamese cats. This tumour, which may be multicentric, is characterised histologically by sheets of histiocyte-like mast cells with scattered lymphoid aggregates and eosinophils. These tumours may regress spontaneously without therapy.

Visceral and systemic mast cell tumours in cats

Lymphoreticular mast cell tumours are occasionally seen in cats. In this condition, also called systemic mastocytosis, the tumour primarily involves the spleen. Presenting signs are usually vomiting and anorexia with common clinical findings of mastocytosis, marked splenomegaly and bone marrow infiltration, the latter often leading to anaemia and other cytopenias. Occasionally mediastinal involvement can lead to a pleural effusion, and lymph nodes elsewhere may also be involved. A diffuse cutaneous infiltration has sometimes been reported with this form of the disease, and this has been the cause of some confusion regarding the clinical behaviour of cutaneous mast cell tumours (most of which are benign). The diagnosis may be confirmed by fine needle aspirates from the enlarged spleen, and splenectomy is the treatment of choice. Long term survival has been reported in cats receiving no other therapy (Liska *et al.* 1979). It has been postulated that the response to splenectomy alone may involve the cat's immune system, hence the use of post-operative corticosteroids in these animals is controversial.

Intestinal mast cell tumour in the cat is distinct from systemic mastocytosis (which does not involve the bowel). This form of feline MCT is malignant, with widespread metastases and carries a poor prognosis.

MULTIFOCAL/DIFFUSE CUTANEOUS NEOPLASIA

As a result of the increasing use of skin biopsies in the investigation of skin disease, disseminated neoplastic infiltration of the skin is assuming increasing importance in the differential diagnosis of ulcerative, nodular or crusting skin lesions. Although MCT and metastases from both carcinomas and sarcomas can present as multiple, nodular skin lesions, lymphoid neoplasms are those most commonly associated with multifocal or diffuse skin lesions. A spectrum of granulomatous to histiocytic skin lesions may also give rise to ulcerative or nodular skin disease in dogs. Some of these may be preneoplastic or neoplastic in nature but our current understanding of these conditions is far from complete.

There are two forms of cutaneous lymphoma, both of T cell origin, which primarily affect the skin: primary and epitheliotropic.

Primary cutaneous (T cell) lymphoma

This is a very aggressive neoplasm. This tumour initially presents with multiple cutaneous nodules, plaques or erythroderma (Figs 4.13 and 4.14). Histologically there is a nodular infiltration of the dermis and subcutis with malignant lymphoid cells (Fig. 4.15). The disease usually has a rapid course and the tumour quickly disseminates to involve other organs such as the liver, spleen and bone marrow.

Treatment and prognosis

In the early stages the cutaneous tumours may respond to chemotherapy schedules used in the treatment of multicentric lymphoma (see Chapter 15); however, periods of remission are usually short and the prognosis is poor with average survival times rarely exceeding 2–3 months.

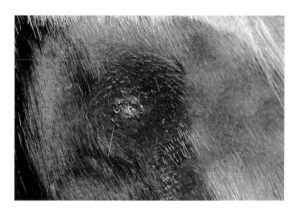

Fig. 4.14 Primary cutaneous T cell lymphoma. Close up of erythematous nodule from a different dog. Note infiltration of surrounding skin. (See also Colour plate 14, facing p. 162.)

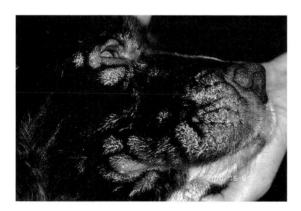

Fig. 4.13 Primary cutaneous T cell lymphoma, generalised erythematous plaques and nodules. (See also Colour plate 13, facing p. 162.)

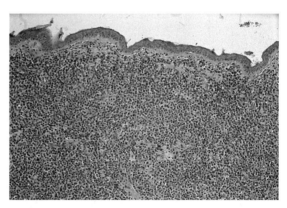

Fig. 4.15 Histological appearance of primary cutaneous lymphoma. The tumour infiltrate affects the dermis; the epidermis is intact. (See also Colour plate 15, facing p. 162.)

Epitheliotropic lymphoma (Mycosis fungoides)

The epitheliotropic form of cutaneous lymphoma is distinct from primary cutaneous (T cell) lymphoma in several important respects. Histological sections show a diffuse infiltration of the epidermis by lymphocytes and other inflammatory cells (Fig. 4.16). In the advanced stages of the disease the tumour cells invade into deeper layers of the dermis, heralding systemic dissemination.

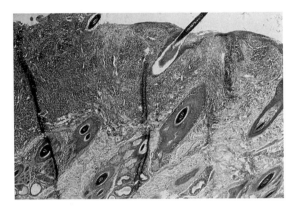

Fig. 4.16 Histological appearance of epitheliotropic lymphoma. In contrast to Fig. 4.15, the tumour cell infiltrate is in the epidermis. (See also Colour plate 16, facing p. 162.)

Mycosis fungoides (MF) runs a very protracted course often spanning many months. In humans mycosis fungoides can be divided into three distinct phases:

- Premycotic
- Mycotic or plaque stage
- Tumour stage.

In dogs these phases are less well defined and may coexist. In the early stage canine MF may present as an erythematous, exfoliative or seborrhoeic skin condition, which is often very pruritic, with lesions that heal in one region and then erupt in another. This gradually progresses with the development of plaques and ulceration of the skin. Finally, the 'tumour stage' is characterised by well defined tumour nodules or plaques. At this stage there is usually a rapid progression of the disease culminating in widespread dissemination to other organs. The mucous membranes of the mouth, eyes and genitalia may be affected at all stages (Figs 4.17 and 4.18).

Treatment

No single treatment has been established as being effective in the control of MF. Topical treatment with nitrogen mustard was once advocated for human patients. This is a very hazardous agent to handle and its use in animals with MF is not rec-

(a)
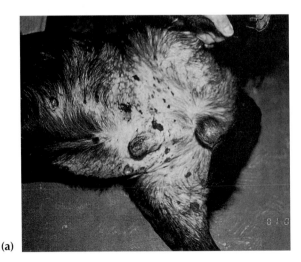

(b)
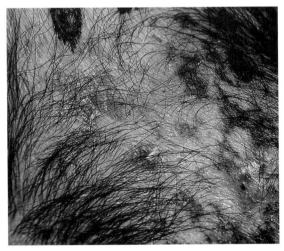

Fig. 4.17 Epitheliotropic lymphoma – (a) shows generalised nature of skin lesions; (b) close up showing erythematous crusting nature of lesions. (See also Colour plates 17 and 18, facing p. 162.)

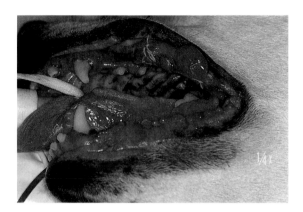

Fig. 4.18 Epitheliotropic lymphoma affecting oral mucocutaneous junctions and mucosae. (Colour plate 19.)

ommended. The response of the disease to systemic chemotherapy is variable but in some cases an improvement in the lesions can be achieved. The disease has been reported to respond favourably to L-asparaginase (MacEwen *et al*. 1987), and to retinoids (White *et al*. 1993). Radiotherapy can be used for localised lesions. Photodynamic therapy is being investigated for localised lesions in human patients.

Histiocytic lymphoma

Cutaneous lesions may also occur as part of a systemic or multicentric lymphoma. 'Large cell' or 'histiocytic' lymphomas are often associated with cutaneous lesions. Although these are relatively infrequent tumours they may respond more favourably to chemotherapy than the more common lymphoblastic or lymphocytic forms of lymphoma.

Lymphomatoid granulomatosis

Lymphomatoid granulomatosis is a rare lympho-histiocytic disorder in humans that has been recognised in the dog. Most human patients primarily have pulmonary lesions but other organs such as kidneys, liver, brain and skin may be affected. It is currently believed that lymphomatoid granulomatosis is not a preneoplastic granulomatous condition (as the name infers) but a rare variant of angiocentric peripheral T-cell lymphoma. In most of the canine cases reported the disease has been described primarily as a pulmonary disorder (Fitzgerald *et al*. 1991) but several canine cases of primary cutaneous lymphomatoid granulomatosis have now been recognised (Smith *et al*. 1996). These dogs have presented with multiple cutaneous nodules, plaques and ulcers, with or without pulmonary involvement. In humans and in some of the canine cases reported the cutaneous and pulmonary lesions can regress in response to immuno-suppressive therapy with cyclophosphamide and corticosteroids but the prognosis is guarded. Most human patients succumb to the development of unresponsive CNS lesions.

Plasmacytoma

Plasma cells are derived from B lymphocytes and can give rise to a spectrum of neoplastic conditions. Multiple myeloma is a systemic condition, often associated with inappropriate secretion of immunoglobulins from neoplastic plasma cells sited in the medullary cavity of bone (Chapter 15). Extramedullary plasma cell tumours may arise in soft tissues and are usually solitary soft tissue tumours although potentially might represent metastasis from a primary multiple myeloma.

Plasmacytomas are common in dogs but rare in cats (Lucke 1987; Rakich *et al*. 1989). They usually affect older dogs but no breed predilection has been established. In dogs they usually present as a solitary skin or mucocutaneous tumour. They can arise at any site but the oral cavity, feet, trunk and ears are most common. Plasmacytoma may also affect mucocutaneous junctions and occasionally arise in the gingiva. Their gross appearance is usually of a raised red or ulcerated, quite well defined mass. They do not usually attain large size, varying from 2–5 cm in diameter. Histological diagnosis can be difficult if the tumour cells are lacking clear differentiation and special staining techniques may be required to differentiate plasmacytoma from poorly differentiated sarcoma and other round cell tumours.

Behaviour/treatment/prognosis

Cutaneous and oral forms of plasmacytoma are usually benign and are rarely associated with systemic signs. Surgical resection is usually curative.

HISTIOCYTIC AND GRANULOMATOUS SKIN CONDITIONS

Canine cutaneous histiocytoma (CCH)

CCH is a benign cutaneous tumour, unique to the skin of the dog and representing up to 10% of all canine cutaneous tumours. CCH is more common in young dogs with 50% of these tumours occurring in animals under two years of age. The tumour typically arises on the head (especially the pinna), the limbs, feet and trunk and presents as a rapidly growing, intradermal lesion. The surface may become alopecic and ulcerated. The boxer and dachshund are reported to be predisposed to CCH and it also appears to be common in the flat-coated retriever.

Histological sections show infiltration of the epidermis and dermis by neoplastic histiocytic cells. Numerous mitotic figures and an indistinct boundary give this lesion the appearance of a highly malignant neoplasm. (This may lead to CCH being misdiagnosed by non-veterinary pathologists who are unfamiliar with this canine tumour.)

Behaviour/treatment/prognosis

Despite the histological appearance and the rapid growth rate, CCH is a benign tumour which usually regresses spontaneously. Regression is associated with infiltration of the tumour by cytotoxic T cells. Lymphocytic infiltration is a feature often described in histological reports. Surgical excision is usually curative and the prognosis is good.

Other histiocytic/granulomatous skin conditions

A group of 'histiocytic' skin lesions are recognised, particularly in dogs, which have yet to be fully characterised. In such cases there is a diffuse or nodular infiltration of the dermis by mononuclear cells that have a histiocytic appearance. In some cases these cells may be a variant of lymphoid neoplasia (i.e. 'histiocytic' lymphoma) as demonstrated through the use of canine lymphocyte cell surface markers (Baines et al. 2000) but conditions

termed 'cutaneous histiocytosis' or 'granulomatous dermatoses' are also recognised where the cells involved are not morphologically malignant (Panich et al. 1991).

Cutaneous histiocytosis/sterile pyogranulomatous skin conditions

Granulomatous and pyogranulomatous dermatoses appear clinically as skin nodules. These may be solitary or multiple, localised or diffuse, haired, alopecic or ulcerated (Figs 4.19 and 4.20). Clinically it can be difficult to differentiate these lesions from certain tumours. These dermatoses may be divided into infectious and non-infectious categories. Overall, 'infectious' agents such as bacteria, fungi, protozoa and algae are probably the most common cause of such lesions and these should be excluded by culture, special staining of skin biopsies and response to antimicrobial therapy. Conditions where no inciting cause can be identified are termed idiopathic sterile granulomas and several variants are described, as shown in Table 4.6.

Some of these conditions (e.g. sterile panniculitis) have a characteristic histological appearance, others (e.g. sterile pyogranuloma and cutaneous histiocytosis) are harder to differentiate by light microscopy; indeed, cutaneous histiocytosis may be an extension of the pyogranuloma/granuloma syndrome. In all cases the infiltrating inflammatory cells are morphologically normal and do not show any characteristics of neoplastic transformation. Most of these conditions are potentially immune-mediated, or at least related to dysregulation of the immune system, and some (e.g. sterile pyogranuloma/granuloma syndrome) show a favourable response to immunosuppressive therapy. In cutaneous histiocytosis and systemic histiocytosis the lesions typically wax and wane over a variable period of time. The response of cutaneous histiocytosis to immunosupressive doses of prednisolone is variable and the response of systemic histiocytosis is poor. It is difficult to make specific recommendations about the treatment of these two conditions and the long-term prognosis is guarded to poor.

Table 4.6 Granulomatous and pyogranulomatous dermatoses.

Condition	Clinical features
Sterile pyogranuloma/granuloma syndrome (Panich *et al.* 1991)	Uncommon in dogs, rare in cats Reported in collie, boxer, great Dane, Weimaraner, golden retriever ? Male predisposition in dogs Papules, nodules and plaques located on the head (periocular, muzzle and bridge of nose) and feet Affected animals are systemically healthy
Sterile panniculitis (Scott & Anderson 1988)	Uncommon in dogs and cats Associated with both infectious and non-infectious aetiologies Lesions often solitary, subcutaneous, fluctuant. May ulcerate and result in discharging fistulae
Granulomatous sebaceous adenitis (Scott 1986)	Rare condition, usually affects young adult dogs, reported in vizsla, akita, samoyed and standard poodle Pyogranulomatous inflammation destroys sebaceous glands resulting in alopecia and scaling. May be focal or generalised
Cutaneous histiocytosis	Rare disorder of dogs Nodular skin lesions may be alopecic and ulcerated. Usually affect face, neck and trunk. Nasal mucosa may be involved resulting in respiratory stridor. Affected animals are usually systemically healthy
Systemic histiocytosis (Paterson *et al.* 1995)	Rare familial condition affecting young adult Bernese mountain dogs. Skin lesions comprise papules, nodules and plaques and are most common on the flanks, muzzle, nasal planum, eyelids and scrotum. Ocular lesions, uveitis, chemosis, episcleritis and scleritis are also common. Variable lymphadenopathy. Affected animals may also show anorexia, weight loss and lethargy.

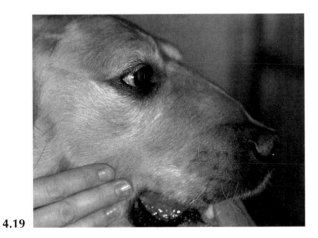
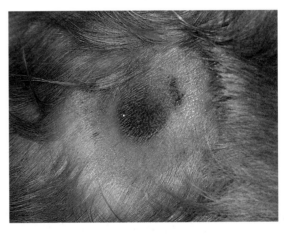

4.19 **4.20**

Figs 4.19 and 4.20 Cutaneous histiocytosis/pyogranulomatous skin condition in a retriever. Figure 4.19 The dog presented with a soft tissue swelling over the bridge of the nose. Figure 4.20 Several other dermal masses were noted. (See also Colour plates 20 and 21, facing p. 162.)

References

Baines, S.J., McCormick, D., McInnes, E., Dunn, J.K., Dobson, J.M. & McConnell, I. (2000). Cutaneous T-cell lymphoma mimicking cutaneous histiocytosis: differentiation by flow cytometry. *Veterinary Record*.

Bostock, D.E. (1986) Neoplasms of the skin and subcutaneous tissues in dogs and cats. *British Veterinary Journal*, (142), 1–18.

Bostock, D.E., Crocker, J., Harris, K. & Smith, P. (1989) Nucleolar organiser regions as indicators of post-surgical prognosis in canine spontaneous mast cell tumours. *British Journal of Cancer*, (59), 915–18.

Fitzgerald, S.D., Wolf, D.C. & Carlton, W.W. (1991) Eight cases of canine lymphomatoid granulomatosis. *Veterinary Pathology*, **28** (3), 241–5.

Freeman, W.H. & Bracegirdle, B. (1976) *An Advanced Atlas of Histology*. Heinemann Educational Books Ltd, London.

Goldschmidt, M.H. & Shofer, F.S. (1992) *Skin Tumours of the Dog and Cat*. Pergamon Press, Oxford.

Hayes, H.M. & Wilson, G.P. (1977) Hormone dependent neoplasms of the canine perianal gland. *Cancer Research*, (37), 2068–71.

Henfrey, J.I. (1991) Treatment of multiple intracutaneous cornifying epitheliomata using isotretinoin. *Journal of Small Animal Practice*, (32), 363–5.

Jaffe, M.H., Hosgood, G., Kerwin, S.C., Hedlund, C.S. & Taylor, H.W. (2000) Deionised water as an adjunct to surgery for the treatment of canine cutaneous mast cell tumours. *Journal of Small Animal Practice*, (41), 7–11.

Liska, W.D., MacEwen, E.G., Zaki, F.A. & Garvey, M. (1979) Feline systemic mastocytosis: a review and results of splenectomy in seven cases. *Journal of the American Animal Hospital Association*, (15), 589–97.

Lucke, V.M. (1987) Primary cutaneous plasmacytomas in the dog and cat. *Journal of Small Animal Practice*, (28), 49–55.

MacEwen, E.G., Rosenthal, R., Matus, R. *et al.* (1987) An evaluation of asparaginase: polyethylene glycol conjugate against canine lymphosarcoma. *Cancer*, (59), 2011–15.

Molander-McCrary, H., Henry, C.J., Potter, K., Tyler, J.W. & Buss, M.S. (1998) Cutaneous mast cell tumours in cats: 32 cases (1991–1994). *Journal of the American Animal Hospital Association*, (34), 281–4.

Nielsen, S.W. & Cole, C.R. (1960) Cutaneous epithelial neoplasms of the dog. A report of 153 cases. *American Journal of Veterinary Research*, (21), 931–48.

Owen, L.N. (1980) *TNM Classification of Tumours in Domestic Animals*. World Health Organization, Geneva.

Paradis, M., Scott, D.W. & Breton, L. (1989) Squamous cell carcinoma of the nail-bed in three related giant schnauzers. *Veterinary Record*, (125), 322–4.

Panich, R., Scott, D.W. & Miller, W.H. (1991) Canine cutaneous sterile pyogranuloma/granuloma syndrome: a retrospective analysis of 29 cases (1976 to 1988). *Journal of the American Animal Hospital Association*, (27), 519–28.

Paterson, S., Boydell, P. & Pike, R. (1995) Systemic histiocytosis in the Bernese mountain dog. *Journal of Small Animal Practice*, (36), 233–6.

Al-Sarraf, R., Maudlin, G.N., Patnaik, A.K. & Meleo (1996) A prospective study of radiation therapy for the treatment of grade 2 mast cell tumours in 32 dogs. *Journal of Veterinary Internal Medicine*, (10), 376–8.

Rakich, P.M., Latimer, K.S., Weiss, R. & Steffens, W.L. (1989) Mucocutaneous plasma cytomas in dogs: 75 cases (1980–1987). *Journal of the American Veterinary Medical Association*, (194), 803–10.

Scott, D.W. (1986) Granulomatous sebaceous adenitis in dogs. *Journal of the American Animal Hospital Association*, (22), 631–34.

Scott, D.W. & Anderson, W. (1988) Panniculitis in dogs and cats: a retrospective analysis of 78 cases. *Journal of the American Animal Hosptial Association*, (24), 551–59.

Scott-Moncrieff, J.C., Elliott, G.S., Radovsky, A. & Blevins, W.E. (1989) Pulmonary squamous cell carcinoma with multiple digital metastases in a cat. *Journal of Small Animal Practice*, (30), 696–9.

Smith, K.C., Day, M.J., Shaw, S.C., Littlewood, J.D. & Jeffery, N.D. (1996) Canine lymphomatoid granulomatosis: and immunophenotypic analysis of three cases. *Journal of Comparative Pathology*, (115), 129–38.

White, S.D., Rosychuk, R.A., Scott, K.V., Trettien, A.L., Jonas, L. & Denerolle, P. (1993) Use of isotretinoin and etretinate for the treatment of benign cutaneous neoplasia and cutaneous lymphoma in dogs. *Journal of the American Veterinary Medical Association*, (202), 387–91.

Further reading

Goldschmidt, M.H. & Shofer, F.S. (1992) *Skin Tumours of the Dog and Cat*. Pergamon Press, Oxford.

5
Soft Tissues

Definition

Soft tissue tumours are those that arise from the mesenchymal connective tissues of the body. Benign tumours of this group usually carry the suffix 'oma' and their malignant counterparts are termed 'sarcoma'. Tumours of fibrous, adipose, muscular and vascular tissues are included in this definition and by convention it also includes tumours of the peripheral nervous system because tumours arising from nerves present as soft tissue masses and pose similar problems in differential diagnosis and management.

Although the term 'soft tissue sarcoma' would appear to cover a diverse collection of tumours, these may be considered as a group not only because they share overlapping histological features but also because they share several important clinical and behavioural features.

Epidemiology

Soft tissue tumours are relatively common tumours in both the dog and cat. In the dog the majority of soft tissue tumours are benign whereas in the cat benign soft tissue tumours are uncommon. The malignant counterpart, soft tissue sarcomas, are important tumours in both the cat and the dog. Collectively they comprise approximately 15% of all canine and 7% of all feline 'skin' and subcutaneous tumours, but they can arise in other sites, for example oral, nasal and urogenital, hence the actual incidence of soft tissue tumours may be higher than indicated in many studies.

Soft tissue tumours are typically solitary and tend to arise in older animals.

Dogs

Benign soft tissue tumours are common and show no particular breed or sex predisposition, although lipoma, which is probably the most common benign soft tissue tumour of the dog, does seem to be more common in animals that are overweight. Soft tissue sarcomas are more common in the larger breeds and some breeds may be predisposed to develop certain soft tissue tumours:

- Bernese mountain dogs – malignant histiocytosis (see Chapter 17)
- Flat-coated retrievers – anaplastic sarcomas (Morris *et al.* 2000)
- Golden retrievers – fibrosarcoma
- German shepherd dogs – haemangiosarcoma.

Although the average age of onset of canine soft tissue sarcoma is 8–9 years, it is not unknown for younger animals of these and other large breeds to be affected. For example, in our clinic we quite frequently see golden retrievers 4–6 years of age with fibrosarcoma. On occasion rhabdomyosarcoma and anaplastic sarcomas may occur in juveniles as young as four months. For most soft tissue sarcomas there is no clear sex predisposition although a higher incidence of synovial sarcoma and malignant histiocytosis has been reported in males.

Cats

Benign soft tissue tumours are uncommon. There is no breed or sex predisposition to soft tissue sarcoma reported and most tumours are solitary and occur in the older animal. There are two notable exceptions:

- Feline sarcoma virus-induced tumour – This is very rare and has not been reported in the UK. It occurs in young animals which usually present with multiple subcutaneous tumours.
- 'Vaccine-site' sarcomas – These have been reported in younger animals (see later).

Aetiology

With few exceptions, the cause of soft tissue sarcomas in cats and dogs is not known. Those tumours where an aetiology is known or proposed tend to be very rare but include the following.

Feline sarcoma virus-induced sarcoma

FeSVs are recombinant viruses generated by interaction of FeLV DNA provirus with endogenous oncogenes in the feline genome (Chapter 1). FeSV-induced fibrosarcomas are rare (probably accounting for less than 2% of all feline fibrosarcomas) and only arise in young, FeLV positive cats, most of which are under three years of age. Tumours are usually multicentric and present as multiple subcutaneous masses on limbs and trunk. These are aggressive tumours which may metastasise to internal organs. Histologically they are often anaplastic but may show partial differentiation with areas of osteosarcoma or chondrosarcoma.

Vaccine-site sarcomas in cats

In the early 1990s an increase in the incidence of feline fibrosarcomas that appeared to coincide with an increase in vaccination with rabies and FeLV vaccines was reported in North America (Kass *et al.* 1993; Hendrick & Brooks 1994). Possible vaccine-associated sarcomas have since been reported in North America and in Europe with tumours arising at classical injection sites, especially in the interscapular space. The age of onset is variable but it is often younger animals that are affected. Histologically, most of these tumours are fibrosarcoma although they are reported to have a characteristic morphology with more cellular pleomorphism, central necrosis and sclerosis than non vaccine-site fibrosarcomas. In many the peripheral

macrophages contain adjuvant (Doddy *et al.* 1996). While no definitive proof has shown that vaccines or the act of vaccination cause the sarcoma, and in fact the incidence of such tumours is low (the annual incidence is estimated to be 0.13% of all cats vaccinated (Lester *et al.* 1996)), recommendations have been established in North America regarding sites for vaccination, avoidance of simultaneous injections at one site and accurate record keeping.

Spirocerca lupi-induced sarcoma

Sarcomas of the oesophagus have been reported in areas where the helminth parasite *Spirocerca lupi* is indigenous (Africa and south-eastern USA).

Trauma and inflammation

The development of a sarcoma at a site of previous trauma or inflammation has been documented in animals and people, although rarely. Examples of such sites include scar tissue following surgical procedures, thermal or chemical burns, fracture sites and sites in the vicinity of plastic or metallic implants, usually after a latent period of several years. Feline ocular sarcomas may be associated with trauma to the lens and chronic ocular inflammation (Chapter 16).

Radiation

Radiation has been related to the development of sarcomas and there certainly is a risk that a very small proportion of human cancer patients (0.1%) who survive over five years following radiotherapy will develop a sarcoma of either bone or soft tissue. In dogs a 10–20% incidence of sarcoma development has been reported following irradiation of acanthomatous epulis/basal cell carcinoma of the oral cavity (White *et al.* 1986).

Pathology

Soft tissue tumours of cats and dogs may be classified according to their tissue of origin, as shown in Table 5.1. In some soft tissue sarcomas the component cells are so poorly differentiated that it is difficult to determine the tissue of origin and, in the absence of further cytochemical and

Table 5.1 Classification of soft tissue tumours.

Tissue of origin	Benign tumour	Malignant tumour
Fibrous tissue	Fibroma	Fibrosarcoma Canine haemangiopericytoma
Fibro-histiocytic	–	Malignant fibrous histiocytoma/ malignant histiocytosis
Adipose	Lipoma (Infiltrative lipoma)	Liposarcoma
Muscular-skeletal -smooth	(Rhabdomyoma) Leiomyoma/ fibroleiomyoma	Rhabdomyosarcoma Leiomyosarcoma
Synovial	–	Synovial (cell) sarcoma
Vascular	Haemangioma (Lymphangioma)	Haemangiosarcoma (Lymphangiosarcoma)
Peripheral nerve	'Peripheral nerve sheath tumours'* Neurofibroma Schwannoma Neurilemmoma	Neurofibrosarcoma Malignant Schwannoma
Other	Myxoma	Myxosarcoma

The terminology for tumours of peripheral nerves is not resolved in veterinary medicine. The different terms listed essentially describe the same tumours.

immunohistochemical evaluation, such tumours may be described by their morphology, i.e. spindle cell sarcoma, round cell sarcoma, anaplastic sarcoma.

Presentation/signs

Both benign and malignant soft tissue tumours are usually bulky, fleshy tumours, as opposed to invasive and ulcerative masses as seen with carcinomas. They may arise from any anatomic site but most commonly present as a soft tissue mass of the subcutis although they can arise in deeper soft tissues or within body cavities and internal organs (Figs 5.1 and 5.2). The tumour itself is usually painless. Pain or discomfort may occur, however, when the tumour involves or abuts sensitive structures. A classical example of this is the neurofibrosarcoma of the brachial plexus as seen in the dog that presents with a progressive forelimb lameness and marked muscle wastage. A painful mass may sometimes be palpated deep in the axilla.

Tumours often appear well circumscribed or even encapsulated; however, in reality these soft tissue sarcomas have poorly defined histological margins and often infiltrate through fascial planes (see below).

Tumour behaviour

Primary tumour

Benign soft tissue tumours are usually slowly growing, non-invasive, well circumscribed masses. On occasion growth may cease but some tumours, for example lipomas, may attain massive proportions.

A rare variant of the common lipoma is the infiltrating lipoma. Histologically the tumour is comprised of mature adipose tissue with no features of malignancy and yet the tumour is characterised by an infiltrating pattern of growth around and within surrounding muscles and nerves (Fig. 5.3).

Soft tissue sarcomas enlarge in a centrifugal fashion and compress normal tissue so as to give the appearance of encapsulation. This pseudocapsule is actually composed of an inner compressed rim of normal tissue (compression zone) and an outer rim of oedema and newly formed vessels (reactive zone). Finger-like extensions of tumour

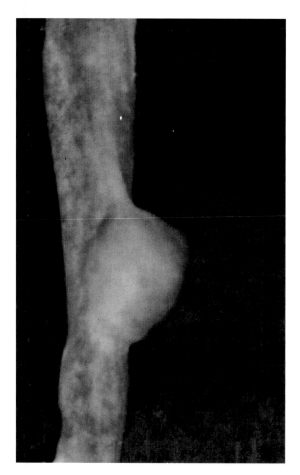

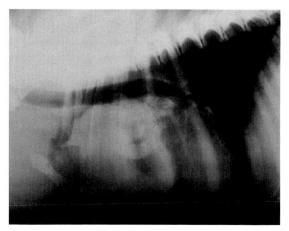

Fig. 5.2 Rhabdomyosarcoma presenting as a lung mass.

Fig. 5.1 Haemangiopericytoma on the distal limb/carpus of a dog.

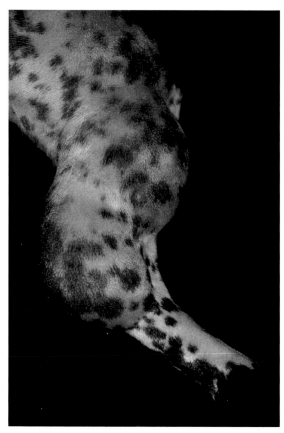

can extend into and through this pseudocapsule and give rise to satellite lesions (Fig. 5.4). Because of this pattern of growth, local tumour recurrence after surgical excision is common. The pseudocapsule provides a tempting plane for resection – 'the tumour shelled out nicely'; however, such a procedure leaves microscopic and even gross tumour in the wound. Excision of any sarcoma within the pseudocapsule is inadequate therapy and will result in local tumour recurrence.

Metastasis

Overall it is estimated that metastasis occurs in up to 25% of all soft tissue sarcomas. Whilst there is some variation in the incidence of metastasis

Fig. 5.3 Infiltrating lipoma. Extending from the stifle to the hock.

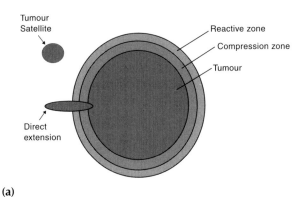
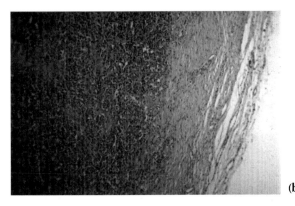

(a)

(b)

Fig. 5.4 Pseudoencapsulation of a soft tissue sarcoma – (a) diagrammatic representation of the reactive and compression zones comprising the 'pseudocapsule' of a soft tissue sarcoma. Tumour cells may exend into and through both these layers as shown in (b) histological section at the 'edge' of an anaplastic soft tissue sarcoma.

between tumours of different histological types, it is now recognised that the risk of metastasis for a particular tumour type correlates with the grade of tumour. Histological grading is an assessment of the tumour based on:

- Degree of tumour differentiation (poor differentiation = high grade)
- Cellularity (increases with higher grade)
- Cellular pleomorphism (increases with higher grade)
- Amount of stroma (decreases with increasing grade)
- Mitotic activity (increases with increasing grade)
- Tumour necrosis (present in high grade tumours).

Using such criteria, sarcomas may be described as low, intermediate or high grade. A high grade tumour of any histological type will carry a higher risk of metastasis than its low grade counterpart. Prediction of likely behaviour of an individual sarcoma will therefore depend on consideration of both histological type and grade of tumour, as shown in Table 5.2.

Metastasis is usually via the haematological route with blood borne metastases favouring the lung as the predominant site for the development of secondary tumours. Other sites for metastasis include internal viscera, skin and bone. The incidence and pattern of distant metastasis depend on the site and type of the primary tumour, for example animals with splenic haemangiosarcoma show a higher incidence of disseminated disease throughout the abdomen. Regional lymph node metastasis is less

common although it is reported for synovial cell sarcoma and, may occur with 'anaplastic' tumours.

Paraneoplastic syndromes

Paraneoplastic syndromes are not common in soft tissue sarcoma although the occasional tumour may be associated with hypercalcaemia, and masses in the thorax may cause hypertrophic osteopathy. Haemangiosarcoma may be associated with haematological complications including microangiopathic anaemia, thrombocytopenia and DIC.

Investigations

Bloods

Routine haematological/biochemical analyses are not generally very helpful in the diagnosis of most soft tissue tumours. Some soft tissue tumours, e.g. haemangiosarcoma, may be associated with haematological or paraneoplastic complications (as above) and blood samples would be indicated in the evaluation of cases such as these.

Imaging techniques

Radiography of the primary tumour may be indicated if the lesion is invasive and sited close to bone (e.g. synovial sarcoma). Radiography of the thorax to look for pulmonary metastases is required in the clinical staging of all malignant tumours and ultra-

Table 5.2 Relationship between histological type and grade for soft tissue sarcomas.

Histological type	Low grade	Intermediate grade	High grade
Haemangiopericytoma	+		
Fibrosarcoma	+	+	(+)
Neurofibrosarcoma	+		
Myxosarcoma	+	+	
Malignant fibrous histiocytoma	+	+	?
Synovial cell sarcoma		+	(+)
Liposarcoma		+	(+)
Rhabdomyosarcoma		+	(+)
Anaplastic sarcoma		+	+
Haemangiosarcoma	(+)*		+

Low grade = low risk of metastasis, i.e. less than 10%
Intermediate = moderate risk of metastasis, i.e. 25–50%
High grade = strong possibility of metastasis i.e. 75–100%
* A low grade haemangiosarcoma of the skin is recognised, with low metastatic potential.

sound evaluation of abdominal organs is important in the clinical staging of internal tumours and high grade or anaplastic tumours.

CT and MRI of the primary tumour mass is widely used in pre-operative evaluation of human sarcoma patients to assess the deep relationships of such tumours and to plan therapy. It is likely that use of these techniques will increase in veterinary medicine.

Biopsy/FNA

The clinical presentation of a soft tissue mass with variable rate of growth may be suggestive of a soft tissue sarcoma; however, histological examination of biopsy material is essential for diagnosis of tumour type and assessment of histological grade. Although fine-needle aspiration cytology may be helpful in distinguishing differential diagnoses such as lipoma, mast cell tumour or abscess, cytology is of limited value in the diagnosis of soft tissue sarcoma. Often these tumours do not exfoliate well (Fig. 5.5) and furthermore, their variable tissue components mixed with areas of necrosis and inflammation complicate cytological diagnosis.

Knowledge of tumour type is vital prior to definitive treatment and an incisional biopsy is preferable to an excisional technique in all but the most exceptional case. The biopsy site and tech-

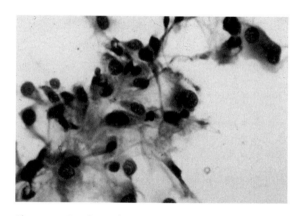

Fig. 5.5 Cytological preparation of sarcoma. The spindle shaped cells collected by FNA are suggestive of a tumour of mesenchymal origin but do not provide sufficient information to type or grade the tumour.

nique should be planned to minimise tissue trauma and haemorrhage (which may disseminate tumour cells locally) and should be performed at a location which will be within a future surgical excision.

Staging

Clinical staging of soft tissue tumours is by clinical examination, radiography and ultrasonography. CT and MRI are useful if available. The primary

Table 5.3 TNM classification for soft tissue sarcoma. Owen (1980).

T	*Primary tumour*			
	T1	Tumour <2 cm maximum diameter		
	T2	Tumour 2–5 cm maximum diameter		
	T3	Tumour >5 cm maximum diameter		
	T4	Tumour invading other structures such as fascia, muscle, bone or cartilage.		
N	*Regional lymph nodes (RLN)*			
	N0	No histologically verified metastasis		
	N1	Histologically verified metastasis		
M	*Distant metastases*			
	M0	No evidence of distant metastasis		
	M1	Distant metastasis detected (specify sites)		
Stage grouping		T	N	M
I				
IA		T1	N0	M0
IB		T2	N0	M0
II				
IIA		T3	N0	M0
IIB		T4	N0	M0
III				
IIIA		Any T	N1	M0
IIIB		Any T	any N	M1

tumour is assessed on the basis of its size, infiltration and involvement of other structures such as fascia, muscle and bone, as shown in Table 5.3.

Treatment

Surgery

Surgery is the most effective treatment for soft tissue sarcomas. Cures can be achieved in low grade sarcomas with aggressive surgery. The surgical margin should be as large as necessary to obtain a complete excision and in most cases this will require a compartmental or 'en bloc' resection. This aims to remove the tumour in one piece with all dissection in a separate fascial plane or tissue type to the tumour. If there is any concern that the surgical instruments have penetrated the tumour pseudocapsule, the surgeon should change instruments and gloves before proceeding with the dissection in a wider tissue plane. For tumours sited on the limb an amputation may be required for complete tumour removal. Careful planning is necessary to achieve the aim of complete excision, and imaging techniques such as CT can be helpful in this process.

The best opportunity for a surgical cure is the first time the tumour is removed surgically. Not only does inadequate surgical resection result in local tumour recurrence, it also selects for the most aggressive component of the tumour, i.e. those invasive cells at the periphery of the main mass. Hence locally recurrent tumours tend to be more aggressive in terms of growth rate and invasion than the original mass. Second surgeries should include the whole scar and the sites of any surgical drains, and dissection should be extremely radical.

Excisional samples should be sent for histopathology to confirm the biopsy diagnosis and to assess the margins of the resected tumour for evidence of incomplete excision.

Radiotherapy

Sarcomas are generally considered to be resistant to radiotherapy, although with the use of megavoltage irradiation allowing more sophisticated fractionation schemes and treatment planning, results of radiotherapy for soft tissue sarcomas have been more encouraging. Radiotherapy is of little value in the management of large, bulky tumours and when used as a sole treatment will only achieve low control rates for such tumours. Radiotherapy is best combined with cytoreductive surgery. Post-operative radiotherapy has been shown to increase the disease-free survival of dogs with haemangiopericytoma and other low grade sarcomas (McChesney *et al.* 1989). A detailed plan of the tumour site pre and post operatively is needed for treatment planning purposes, especially if the area to be irradiated is in a complex anatomic region. The entire surgical field should be considered contaminated and included in the radiation field, as well as any entry or exit holes from drains placed at closure. Thus the tumour should be assessed pre-operatively by the radiotherapist, and the treatment plan constructed in consultation with the surgical team.

Chemotherapy

The role of chemotherapy in treatment of soft tissue sarcomas is poorly defined at this time but theoretically chemotherapy would be a rational

Table 5.4 Chemotherapy protocols used in the treatment of haemangiosarcoma and other high grade sarcomas in dogs.

Protocol	Agents
Doxorubicin (single agent)	Doxorubicin* 30 mg/m^2 IV every three weeks (maximum recommended cumulative dose of doxorubicin = 240 mg/m^2)
AC**	Doxorubicin* 30 mg/m^2 IV day 1 Cyclophosphamide 100–150 mg/m^2 IV day 1 or 50 mg/m^2 PO days 3,4,5,6 Repeat at 21 day cycles
VAC**	Doxorubicin* 30 mg/m^2 IV day 1 Cyclophosphamide 100–150 mg/m^2 IV day 1 Vincristine 0.7 IV days 8 and 15 Repeat at 21 day cycles

* Recommended dose for doxorubicin in cats is 20 mg/m^2.
** The combination of doxorubicin and cyclophosphamide is very myelosuppressive and prophylactic antibiotics may be required in these protocols.

choice for high grade and multifocal tumours. There have been reports of response rates of 20% or greater to doxorubicin as a single agent or in combination with vincristine and/or cyclophosphamide (VAC protocol). Mitoxantrone, vincristine, dacarbazine (DTIC) and carboplatin have also been used with varying degrees of success but the role of chemotherapy in the treatment of measurable soft tissue tumours is, at best, palliative.

Chemotherapy may be of greater value in the post-surgical management of high grade sarcoma, such as haemangiosarcoma, where the actions of drugs are directed against microscopic disease residual at the tumour site or elsewhere in the body in the form of micrometastases. For example doxorubicin may be used as a single agent, with cyclophosphamide (AC) or in the VAC protocol (see Table 5.4) following splenectomy for removal of splenic haemangiosarcoma, to increase post-operative survival time (Hammer et al. 1991). It is possible that similar benefit may be achieved through the use of these agents in other high grade sarcomas following aggressive surgical management of the primary tumour by amputation, chest wall resection etc, but this has yet to be established in controlled clinical trials. Mitoxantrone has also been shown to have

anti-tumour activity in soft tissue sarcomas and may be a good alternative to doxorubicin in cats (Ogilvie et al. 1993).

Other

In North America an 'immunomodulating' agent called 'Acemannan Immunostimulant' has been marketed for treatment of canine and feline fibrosarcomas in combination with surgery and radiotherapy (King et al. 1995). It is used prior to surgery, to promote an inflammatory response which causes necrosis of the tumour leading to a more resectable tumour. Controlled studies indicating that it is any more effective than radiation and surgery have not been performed.

Prognosis

The prognosis for soft tissue sarcoma is dependent on many factors including size, site and histological grade. The main causes of treatment 'failure' are:

- Local recurrence of the tumour – may occur with both high and low grade tumours as a result of inadequate surgical resection.
- Metastasis – irrespective of management of the primary tumour, high grade sarcomas carry a significant risk of metastases.

References

Doddy, F.D., Glickman, L.T., Glickman, N.W. & Janovitz, E.B. (1996) Feline fibrosarcomas at vaccination sites and non-vaccination sites. *Journal of Comparative Pathology*, (114), 165–74.
Hammer, A.S., Couto, C.G., Filppi, J. et al. (1991) Efficacy and toxicity of VAC chemotherapy (vincristine, doxorubicin and cyclophosphamide) in dogs with haemangiosarcoma. *Journal of Veterinary Internal Medicine,* (5), 160–66.
Hendrick, M.J. & Brooks, J.J. (1994) Post vaccinal sarcomas in the cat: histology and immunohistochemistry. *Veterinary Pathology*, (31), 126–9.
Kass, P.H., Barnes, W.G., Spangler, W.L., Chomel, B.B. & Culbertson, M.R. (1993) Epidemiologic evidence for a causual relation between vaccination and fibrosarcoma tumorigenesis in cats. *Journal of the American Veterinary Medical Association*, (203), 396–405.
King, G.K., Yates, K.M., Greenlee, P.G., Pierce, K.R., Fors, C.R., McAnalley, B.H. & Tizard I.R. (1995) The effect of Acemannan Immunostimulant in combination with surgery and radiation therapy

on spontaneous canine and feline fibrosarcomas. *Journal of the American Animal Hospital Association*, (31), 439–47.

Lester, S., Clemett, T. & Burt, A. (1996) Vaccine site-associated sarcomas in cats: clinical experience and a laboratory review (1982–1993). *Journal of the American Animal Hospital Association*, (32), 91–5.

Ogilvie, G.K., Moore, A.J., Obradovich, J.E. *et al.* (1993) Toxicoses and efficacy associated with the administration of mitoxantrone to cats with malignant tumours. *Journal of the American Veterinary Medical Association*, (2023), 1839–44.

Owen, L.N. (1980) TNM Classification of tumours in domestic Animals. World Health Organisation, Geneva.

McChesney, S., Withrow, S.J., Gillette, E.W., Powers, B.E. & Dewhirst, M.W. (1989) Radiotherapy of soft tissue sarcomas in dogs. *Journal of the American Veterinary Medical Association*, (194), 60–63.

Morris, J.S., Bostock, D.E., McInnes, E.F., Hoather, T.M. & Dobson, J.M. (2000) A histopathological survey of neoplasms in flat-coated retrievers 1990–1998. *Veterinary Record*, (147), 291–95.

White, R.A.S., Jefferies, A.R. & Gorman, N.T. (1986) Sarcoma development following irradiation of acanthomatous epulis in two dogs. *Veterinary Record*, (118), 668.

6
Skeletal System

■ Bone and cartilage, 78
■ Joints and associated structures, 89

For the purposes of this book, the 'skeletal system' is defined as comprising bone, cartilage and joints. Tumours affecting muscle are included in Chapter 5, Soft tissues. A variety of tumours may affect the skeletal system. These may be primary tumours arising from elements of bone or cartilage, soft tissue tumours which invade into bone, or malig-nant tumours which metastasise to bone. Multiple myeloma and other lymphoid tumours may also affect bone and cause painful, osteolytic lesions (see Chapter 15). Tumours of bone and cartilage may affect both the appendicular and axial skeleton; those affecting the skull are given more detailed consideration in Chapter 7, Head and neck.

BONE AND CARTILAGE

Epidemiology

Tumours of bone and cartilage are relatively un-common in the dog and cat population as a whole, representing less than 5% of all tumours. Bone tumours in the dog and cat are usually malignant; benign tumours are rare in both species. In the dog, bone tumours of the appendicular skeleton occur with increasing frequency with increasing size/body weight and predominantly affect large–giant breeds. So great is this size relationship that primary bone tumours are rare in dogs less than 15 kg, yet common in breeds such as the Irish wolfhound, great Dane, rottweiler and St Bernard. Bone tumours tend to affect middle-aged to old animals, although they may occur in young dogs of giant breeds. It has been suggested that males are predisposed.

Primary bone tumours are uncommon in cats. They tend to affect older cats (mean age 10 years) and there is no sex or breed predisposition reported. Tumours of the appendicular skeleton are more common than those of the axial skeleton and are most frequent in the pelvic limb.

Tumours of cartilage are rare in both species; benign and malignant variants have been described.

Aetiology

The aetiology of most tumours of bone and cartilage is not known. However, the pattern of development of primary malignant bone tumours (osteosarcoma) suggests some contributory factors which may play a role in their development. Primary bone tumours have a predilection for the metaphyseal regions of long bones especially the distal radius, proximal humerus, distal femur and proximal tibia and are more frequent in the forelimb than the hind limb. The increased frequency in the forelimb and increased frequency with size, seems to correlate with weight bearing. Rapid bone growth during early development and bone stress due to weight bearing, possibly

Table 6.1 Classification of tumours affecting the skeleton of the dog and cat.

Primary tumours of bone	
Benign	*Malignant*
Osteoma	**Osteosarcoma**[*]
Chondroma (rare)	Parosteal osteosarcoma
Enchondroma	Chondrosarcoma
Monostotic osteochondroma (dog)	Fibrosarcoma
	Haemangiosarcoma
Polyostotic osteochondroma (multiple cartilagenous exostoses) (dog)	Liposarcoma
	Anaplastic sarcoma
Osteochondromatosis (cats)	Giant cell tumour (of bone)
Other primary tumours	Multiple myeloma (Lymphoma)
Tumours which invade bone	Soft tissue sarcomas
	Squamous cell carcinoma (digit, jaw)
	Malignant melanoma digit
Tumours which metastasise to bone	Carcinomas, mammary, prostatic (pulmonary carcinoma in cat – digit)

[*] various histological subtypes, see text.

resulting in microfractures, are implicated as important factors. There may also be a genetic predispostion in the large and giant breed dogs and a familial incidence has been reported in rottweilers and St Bernards. Tumours may occasionally develop at the sites of old fractures (especially those with a history of delayed healing) and in bone that has been included in treatment fields during radiotherapy.

Pathology

Primary tumours of bone may arise from any tissue within the bone 'organ' and may develop at any site, i.e. periosteum, endosteum or the medullary cavity. The most common tumours arise in the mesenchymal precursors of osseus and cartilagenous tissues, giving rise to osteosarcoma and chondrosarcoma respectively. Osteosarcoma is the most common primary bone tumour in the dog and accounts for 80–90% of bone tumours in large dogs and 50% of bone tumours in small dogs. Tumours of fibrous connective tissue (fibrosarcoma) and vascular tissue (haemangiosarcoma) are less common. Osteosarcoma is the most common primary bone tumour of cats; fibrosarcoma is the

second most common. Bone may also be affected by lymphoproliferative conditions (notably multiple myeloma), may be invaded by soft tissue tumours and may be the site of metastasis for other malignant tumours. Tumours which may affect the bone are summarised in Table 6.1.

Benign

Benign tumours of bone (osteoma) and cartilage (chondroma) are rare in cats and dogs and are of little clinical importance. Several benign conditions which affect the skeleton of cats and dogs are worthy of note, although uncommon.

Osteochondroma/multiple cartilagenous exostoses
Osteochondroma is a benign 'tumour' formed by endochondral ossification from the surface of a bone, and is capped with hyaline cartilage. These 'growths' result from developmental disturbances in the growing animal, and they cease to enlarge at skeletal maturity. They may form in any bone of endochondral origin; the scapulae, ribs, vertebrae and pelvis are the most common sites. These tumours may be monostotic lesions which are of little clinical consequence, except that they may be hereditary in the dog. They are usually incidental

findings on radiographic examination. Polyostotic lesions (also referred to as osteochondromatosis or multiple cartilagenous exostosis) have, on rare occasions, been reported to undergo malignant transformation in the dog.

Osteochondromatosis in cats is a different entity in that the lesions show progressive enlargement with time, and have a random distribution, including bones of the skull (formed by intramembranous ossification). The condition is usually diagnosed in young adult cats (2–4 years). There is no evidence of breed or sex predilection, nor is there any hereditary pattern, but viral particles have been found consistently in the cartilage caps of the lesions. The significance of the virus in the pathogenesis of the condition is not known.

Enchondroma

Enchondroma is a benign cartilagenous tumour which originates within the medullary cavity of a bone. Histologically the tumour resembles hyaline cartilage and is thus distinct from chondrosarcoma. The expansile growth of the tumour within the bone eventually erodes the cortex and results in a well-defined, firm palpable mass. The growth of the tumour can be associated with pain and in some cases can precipitate a pathological fracture. Lesions may be monostotic or polyostotic; the latter may be termed enchondromatosis. The condition is distinct from osteochondromatosis in that the lesions originate within the bone as opposed to on the surface.

Multilobular osteoma/chondroma/ osteochondrosarcoma, 'chondroma rodens'

This is an uncommon tumour which classically arises in the bones of the skull and has a characteristic radiographic appearance (see Chapter 7). It has been given many names (as above) but is now regarded as a low grade malignancy, because although the rate of growth is often quite slow, metastasis can occur.

Other benign tumours – like lesions including bone cysts, aneurysmal bone 'cysts' and fibrous dysplasia of bone – are occasionally encountered but because of their rarity have not been well characterised in veterinary medicine and their behaviour is not well documented.

Malignant

Primary bone tumours

Malignant tumours arising within bone are listed in Table 6.1. In addition to osseus and cartilagenous elements, which give rise to the majority of tumours occurring at this site, bone also contains fibrous, vascular and other mesenchymal elements, all of which may undergo neoplastic transformation and give rise to sarcomas within the bone, e.g. fibrosarcoma, haemangiosarcoma. Osteosarcoma is the most common primary sarcoma of bone and accounts for 80–90% of tumours at this site. Chondrosarcoma is the second most common primary bone tumour in dogs, accounting for approximately 5–10% of all canine primary bone tumours; the other sarcomas account for the remaining primary bone tumours.

Osteosarcoma may vary considerably in the histological pattern and the amount and type of matrix produced. Tumours may be classified as poorly differentiated, osteoblastic, chondroblastic, fibroblastic, telangiectatic, giant cell type or combined type, on the basis of the predominant histological features within the lesion. In contrast to human osteosarcoma, the clinical relevance of histological classification of canine osteosarcoma has not been established. Of more relevance is the site of development of the tumour. Osteosarcoma of central or medullary origin (Fig. 6.1) exhibits more aggressive and malignant behaviour than parosteal (or juxtacortical) osteosarcoma, which grows outward from the periosteal side of the cortex and causes minimal cortical lysis (Fig. 6.2). However, also recognised is a high grade periosteal osteosarcoma which arises on the outside surface of a bone but has the invasive and malignant character of the intraosseus osteosarcoma.

Giant cell tumour of bone

This is a rare tumour affecting bone, whose histogenesis is uncertain. Tumours appear to arise from stromal cells of the bone marrow and produce expansile, osteolytic lesions.

Metastatic and other tumours involving bone

Bone may be a site for secondary, metastatic tumour development, and carcinomas, in particular mammary, prostatic and pancreatic carcinoma,

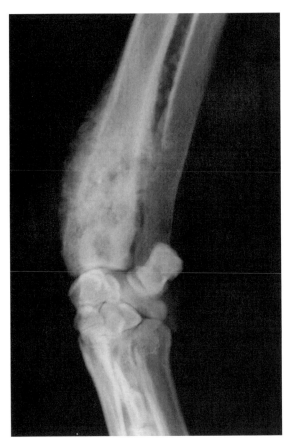

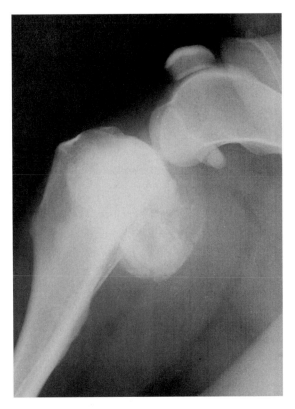

Fig. 6.2 Parosteal osteosarcoma. The tumour is growing out from the cortex of the bone with very little invasion of normal bone.

Fig. 6.1 Typical radiographic appearance of medullary osetosarcoma (of the distal radius).

show a tendency to metastasise to bone where they give rise to painful, osteolytic lesions (Fig. 6.3). Several reports have described a primary lung adenocarcinoma in the cat with a metastatic predilection for the digits (Scott-Moncrieff *et al.* 1989). Multiple myeloma and, on occasion, lymphoma may also give rise to osteolytic bone lesions (Fig. 6.4) (see Chapter 15).

Locally invasive soft tissue tumours may invade into adjacent bone. Squamous cell carcinoma of gingiva is often associated with marked destruction of the adjacent maxillary or mandibular bone, especially in the cat (Fig. 6.5) (see Chapter 7) and that arising in the digit can lead to total destruction of the phalanx (Chapter 4, Fig. 4.9). Soft tissue tumours arising in the periarticular tissues also show a tendency to local bone involvement (see later in this chapter under tumours of joints).

Tumour behaviour

Osteosarcoma is a rapidly growing, invasive and destructive tumour. Its presence within the bone causes pain, and the destruction of normal structural bone leads to weakening of the bone, predisposing to pathological fracture (Fig. 6.6). The tumour tends to spread along the medullary cavity and may invade through the periosteum and deep fascia to involve adjacent soft tissues, although they rarely invade or cross joints (Fig. 6.7).

Osteosarcoma (of long bones) in the dog is a highly malignant tumour which metastasises early in the course of the disease. In most cases microscopic metastatic disease is present at the time of presentation or diagnosis of the primary lesion. Metastasis is haematogenous and the lungs are the most common site for the development of secondary tumours. Other sites of distant metastases

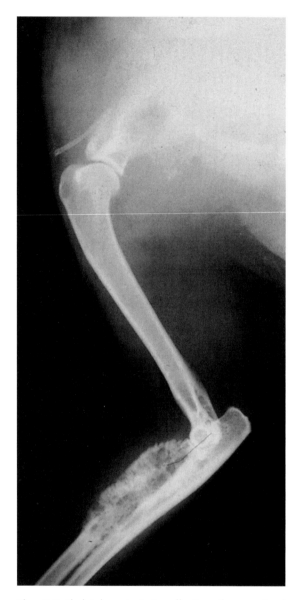

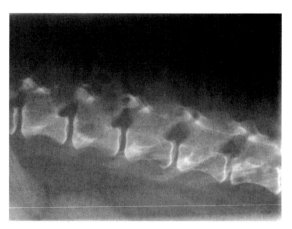

Fig. 6.4 Multiple 'punched-out' osteolytic lesions in the dorsal spinous processes of the lumbar vertebrae in a dog with multiple myeloma.

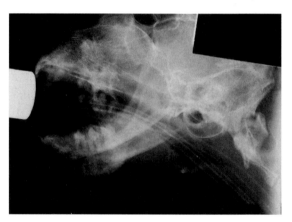

Fig. 6.5 Squamous cell carcinoma of the mandible in a cat; there is a massive bony reaction to the invading tumour.

Fig. 6.3 Skeletal metastasis affecting the proximal radius in a cat with a primary lung carcinoma. The cat had similar lesion in other limbs.

include kidney, liver, spleen and the skeleton itself.

Osteosarcoma of the axial skeleton, for example the skull, is usually less aggressive in terms of local growth rate and in terms of the incidence and the rate of metastasis.

Osteosarcoma in cats also behaves less aggressively with an estimated metastatic rate less than 20%.

Chondrosarcoma and fibrosarcoma are generally slower growing tumours in both species with a lower incidence of metastasis. Giant cell tumour of bone may follow a benign or malignant course.

Paraneoplastic syndromes

No specific paraneoplastic syndromes are associated with osteosarcoma or other primary bone tumours. Hypercalcaemia is rarely associated with primary bone tumours although it may occur with extensive skeletal metastases from soft tissue

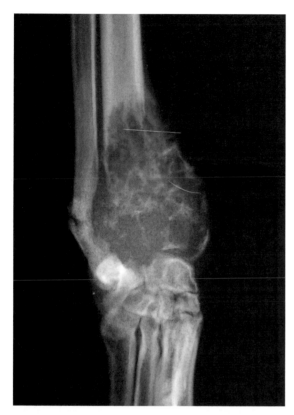

Fig. 6.6 Extreme destruction of the distal radius by an aggressive osteosarcoma has led to collapse of the radius and pathological fracture of the ulna.

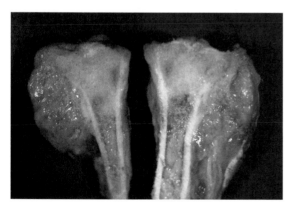

Fig. 6.7 Gross appearance of an osteosarcoma of the proximal tibia. The sectioned limb shows how the tumour has invaded through the cortex and into the surrounding soft tissues, but has not crossed into the joint. (Picture courtesy of Mr D. Bostock.)

tumours and in association with multiple myeloma and lymphoma. Primary tumours of the axial sketeton may give rise to local site-specific complications, as detailed below.

Presentation/signs

Long bone osteosarcoma

Affected animals usually present with lameness (gradual or acute onset) with or without painful swelling of the affected area of the limb. The lameness is usually progressive but can become acute if associated with a pathological fracture.

The tumour has a predilection for the metaphyseal regions of long bones especially:

- Proximal humerus
- Distal radius
- Distal femur
- Proximal tibia.

Axial osteosarcoma

The presenting signs of tumours sited in the axial skeleton are site specific. An enlarging mass with or without pain may be the only clinical sign of tumours affecting the skull but in other cases the tumour mass may not be obvious on physical examination and the animal will present with signs relating to the physical presence of the tumour or collapse of the affected bone. For example:

- Oral, mandibular, maxillary and orbital tumours may present with dysphagia, pain on opening the mouth or exophthalmos (Chapter 7)
- Nasal sinus tumours may present with nasal discharge and epistaxis (Chapter 7)
- Tumours affecting the spine may present with neurological signs (Chapter 13).

Investigations

Bloods

Routine haematological/biochemical analyses are not generally very helpful in the diagnosis of primary bone tumours. Total serum alkaline phosphatase and bone-specific alkaline phosphatase are elevated in dogs with primary osteosarcoma, but whilst this may be of prognostic significance

(Ehrhart *et al.* 1998), it is not really a useful diagnostic test.

Imaging techniques

Radiography is valuable in the diagnosis of primary bone tumours. Radiography of the affected area (Figs 6.8 and 6.9) will show a variable mixture of:

- Osteolysis – destruction of both medullary and cortical bone; this may be focal or disseminated.
- Irregular, haphazard new bone formation, often spiculated and at right angles to the original cortex ('sun-burst' appearance), sclerosis of medullary areas, and periosteal new bone at the periphery of the lesion – 'Codman's triangle'.
- Soft tissue swelling with or without calcification.

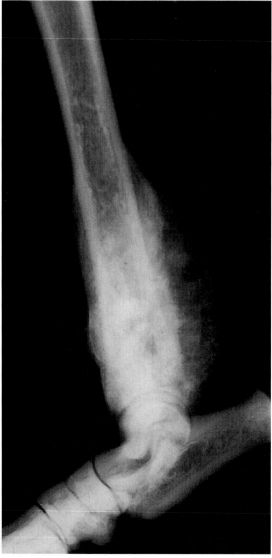

6.8

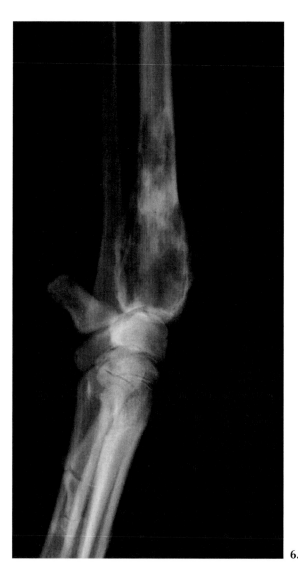

6.9

Figs 6.8 and 6.9 Radiographic appearance of osteosarcoma. Fig. 6.8 A tumour of the distal femur, showing typical features of Codman's triangle and 'sunburst' periosteal new bone. Fig. 6.9 A tumour of the distal radius is more osteolytic in nature.

The combination of these changes, along with the presenting history and clinical signs, will lead to a high index of suspicion of a diagnosis of osteosarcoma; however 'osteosarcoma' is a histological diagnosis. The radiographic diagnosis should be described as a 'primary malignant bone tumour'.

Radiography of the thorax is important in clinical staging. Ultrasound, CT and MRI are of little to no value in the diagnosis of primary tumours of the appendicular skeleton, although CT or MRI may be useful for those tumours involving the axial skeleton. Scintigraphy may be useful in clinical staging to detect the presence of skeletal metastases.

Biopsy/FNA

Fine needle aspirate cytology is of limited value in the diagnosis of primary bone tumours, not least because of the hard, calcified nature of the tissues. FNA of local lymph nodes should be performed if they are enlarged but local lymphatic metastasis is unusual.

A biopsy of the lesion is required to reach a histological diagnosis but this can be problematic for a number of reasons:

- The hard/bony nature of the lesion limits choice of biopsy techniques and the need for decalcification of the tissue prior to sectioning for histological examination introduces a delay in obtaining the results.
- These are aggressive tumours and often contain areas of haemorrhage and necrosis; furthermore bone tumours induce a response from normal bone cells. Thus selection of the site for collection of representative tissue can be a problem.
- It usually requires general anaesthesia of the patient.
- There is a risk of precipitating a pathological fracture.

A Jamshidi core biopsy technique is probably the best method for biopsy of primary bone tumours (Fig. 6.10), although open biopsy techniques may also be used. Two or three needle samples should be taken from different angles or at different sites to ensure collection of representative tissue.

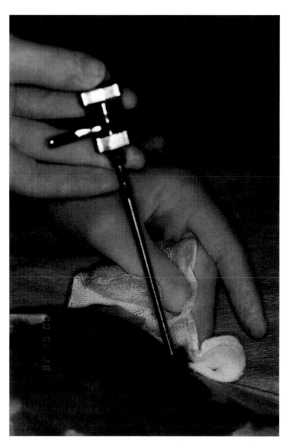

Fig. 6.10 Jamshidi biopsy needle.

Staging

The extent of the primary tumour can be assessed by radiography. Right and left lateral inflated thoracic radiographs are essential to assess the lungs for the presence of metastases but will not detect microscopic disease. Scintigraphy ('bone scan') may be used to look for skeletal metastases.

Primary malignant bone tumours may be staged clinically according to the World Health Organization TNM Classification (Table 6.2); tumours arising at other sites, e.g. oral cavity, could be staged according to the relevant system.

Treatment

The major dilemma following diagnosis of appendicular osteosarcoma in a dog is whether to treat or

Table 6.2 World Health Organization TNM classi-fication of canine/feline tumours of the bone (Owen 1980).		

T	*Primary tumour*	
	T0	No evidence of tumour
	T1	Tumour confined within the medulla and cortex
	T2	Tumour extends beyond the periosteum
	Multiple tumours should be classified independently	
M	*Distant metastases*	
	M0	No evidence of distant metastasis
	M1	Distant metastasis detected (specify sites)

No stage grouping is at present recommended.

not. The options for treatment, as set out below, are limited and in the majority of cases do not alter the fatal outcome of the disease. Dogs with osteosarcoma are lame because they are in pain. If this pain cannot be relieved through treatment of the primary tumour then euthanasia should be carried out on humane grounds. Non-steroidal anti-inflammatory agents can be used for short term relief of pain to allow the owners time to come to terms with the imminent loss of their pet.

Bone tumours at other sites of the body which are amenable to surgical management may carry a more favourable prognosis as these tumours are usually less aggressive and slower to metastasise.

Surgery

Surgery is the most effective means of treatment for the primary tumour but the locally invasive nature of bone tumours means that removal of the tumour requires a wide margin of excision within and including the bone. This may be feasible for some tumours of the skull or axial skeleton, for example removal of a hemi-mandible may achieve a compartmental resection of a tumour sited within this bone. For most appendicular tumours a wide surgical margin requires amputation of the affected limb. Forequarter or hindlimb amputation is actually quite well tolerated in animals up to 45–50 kg and in some cases in dogs much larger than this (Kirpensteijn *et al.* 1999). Amputation is probably the treatment of choice for pain relief and for effective removal of the primary tumour, but post-

amputation survival times are short, on average three to four months.

Limb salvage

In carefully selected cases it may be possible to salvage the limb by local surgical resection of the affected segment of bone and replacement by a cortical allograft supported by a plate (LaRue *et al.* 1989) (Figs 6.11 and 6.12). Limb salvage is not possible in all cases of osteosarcoma. The procedure is restricted to animals with relatively small, early tumours which are contained within the deep periosteal fascia and have not invaded the soft tissues of the limb. The distal radius is the most favourable site to attempt limb salvage because it is relatively simple to arthrodese the carpus compared to other joints. Limb salvage is not without complications:

- The dog has to be severely restricted for several months after surgery while the leg is maintained in a cast (this may represent a substantial portion of its remaining life).
- Surgical complications are frequent, ranging from loosening of the screws which hold the plate and graft in place to osteomyelitis and failure of the graft. Further surgical and or medial intervention is inevitable.
- Local tumour recurrence occurs in a significant number of cases.
- Limb salvage does not affect the progression of metastatic disease which is the ultimate cause of death in these patients.

Radiotherapy

Radiotherapy may be of short term value as a palliative for pain relief in a small proportion of cases but should not be viewed as an effective means of treatment of the tumour. Pre or post-operative radiotherapy may be used in conjunction with limb sparing surgery to improve local tumour control in cases where only marginal resection of the primary tumour is possible.

Chemotherapy

Systemic chemotherapy usually has little effect on the growth of the primary tumour, although it has

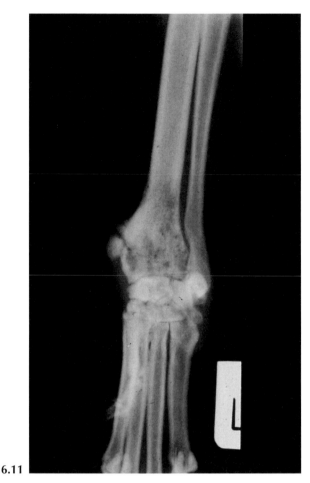

6.11

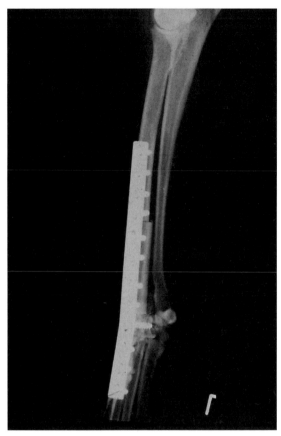

6.12

Figs 6.11 and 6.12 Limb salvage. Fig. 6.11 shows a localised osteosarcoma of the distal radius with virtually no soft tissue involvement. It was possible to surgically remove the affected area of bone, with the tumour contained within the deep fascia. Fig. 6.12 shows replacement of the diseased bone with an allograft, held in place by a large compression plate.

been used on occasion in a neo-adjuvant setting to temporarily arrest tumour growth prior to surgical resection/limb salvage. Intralesional or regional (limb perfusion/intra-arterial) adminstration of cytotoxic drugs has met with little success.

Chemotherapy is indicated as an adjuvant to surgical management of the primary disease in an attempt to prevent or at least delay the onset of metastatic disease (Table 6.3). The most commonly used agent for the treatment of micrometastatic disease in canine osteosarcoma is cisplatin. (This agent should never be used in cats. There is no indication for its use in osteosarcoma in this species and

the drug is highly toxic to cats). Cisplatin is nephrotoxic in the dog and has to be administered with fluids to protect against renal damage. A variety of protocols have been described for the administration of cisplatin (Table 6.4). Carboplatin has also been used at a dose rate of $300\,mg/m^2$ every 21 days for four cycles (Bergman *et al*. 1996) and although carboplatin is more expensive than cisplatin, it is less nephrotoxic and can be administered without diuresis.

There is no evidence that adjuvant chemotherapy is of any benefit in preventing metastases with chondrosarcoma or other bone sarcomas.

Table 6.3 Post-amputation survival times for dogs with appendicular osteosarcoma with adjuvant chemotherapy.

Protocol	Median survival (days)	One year survival rate (%)	Reference
Cisplatin 60 mg/m^2 q 21 days × 1–6	300–325	45.5	Berg *et al.* 1992
Carboplatin 300 mg/m^2 q 21 days × 4	321	35.4	Bergman *et al.* 1996
Doxorubicin 30 mg/m^2 q 14 days × 5	278	50	Berg *et al.* 1995

Table 6.4 Protocols for administration of cisplatin (See also Appendix IV).

Cisplatin dose: 50–70 mg/m^2 every 3–4 weeks, usually for 4–6 treatments

Six hour infusion with saline diuresis
Prehydration – intravenous saline (0.9%) at rate of 25 ml/kg/hour for 3 hours
Antiemetic – metoclopramide 1 mg/kg prior to administration of cisplatin
Cisplatin 50–70 mg/m^2 – given as a slow intravenous infusion over 15 minutes
Diuresis – intravenous saline (0.9%) continued at 15 ml/kg/hour for 3 hours
Frusemide – may be administered if urine production is not adequate

Infusion with mannitol diuresis
Prehydration – intravenous saline (0.9%) at rate of 10 ml/kg/hr for 4 hours
0.5 g/kg mannitol iv in saline over 20–30 minutes
Antiemetic – metoclopramide 1 mg/kg prior to administration of cisplatin
Cisplatin 50–70 mg/m^2 – given as slow intraveous infusion over 15 minutes
Continue saline infusion (0.9%) at 10 ml/kg/hr for 2 hours.

Handling precautions
Cisplatin should be regarded as a very hazardous substance and handled accordingly. Ideally the drug should be
    prepared in a flow cabinet. Face masks, protective clothing and gloves should be worn by any person handling the
    agent or the patient. Following administration, cisplatin is excreted, unchanged, in the urine and this presents a
    potential hazard. All contaminated equipment and bedding should be incinerated. Cisplatin should not be handled
    by pregnant staff.

Other

Non-specific immunotherapy with liposome-encapsulated muramyl tripeptide has been used post-amputation for treatment of dogs with osteosarcoma and has been shown to extend survival times compared with dogs receiving amputation only (MacEwen *et al.* 1989). MTP-PE may also be used in conjunction with cisplatin chemotherapy to extend post-amputation times further. Unfortunately this is an investigational product and is not available routinely in the UK.

Prognosis

The prognosis for appendicular osteosarcoma in dogs is universally poor. In 90% of cases micrometastatic disease is present at the time of presentation/diagnosis of the primary tumour and irrespective of method of treatment almost all patients are eventually euthanased as a result of metastatic disease and/or local tumour recurrence. The prognosis for cats with osteosarcoma is more favourable as such tumours in this species appear to be less aggressive and carry a far lower risk of metastasis. Osteosarcoma of the axial skeleton in both the cat and dog is usually less aggressive than that of the long bones, and although long-term follow-up of such cases has shown that some of these tumours do eventually metastasise, if effective treatment of the primary tumour is possible, post-operative survival times can exceed 12 months.

Haemangiosarcoma of bone is also highly malig-nant but the prognosis for other tumours arising in bone is generally more favourable. Chondrosar-coma is slow to metastasise and at some sites, e.g. rib, an en bloc resection may result in cure or at least prolonged survival (Pirkey-Ehrhart et al. 1995). Complete surgical resection may also be curative for fibrosarcoma, although metastases have been reported in some cases.

JOINTS AND ASSOCIATED STRUCTURES

Epidemiology

Tumours affecting the joints and the adjacent tendon sheaths, bursae and fascia are rare in both the cat and the dog. Most of the lesions described in small animals at this site are malignant and tumours of the canine joints are the most common of this rare group. Large (but not giant) breed dogs appear to be predisposed, and the average age at presentation is eight years with a range of 1–12 years (Madewell & Pool 1978).

Aetiology

The aetiology of tumours of joints and associated structures is not determined. Metabolic and inflammatory lesions may occur in the synoviae, which have to be distinguished from synovial tumours.

Pathology

The most commonly reported primary joint tumour in the dog is the synovial sarcoma, a malignant tumour that is thought to arise from undifferentiated mesenchymal cells in the deep connective tissue associated with synovial joints, which differentiate into synovioblasts. Histo-logically this tumour is composed of two cellular elements:

• Fibroblastic component
• Synovioblastic or epithelioid component.

The proportion of these two, intermingled com-ponents varies considerably both within and between tumours. A variety of other soft tissue sarcomas may arise in the periarticular soft tissues (Table 6.5) and these can be difficult to distinguish clinically or radiologically from true synovial sarcoma. As with all soft tissue sarcomas that lack clear differentiation, histological classi-fication can be problematic and is open to individ-ual interpretation. In humans the classification of soft tissue tumours affecting joints or tendons is complex and detailed but the relevance of such classification systems in veterinary medicine is not established. In practice all these tumours share common clinical features and prediction of their likely behaviour may be better made according to the grade of the tumour rather than histological type (see also Chapter 5).

Synovial 'cysts' have been reported in both cats and dogs and a number of proliferative conditions of the synovium may also present with nodular or hyperplastic tumour-like lesions. None of these conditions show bony involvement.

Tumour behaviour

Synovial sarcomas are locally aggressive tumours which invade into the subchondral bone at the articular margins, causing osteolysis of the periar-ticular bone and destruction of the joint. They tend not to affect articular cartilage directly. The rate of local progression of the tumour is variable and the clinical course of the disease can vary from acute to protracted over several months, on occasion exceeding one year. The reported metastatic rate for canine synovial sarcoma varies from 25–40% (Madewell & Pool 1978; Vail et al. 1994), and the pattern of metastasis is to regional lymph nodes, lungs and other organs. However, many animals are euthanased as a result of the primary tumour and there are few reports of long-term follow-up in treated animals.

Table 6.5 Tumours affecting joints (Whitelock *et al.* 1997).

Tumour type	Number	Joint affected	Number
Synovial cell sarcoma	8	Stifle	3
		Hock	2
		Elbow	2
		Shoulder	1
Fibrosarcoma	5	Stifle	2
		Elbow	2
		Temporo-mandibular joint	1
Osteosarcoma	3	Elbow	3
Rhabdomyosarcoma	3	Stifle	1
		Elbow	1
		Shoulder	1
Undifferentiated sarcoma	2	Stifle	1
		Elbow	1
Liposarcoma	2	Stifle	1
		Elbow	1
Malignant fibrous histiocytoma	1	Elbow	1
Haemangiosarcoma	1	Shoulder	1
Haemangiopericytoma	1	Carpus	1
Mast cell tumour	1	Stifle	1
Squamous cell carcinoma	1	Metacarpophalangeal and interphalangeal joints	1
Amelanotic melanoma	1	Metacarpophalangeal joint	1

Paraneoplastic syndromes

No specific paraneoplastic syndromes are associated with synovial sarcoma, or other periarticular sarcomas.

Presentation/signs

Most affected animals present with a progressive lameness of the affected limb with a mild to pronounced peri-articular soft tissue swelling (Fig. 6.13). The stifle is the joint most frequently affected, followed by the elbow and the hock.

Investigations

Bloods

Routine haematological/biochemical analyses are not generally very helpful in the diagnosis of tumours of the joints.

Imaging techniques

Radiography of the affected joint (Fig. 6.14) will generally show:

- A quite well-defined periarticular soft tissue swelling
- Permeative or punctate osteolysis of the metaphyses and epiphyses adjacent to the joint
- Multiple bone involvement
- Irregular, spiculated periosteal new bone is a feature in some cases.

These radiological findings of periarticular soft tissue swelling and osteodestruction on both sides of a joint in an older, large breed dog are highly suggestive of synovial sarcoma but other soft tissue tumours may present in a similar manner (see Table 6.5) and these cannot be distinguished without histopathological examination.

Ultrasonography is not useful in most cases.

CT/MR imaging of synovial tumours has become standard in human clinical practice and is useful in determining the anatomic extent of the tumour and its relationship with the joint space and other structures such as tendon sheaths or bursae.

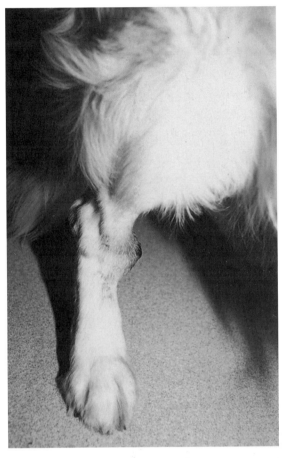

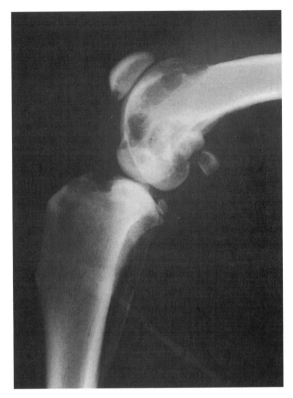

Fig. 6.14 Radiographic appearance of a synovial sarcoma of the stifle, showing osteolytic lesions on either side of the joint.

Fig. 6.13 Peri-articular swelling due to a synovial sarcoma of the hock.

punch biopsies may be appropriate in certain tumours.

Radiography of the thorax would be required for clinical staging, although most cases do not have demonstrable metastases at the time of first presentation.

Staging

Clinical, surgical and radiographic examination are required for clinical staging of tumours of the joints and associated structures and the TNM system is outlined in Table 6.6.

Biopsy/FNA

As with all soft tissue sarcomas, fine needle aspirate cytology is of limited value in the diagnosis of synovial tumours, although an aspirate could help to distinguish between neoplastic and non-neoplastic causes of periarticular swelling. FNA of local lymph nodes should be performed if they are enlarged but local lymphatic metastasis is unusual.

A biopsy of the lesion is required to reach a histological diagnosis, and an incisional biopsy is probably the preferred technique. Needle or

Treatment

Surgery

Surgical resection is the treatment of choice for synovial sarcoma and other sarcomas involving the joints; however, because of the close proximity of these tumours to the joint and the invasion of bone,

Table 6.6 Clinical stages (TNM) of canine and feline tumours of joints and associated structures (Owen 1980).

T	*Primary tumour*
	T0 No evidence of tumour
	T1 Tumour well-defined, no invasion of surrounding tissues
	T2 Tumour invading soft tissues
	T3 Tumour invading joints and/or bones
	Multiple tumours should be classified independently
N	*Regional lymph nodes (RLN)*
	N0 No evidence of RLN involvement
	N1 RLN involved
	(−) histologically negative, (+) histologically positive
M	*Distant metastases*
	M0 No evidence of distant metastasis
	M1 Distant metastasis detected (specify sites)

No stage grouping is at present recommended.

surgical resection usually requires an amputation of the affected limb.

Radiotherapy

Radiotherapy may be of short term value as a palliative for pain relief in a small proportion of cases but there is no clinical evidence to support the use of radiotherapy as an effective treatment for synovial sarcoma. It is not usually possible to use radiotherapy in an adjuvant, post-operative setting for such tumours as the only surgical approach is an amputation.

Chemotherapy

Chemotherapy is unlikely to be of benefit in treatment of the primary tumour, although the use of doxorubicin alone or in combination with cyclophosphamide (see Table 5.4) has been reported to delay the progression of the disease in cases where amputation is not deemed acceptable (Tilmant *et al.* 1986). Larger scale studies are required to validate this observation.

As with other soft tissue sarcomas, theoretically chemotherapy would be indicated as an adjuvant to surgical management of high grade, malignant tumours in an attempt to prevent or at least delay the onset of metastatic disease, but the role of chemotherapy in this context has not been fully evaluated in veterinary medicine.

Prognosis

Despite the fact that between a quarter to a third of these tumours may metastasise, most dogs treated by amputation have disease-free survival times in excess of three years (Vail *et al.* 1994). The prognosis with amputation is therefore quite good.

References

Berg, J., Weinstein, J., Schelling, S.H. & Rand, W.M. (1992) Treatment of dogs with osteosarcoma by administration of cisplatin after amputation of limb sparing surgery: 22 cases (1987–1990). *Journal of the American Veterinary Medical Association*, (200), 2005–2008.

Berg, J., Weinstein, J., Springfield, D.S. & Rand, W.M. (1995) Results of surgery and doxorubicin chemotherapy in dogs with osteosarcoma. *Journal of the American Veterinary Medical Association*, (206), 1555–9.

Bergman, P.J., MacEwen, E.G., Kurzman, I.D. *et al.* (1996) Amputation and carboplatin for treatment of dogs with osteosarcoma: 48 cases (1991–1993). *Journal of Veterinary Internal Medicine*, 10 (2), 76–81.

Ehrhart, N., Dernell, W.S., Hoffmann, W.E., Weigel, R.M., Powers, B.E. & Withrow, S.J. (1998) Prognostic importance of alkaline phosphatase activity in serum from dogs with appendicular osteosarcoma: 75 cases (1990–1996). *Journal of the American Veterinary Medical Association*, (213), 1002–1006.

Kirpensteijn, J., Van den Bos, R. & Endenburg, N. (1999) Adaption of dogs to the amputation of a limb and their owners' satisfaction with the procedure. *Veterinary Record*, (144), 115–18.

Pirkey-Ehrhart, N., Withrow, S.J., Straw, R.C. *et al.* (1995) Primary rib tumours in 54 dogs. *Journal of the American Animal Hospital Association*, (31), 65–9.

LaRue, S.M., Withrow, S.J., Powers, B.E. *et al.* (1989) Limb sparing treatment for osteosarcoma in dogs. *Journal of the American Veterinary Medical Association*, (195), 1734–44.

Madewell, B.R. & Pool, R.R. (1978) Neoplasms of joints and related structures. *Veterinary Clinics of North America*, (8), 511–21.

MacEwen, E.G., Kurzman, I., Rosenthal, R.C., Smith, B.W., Manley, P.A., Roush, J.K. & Howard, P.E. (1989) Therapy for osteosarcoma in dogs with intravenous injection of liposome-encapsulated muramyl tripeptide. *Journal of the National Cancer Institute*, (81), 935–7.

Owen, L.N. (1980) *TNM Classification of Tumours in Domestic Animals*. World Health Organization, Geneva.

Scott-Moncrieff, J.C., Elliott, G.S., Radovsky, A. & Blevins, W.E. (1989) Pulmonary squamous cell carcinoma with multiple digital metastases in a cat. *Journal of Small Animal Practice*, (30), 696–9.

Tilmant, L.L., Gorman, W.T., Ackerman, N. *et al.* (1986) Chemotherapy of synovial cell sarcoma in a dog. *Journal of American Veterinary Medical Association*, (188), 530–32.

Vail, D.M., Powers, B.E., Getzy, D.M. *et al.* (1994) Evaluation of prognostic factors for dogs with synovial sarcoma, 36 cases (1986–1991). *Journal of the American Veterinary Medical Association*, 205 (9), 1300–1307.

Whitelock, R.G., Dyce, J., Houlton, J.E.F. & Jefferies, A.R. (1997) A review of 30 tumours affecting joints. *Veterinary Comparative Orthopaedics and Traumatology*, (10), 146–52.

7
Head and Neck

The head and neck are important sites for development of tumours in both cats and dogs. Included in this chapter are tumours affecting the nasal planum, nasal cavity, oropharynx (including the tonsils and tongue) and tumours of the skull, ears and salivary glands. Skin and soft tissue tumours may be sited on the head or neck but these are considered in Chapters 4 and 5 respectively. Likewise tumours of the thyroid gland are considered in Chapter 14 and tumours of the eye in Chapter 16.

NASAL PLANUM

Epidemiology

Tumours of the nasal planum are relatively uncommon in the dog but common in the cat, where they are reported to account for 17% of all skin tumours (Bostock 1986). In the cat they affect older animals, especially those with lightly pigmented skin of the nasal region.

Aetiology

Exposure of non-pigmented, lightly haired skin to UV light (especially UVB) (see Chapters 1 and 4) is an important aetiological factor in the development of tumours of the nasal planum in cats. The aetiology of tumours of the nasal planum in dogs is not known.

Pathology

Squamous cell carcinoma (SCC) is by far the most common tumour arising at this site in cats. Depending on the stage of development, the tumour may be described as carcinoma *in situ*, superficial SCC or invasive SCC. Although tumours of the nasal planum are far less common in dogs, SCC is also the most frequent tumour at this site. Mucosal mast cell tumours, plasmacytoma, basal cell carcinoma, fibrosarcoma and multifocal or diffuse tumours of the skin, e.g. epitheliotrophic lymphoma, may also involve the nasal planum in both species. Eosinophilic granuloma should be considered as a differential diagnosis for an ulcerated lesion of the nasal planum/lip in the cat.

Tumour behaviour

In the cat, SCC usually follows a protracted course of development, often progressing over a period of many months through stages of actinic keratosis with erythematous crusting lesions to superficial erosions and ulcers (carcinoma *in situ*) (Fig. 7.1) before becoming invasive (Fig. 7.2) and destructive of underlying tissues (Fig. 7.3). Metastasis from this site is unusual in the cat. In contrast, SCC of the nasal planum in the dog tends to be a more rapidly progressing tumour which is invasive from the outset and may metastasise to the local and regional lymph nodes (Fig. 7.4).

Mucosal mast cell tumours occasionally affect the nasal planum, especially in young dogs (Fig. 7.5). Such tumours seem to follow a relatively benign course.

Paraneoplastic syndromes

No specific paraneoplastic syndromes are associated with tumours of the nasal planum.

Presentation/signs

Affected cats usually present with an obvious crusted, ulcerative lesion of the nasal planum as described above and shown in Figs 7.1–7.3. Where the tumour is invasive there may be a tendency for the lesion to bleed and local irritation can give rise to sneezing. Very extensive tumours may result in obstruction of the nares. Occasionally dogs with nasal planum SCC may present with a swollen nose or narrowed nares without an obvious external lesion.

Investigations

Bloods

Routine haematological/biochemical analyses are not generally very helpful in the diagnosis of SCC of the nasal planum. Such investigations would be indicated in the work up of cases of cutaneous lymphoma or mast cell tumours and also in the pretreatment evaluation of older animals.

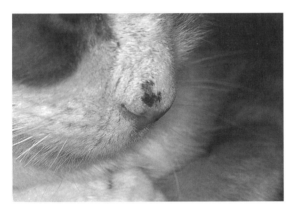

Fig. 7.1 Early crusting lesion of carcinoma on cat's nose. (See also Colour plate 22, facing p. 162.)

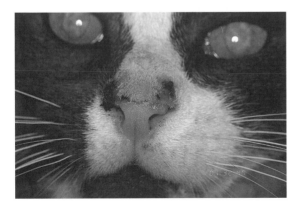

Fig. 7.2 Minimally invasive, early SCC of nasal planum. (See also Colour plate 23, facing p. 162.)

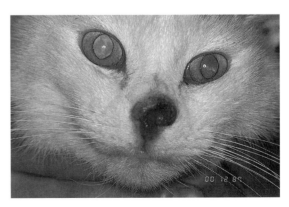

Fig. 7.3 Invasive SCC of nasal planum in cat. (See also Colour plate 24, facing p. 162.)

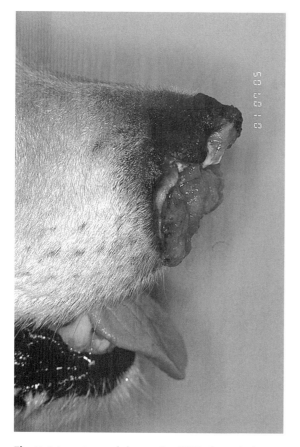

Fig. 7.4 Invasive and destructive SCC of nasal planum in a dog. (See also Colour plate 25, facing p. 162.)

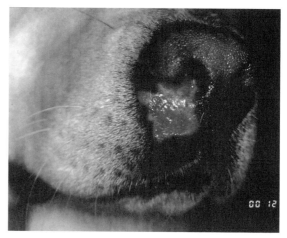

Fig. 7.5 Mucosal mast cell tumour in a young dog.

Imaging techniques

Radiography and ultrasonography are not usually indicated in the investigation of nasal planum tumours in cats. Radiography of the nasal chambers may be indicated in dogs with extensive tumours that may extend into the nasal cartilage and bone.

Radiography of the thorax is indicated in the dog but is of questionable value in the cat.

Biopsy/FNA

Fine needle aspirates or cytological scrapings are of little value in the diagnosis of tumours of the nasal planum; most of these lesions are ulcerated and superficial samples may only reveal haemorrhage

and inflammation. A deep incisional, wedge biopsy is preferred for histological diagnosis and this will also provide information on the degree of invasion of the tumour.

Fine needle aspirate of lymph nodes is indicated if these are enlarged.

Staging

Staging tumours of the nasal planum requires assessment of the degree of invasion and involvement of other tissues by the tumour. A modified staging system is shown in Table 7.1.

Treatment

A variety of techniques have been described for treatment of carcinoma of the nasal planum (SCC) and the choice of treatment really depends on the extent of the lesion. Early, minimally invasive tumours may be managed in a number of ways whereas surgery is the only effective treatment for deeply invasive tumours. Clearly it is always preferable to institute an effective treatment as early as possible in the course of the disease.

Surgery

Surgery is the treatment of choice for invasive tumours which have not invaded extensively into

Table 7.1 Modified staging system for tumours of the nasal planum.

T group	Description
T1	Tumour confined to nasal planum, superficial
T2	Tumour with spread on to adjacent areas, e.g. lip, superficial
T3	Invasion of subcutis
T4	Invasion of other structures, e.g. fascia, muscle, cartilage or bone

the lips or skin. Complete excision of invasive tumours of the nasal planum requires removal of the nasal plate, transecting the nasal turbinates, to ensure an adequate margin to incorporate invasive tumour within the resection. If there is invasion of the lips then these must be included in the resection. Reconstructive techniques may be used to effect wound closure or, in the cat, a technique has been described that uses a single purse string suture to pull the skin edges into an open circle around the airways (Withrow 1996). Functional and cosmetic results are good in the cat. In the dog, where the tumours are often more invasive and extensive at the time of diagnosis, surgery needs to be aggressive with reconstruction, and while the functional results are quite good, the appearance of the animal is significantly altered.

Cryosurgery can be an effective method of treatment for superficial SCC but may not be sufficiently penetrating for control of more invasive tumours.

Radiotherapy

Superficial (orthovoltage or Strontium) radiation is effective for management of superficial tumours in cats but has not been very successful in the management of deeply invasive tumours in either species and the local control rates reported for these are poor (Carlisle & Gould 1982; Thrall & Adams 1982; Lana *et al.* 1997). Post-operative radiotherapy has been used in cases where histological examination of excised samples has shown tumour invasion at the surgical margins.

Chemotherapy

Conventional chemotherapy is not indicated in the management of local SCC.

Other

Photodynamic therapy appears to be an effective treatment for small, superficial (minimally invasive) tumours (Peaston *et al.* 1993). This technique offers the advantage of preserving the anatomy of the nose and unlike radiation can be applied repeatedly without cumulative damage to normal tissues. Photodynamic therapy is not effective for invasive tumours.

Prophylaxis

In sunny climates where the risk of nasal planum SCC is high in cats with non-pigmented noses, topical application of sun blocks or protection of the skin by tattooing may be considered.

Prognosis

The prognosis for SCC of the nasal planum depends on the degree of invasion of the tumour. The prognosis is good for early, non-invasive tumours in cats, although further lesions may develop in adjacent tissues if the underlying cause is not addressed. The prognosis is more guarded for cats with invasive SCC; however a proportion of these can be cured with aggressive surgery. A one year disease-free survival rate of 75% following 'nosectomy' for invasive SCC was reported in one study (Withrow & Straw 1990). The prognosis for dogs with SCC of the nasal planum is guarded, although with aggressive surgery, disease free survival rates in the order of 12 months may be possible.

NASAL CAVITY AND PARANASAL SINUSES

Epidemiology

Tumours of the nasal cavity and paranasal sinuses represent approximately 1% of all neoplasms in both the dog and cat (Madewell *et al.* 1976; MacEwen *et al.* 1977). They tend to affect older animals of both species; an average age of 10 years is reported in the dog. Doliocephalic dogs are at higher risk and most affected dogs are of medium to large breeds such as the collie, Labrador and golden retriever, German shepherd and spaniels. A slight male predilection has been reported in the dog. Siamese cats may be at increased risk of intranasal neoplasia (Cox *et al.* 1991), but no sex predilection has been observed in the cat.

Aetiology

The aetiology of tumours of the nasal cavity and paranasal sinuses is not known. There has been speculation that the incidence of such tumours in long-nosed dogs may be associated with pollutants (in urban environments) or with passive smoking, but such associations have not been proved. In cats, nasal lymphoma may be related to the feline leukaemia virus, although most cases are FeLV negative, and nasopharyngeal polyps may be asso-

ciated with otitis media or inflammation of the eustachian tube.

Pathology

The majority of tumours arising in the nasal cavity and paranasal sinuses are malignant, and various histological types are reported (Table 7.2).

In the dog approximately two thirds of tumours at this site are derived from the nasal epithelium, which is for the most part glandular although squamous cell carcinoma is a relatively common diagnosis. Most of the remainder are sarcomas, arising from cartilage, bone or other connective tissues within the nose. Adenocarcinoma is the most common tumour of the nasal cavity in the cat and lymphoma second. Intranasal sarcomas are rare in the cat.

Tumour behaviour

Malignant tumours of the nasal cavity and paranasal sinuses are locally invasive tumours which cause progressive destruction of both the soft and the bony structures in and surrounding the nasal cavity. These tumours are usually slow to metastasise and most patients succumb to uncontrolled or recurrent local disease rather than metastases.

Table 7.2 Tumours of the nasal cavity and paranasal sinuses in the cat and dog.

Histological type	Comment
Carcinoma Adenocarcinoma Squamous cell carcinoma Undifferentiated carcinoma (including transitional cell carcinoma)	Carcinoma is the most common tumour of the nasal cavity in both cat and dog, representing up to two-thirds of all canine tumours at this site and over half of all feline tumours. Adenocarcinoma is the most common diagnosis in both species
Sarcoma Fibrosarcoma Chondrosarcoma Osteosarcoma Undifferentiated sarcoma	Intranasal sarcomas are less common than carcinomas in the dog and rare in the cat.
Other Lymphoma Transmissible venereal tumour Melanoma Neuroblastoma	Lymphoma is the second most common tumour at this site in the cat but an unusual diagnosis in the dog. Other tumours are rare.

Paraneoplastic syndromes

No specific paraneoplastic syndromes are associated with tumours of the nasal cavity and paranasal sinuses. Most of the problems associated with these tumours are directly due to local growth and invasion by the primary mass as described below.

Presentation/signs

The majority of 'nasal' tumours in cats and dogs are sited in the nasal cavity, and in dogs, radiographically most tumours seem to arise in the region of the ethmoturbinate bones. Tumours affecting the paranasal/frontal sinuses are less common. Tumours at both these sites rarely cause any externally observable swelling until the later stages of the disease. The most common presenting signs for tumours of the nasal cavity are:

- Nasal discharge (watery/mucoid/purulent/ haemorrhagic), often unilateral at first
- Epistaxis
- Sneezing
- Nasal congestion/upper airway obstruction – stertor and stridor
- Epiphora – due to obstruction of the naso-lachrymal duct.

Initially these signs are often intermittent but as the condition progresses, usually over a period of several months, the clinical signs become more severe and persistent and may be accompanied by signs of the tumour erupting out of the nasal cavity resulting in:

- Facial deformity – tumour associated swelling is often seen in the naso-frontal regions of the skull, medial to the eyes (Fig. 7.6)
- Exophthalmos – due to tumour invasion of the orbit
- Bowing of the hard palate
- Neurological signs (usually seizures) due to direct invasion of the cranial vault.

Tumours arising in the frontal sinus may cause few clinical signs in the early stages of growth, although some are associated with occasional epistaxis. The first clinical sign may be associated with pain in the region of the frontal bone and this may manifest as the animal becoming 'head-shy' or showing a change in character leading to depres-

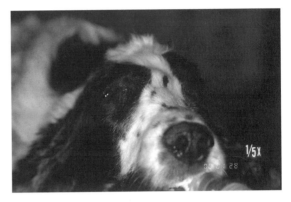

Fig. 7.6 Extensive nasal tumour causing exophthalmos.

sion or aggression. The nature of the problem becomes more obvious when the tumour erodes through the bone to form a firm–soft swelling over the frontal bone (Fig. 7.7).

By virtue of the connections between the nasal and frontal sinuses, tumours of the nasal cavity may invade into the ipsilateral frontal sinus or at least obstruct the flow of mucous from the sinus. Conversely tumours originating in the frontal sinus may give rise to nasal signs, hence there is no clear cut distinction between the two.

Investigations

Bloods

Routine haematological/biochemical analyses are not generally very helpful in the diagnosis of tumours of the nasal cavity and paranasal sinuses; however haematology and clotting studies are important to exclude other causes of epistaxis (thrombocytopenia and coagulopathies) prior to nasal biopsy.

Blood should also be taken for aspergillus serology as aspergillosis is an important differential diagnosis.

Imaging techniques

Radiography is the most useful, widely available means of evaluating the nasal chamber. The best view for assessment of the nasal cavity and turbinate bones is the 'dorso-ventral, intra-oral' (DVIO) view. This is taken using non-screen film placed within the mouth (Fig. 7.8), with the animal

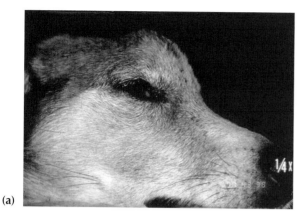

(a)

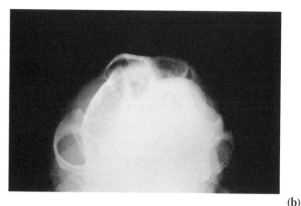

(b)

Fig. 7.7 Frontal sinus tumour – (a) the dog presented with a painful swelling above the right eye; (b) radiographs of the skull show 'sunburst' reaction to tumour invading through the frontal bone.

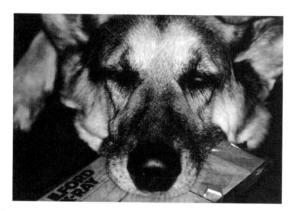

Fig. 7.8 Patient positioned for DVIO radiograph. (Courtesy of Mr M.E. Herrtage, Department of Clinical Veterinary Medicine, University of Cambridge.)

in sternal recumbency and the X-ray beam directed ventrally. The classical radiographic signs of intranasal neoplasia are:

- Loss of the fine trabecular pattern within the nasal cavity due to destruction of the nasal turbinate bones
- Increased soft tissue/fluid density due to the expanding tumour mass and/or accompanying haemorrhage and discharge (Fig. 7.9).

These changes are often easier to appreciate in early cases with unilateral lesions, where the asymmetry of the nasal anatomy may be more obvious than in animals with bilateral involvement.

Lateral skull radiographs are useful for evaluation of the frontal sinuses, although a skyline view

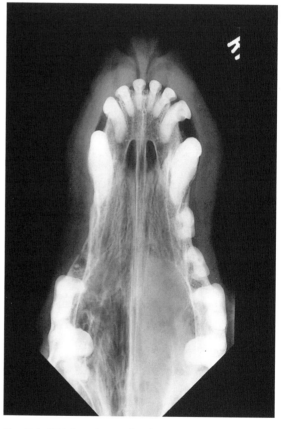

Fig. 7.9 DVIO radiograph of nasal chambers of dog with history of nasal discharge and epistaxis. The film shows loss of fine turbinate detail and increased soft tissue/fluid opacity on the right side. These changes are highly suggestive of intranasal neoplasia.

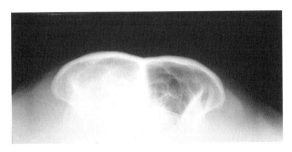

Fig. 7.10 Skyline radiograph of frontal sinuses of the case in Fig. 7.9, showing opacification of right frontal sinus. This may be due to tumour involvement or obstruction of drainage from the sinus.

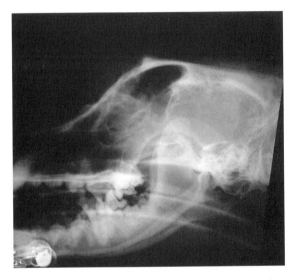

Fig. 7.11 Lateral skull, showing bone disruption due to advanced intranasal tumour.

(using a horizontal beam) provides a better comparison of right and left (Fig. 7.10). Lateral or oblique skull radiographs may also be used to look for destruction of the nasal or frontal bones at sites of facial swelling (Fig. 7.11).

Right and left radiographs of the thorax are important for staging purposes.

MRI and CT offer good alternatives to radiographic imaging of the skull for determination of the extent of tumours within the nasal cavity and paranasal sinuses. Cross-sectional images of the skull provided by these techniques can provide very useful information about the relationships of the tumour, especially in the area of the cribriform plate and orbit, which cannot be ascertained by radiography (Chapter 2, Fig. 2.8) (Thrall *et al.* 1989; Burk 1992). It is likely that the use of such techniques will increase in the future.

Rhinoscopy – the nasal cavity can be visualised by endoscopic techniques and this may assist localisation of lesions for biopsy.

Biopsy/FNA

The relative inaccessibility of the nasal cavity can complicate collection of representative tissue for histological diagnosis of tumours at this site. Cytolological techniques, including nasal washings, are not generally very rewarding although a vigorous flushing technique can be used to collect solid clumps of tumour tissue for histological examination. Various other means of obtaining biopsy samples have been described; probably the most consistently successful are:

- 'Blind' grab technique – crocodile action 'grab' biopsy forceps are inserted via the nostril to the tumour site (determined radiographically); the tumour sample can be collected by grasping tissue and withdrawing the forceps.
- Catheter suction technique – a wide bore urinary catheter, cut down to a predetermined length (long enough to access the tumour but not damage the cribriform plate is inserted via the nares with syringe attached. Tumour tissue is collected by applying negative pressure when the catheter is sited within the tumour mass, and withdrawing. The catheter may be redirected in different angles throughout the tumour to obtain a good tissue sample (Withrow 1996).

All these techniques are likely to cause mild to moderate haemorrhage and it is important that the nasopharynx is packed off to avoid the risk of blood or tissue fragments being aspirated. In none of these techniques is it possible to visualise the tumour at the time of biopsy and because many nasal tumours are accompanied by inflammation and sometimes necrosis, a potential problem is the collection of non-representative tissue and failure to confirm the diagnosis of neoplasia. In this event it is advisable to repeat the biopsy.

Diagnosis of tumours of the frontal sinus requires surgical exploration of the mass and an incisional biopsy.

FNA cytology should be performed on any enlarged lymph nodes.

Staging

Clinical staging of tumours within the nasal cavity requires clinical and radiographic examination. The TNM system for canine and feline tumours of the nasal chamber and sinuses is shown in Table 7.3a. A modified staging system which may be of greater clinical relevance has been suggested in Table 7.3b (Theon *et al.* 1993).

Table 7.3a Clinical stages (TNM) of canine and feline tumours of the nasal chambers and sinuses (Owen 1980).

T	*Primary tumour*
	T0 No evidence of tumour
	T1 Tumour ipsilateral, minimal or no bone destruction
	T2 Tumour bilateral and/or moderate bone destruction
	T3 Tumour invading neighbouring tissues
	The symbol (m) added to the appropriate T category indicates multiple tumours
N	*Regional lymph nodes (RLN)*
	N0 No evidence of RLN involvement
	N1 Movable ipsilateral nodes
	N1a nodes not considered to contain growth
	N1b nodes considered to contain growth
	N2 Movable contralateral or bilateral nodes
	N2a nodes not considered to contain growth
	N2b nodes considered to contain growth
	N3 Fixed nodes
	(−) histologically negative, (+) histologically positive
M	*Distant metastases*
	M0 No evidence of distant metastasis
	M1 Distant metastasis detected (specify sites)

Table 7.3b Proposed stage grouping for canine nasal tumours (Theon *et al.* 1993).

Clinical Stage	Description
I	Unilateral or bilateral neoplasm confined to the nasal passage(s) without extension into frontal sinuses
II	Bilateral neoplasm extending into the frontal sinuses with erosion of any bone of the nasal passages

Treatment

Treatment is principally directed at achieving control of local disease but the inaccessibility of the tumour and its proximity to critical organs such as the brain and eyes restrict treatment options and complicate management.

Surgery

Surgical access to the nasal cavity may be gained via a dorsal rhinotomy through the nasal bones; however, the majority of nasal tumours in cats and dogs are not managed effectively by surgery alone. Indeed the value of surgery in the treatment of such tumours is doubtful. On occasion surgery may be indicated for removal of benign lesions such as nasal polyps or for collection of tumour tissue in cases where repeated 'blind' biopsies have failed to achieve a conclusive diagnosis. It may be possible to 'debulk' a tumour originating in the frontal sinus at the time of surgical exploration but complete removal of all tumour tissue is unlikely to be achieved at this site.

Radiotherapy

Radiotherapy is the treatment of choice for most malignant tumours of the nasal cavity and paranasal sinuses (i.e. carcinomas and sarcomas) and is usually used alone for the treatment of such tumours in both cats and dogs. In the past, radiation was often combined with surgical debulking of the tumour but although post-treatment survival times may be marginally greater for the combined therapy, the benefit of cytoreductive surgery is not really sufficient to justify the additional cost and morbidity of the surgery. With the increasing use of megavoltage radiation (which achieves more even dose distribution within the nasal cavity and sinuses than orthovoltage radiation), the need for surgical debulking of nasal tumours has decreased. A variety of radiotherapy treatment regimes are used for nasal tumours at different centres throughout the world, with dosage and fractionation regimes varying quite widely (as shown in Table 7.4). Rarely is the outcome of treatment curative but most regimes will achieve a symptom-free survival time of over 12 months in 50% of treated animals. A major factor limiting the efficacy of radiotherapy at

Table 7.4 Results of radiotherapy for tumours of the nasal and paranasal cavities in the dog.

Authors	Number of animals	Radiation regime	Results	Toxicity
Adams *et al.* (1987)	67	Various Orthovoltage/ megavoltage +/– surgery Total doses 36–48 Gy	Median survival 8.5 months 1 and 2 year overall survival rates 38% and 30%	Complications reported in 15 dogs (22%), serious in 3 (4%)
Theon *et al.* (1993)	77 (58 carcinomas) (19 sarcomas)	Cobalt 60 unit* 48 Gy in 12 × 4 Gy fractions on M-W-F	Median actuarial survival, 12.6 months 1 and 2 year overall survival rates 60.3% and 25%	Chronic ocular complications in 45% of cases
Morris *et al.* (1994)	12	Linear accelerator 4MV 36 Gy in 4 × 9 Gy weekly fractions	Median survival 63 weeks (14 months) 1 and 2 year actuarial survival 58% and 13%	No severe late reactions (2 dogs subsequently developed aspergillosis)
Adams *et al.* (1998)	21	Cobalt 42 Gy in 9–10 fractions over 11–13 days	Median survival 428 days (14.2 months) 1 year survival rate 60%	Late effects severe in 6/15 dogs (40%) with durable tumour control
LaDue *et al.* (1999)	130	Cobalt 60 Total dose 45–57 Gy in various regimes	Median survival 8.9 months	Late toxicity in 109 evaluable cases. 39% ocular, 6% neurologic, 5% osseus and 1% dermal

* 21 dogs in this study had surgery prior to radiotherapy.

this site is toxicity to the skin, eyes and oral tissues adjacent to the nasal cavity (Fig. 7.12) such that the total dose of radiation administered is a compromise between efficacy and toxicity.

Chemotherapy

Chemotherapy has little role in the treatment of most nasal tumours with the exception of nasal lymphoma, where standard chemotherapy treatment protocols may be used in both the cat and dog (Chapter 15). Lymphoma is radiosensitive but although radiation would be an alternative treatment, chemotherapy is usually preferred because of the potential for any lymphoma to be or become systemic. For example, in the cat renal lymphoma has been observed following radiotherapy of nasal lymphoma (Morris *et al.* 1996a).

Prognosis

Without treatment, the prognosis for nasal tumours is poor and most animals will be euthanased as a result of progressive local tumour-related problems within three to six months of the onset of clinical signs. Even with treatment most animals eventually succumb to the local effects of recurrent tumour, i.e. in most cases therapy is palliative. Surgical treatment alone does not appear to increase survival time. With radiotherapy reported median survival times for canine nasal tumours range from 8 to 14 months (see Table 7.4). Direct comparison of different studies is difficult because of the variability in radiation regimes and defined end points. Some studies have suggested that histological type of tumour does affect the prognosis (Adams *et al.*

1987) but other studies have not supported this. Tumour stage according to the WHO TNM system does not appear to influence prognosis but modified staging systems based on radiographic assessment of the severity of the disease have been shown to correlate with survival time, with more extensive tumours carrying a worse prognosis (Theon *et al.* 1993; Morris *et al.* 1996b; LaDue *et al.* 1999). Tumours originating in the frontal sinuses seem to follow a similar clinical pattern to those of the nasal cavity, in terms of clinical behaviour and radiation response, although their closer proximity to the cranial vault and the orbit may complicate therapy and lead to a more guarded prognosis.

The prognosis is similar in the cat, where radiation treatment for nasal carcinoma and sarcoma resulted in median survival times of 11 months in one study (Theon *et al.* 1994). Response of feline nasal lymphoma to radiotherapy or chemotherapy can be very good and can result in long term remission.

ORAL CAVITY

Epidemiology

The oral cavity is a common site for the development of tumours in small animals, superceded only by the skin and soft tissues, mammary tumours and haematopoietic tumours. Malignant oral tumours account for about 6% of all canine cancers and 3% of feline cancers. Oral tumours generally arise in older animals. Specific age and breed predilections are discussed under individual tumour headings.

Aetiology

The aetiology of most tumours affecting the oral cavity is not known. Infectious (viral) papillomas are rare but may occur in the oral cavity of young dogs. Environmental factors such as pollution may play a role in the development of oral carcinomas such as SCC of the tongue and tonsil in both the cat and dog, and this is supported by observations from the 1950s to 1970s that such tumours had a higher prevalence in urban areas compared to rural areas (Head 1990).

Pathology

A broad spectrum of tumour types arises in the oropharynx in association with the gingiva, oral soft tissues, dental structures and alveolar bone. Tumours range from the benign 'epulides' to the more aggressive squamous cell carcinoma, fibrosarcoma and the highly malignant melanoma (Table 7.5). Because of this wide variation, tumours will be discussed under individual headings.

Presentation/signs

Tumours of the oral cavity and oropharynx may present with a variety of signs including:

- Dysphagia
- Halitosis
- Excessive salivation, purulent/blood stained saliva

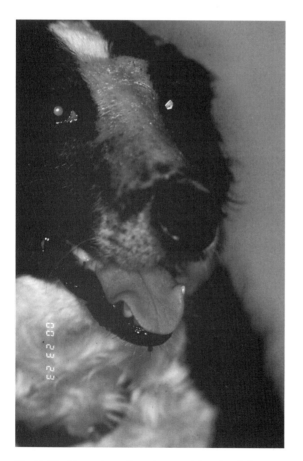

Fig. 7.12 Alopecia and erythema of the skin following orthovoltage radiotherapy for a nasal tumour.

Table 7.5 Tumours of the oropharynx in the dog and cat.

Site	Tumour type
Gingiva and dental arcade	Benign/non-metastatic
	Papilloma
	Peripheral odontogenic fibroma (osseus/
	fibrous epulis)
	(Giant cell epulis)
	Odontoma
	Ameloblastoma
	Basal cell carcinoma (acanthomatous epulis)
	Malignant
	Squamous cell carcinoma
	Malignant melanoma
	Fibrosarcoma
	Other sarcomas
	(Epitheliotrophic lymphoma)
	(Plasmacytoma)
Mandible (maxilla)	Osteosarcoma
	Fibrosarcoma
Tongue	Squamous cell carcinoma
	(Rhabdomyosarcoma, Granular cell
	myoblastoma)
Tonsil	Squamous cell carcinoma
	Lymphoma
Salivary glands	Mixed salivary tumour
	Adenocarcinoma
Cheek and lips	Squamous cell carcinoma
	Mast cell tumour
	Melanoma
	Plasmacytoma
	Epitheliotrophic lymphoma

- Oral haemorrhage
- Displacement or loss of teeth
- Facial swelling.

Because many owners do not routinely inspect their pet's mouth, such tumours can become quite extensive before detection.

Paraneoplastic syndromes

No specific paraneoplastic syndromes are associated with tumours of the oral cavity and oropharynx.

Investigations

Bloods

Routine haematological/biochemical analyses are not generally very helpful in the diagnosis of tumours of the oral cavity and oropharynx.

Imaging techniques

Between 60 and 70% of malignant oral tumours involve bone. Good quality radiographs of the tumour site are essential to evaluate the extent of such tumours. Lateral and dorso-ventral/ventro-dorsal views of the skull may be useful but non-screen, intra-oral films provide better detail. A variety of bony changes occur in association with oral tumours including:

- Osteolysis (may be punctate or permeative, or occasionally expansile bony lesions)
- Irregular periosteal new bone
- Mineralisation of soft tissue tumours.

These radiographic changes are rarely specific for a particular tumour type (Fig. 7.13) but the extent of the changes is important in planning therapy.

Ultrasound is not generally very helpful for imaging tumours of the oral cavity but it is likely

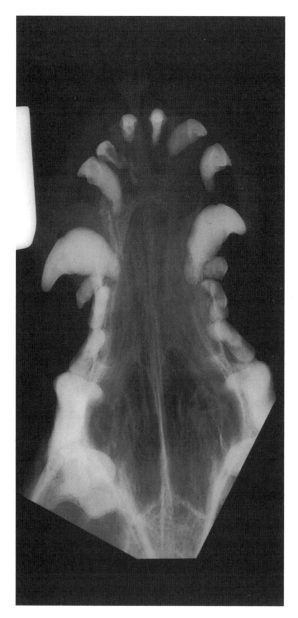

Fig. 7.13 Intraoral radiograph of invasive tumour of the maxilla resulting in dental displacement and bone lysis.

that CT and MRI will be used increasingly for evaluation of such tumours.

Biopsy/FNA

Although gross inspection of an oral neoplasm may give some indication of histiogenisis (see below), a definitive diagnosis can only be made upon histological examination of tumour tissue.

Cytology is of little value in the diagnosis of oral tumours but important for evaluation of enlarged submandibular lymph nodes.

Most intra-oral neoplasms are accessible for biopsy. However, their surface may be infected or necrotic, and hyperplastic or inflammatory reactions in the adjacent tissues are common; thus care must be taken to ensure a representative sample. Small, superficial biopsies can be misleading. As many oral tumours involve the underlying bone a deep wedge or Jamshidi needle-type biopsy is recommended.

Staging

Clinical staging of tumours of the oral cavity and oropharynx is primarily by physical examination and radiography. More than half the tumours occurring at this site are malignant and consideration must be given to the possibility of metastasis via the lymphatic or haematogenous routes. The lymphatic drainage of the oral cavity is primarily to the submandibular lymph nodes. Regional drainage is to the retropharyngeal nodes and via the cervical chain to the prescapular and anterior mediastinal nodes. The tonsils should also be evaluated, especially in the case of malignant melanoma.

The primary tumour is assessed on the basis of its size and invasion of other structures, especially bone, as shown in Tables 7.6. and 7.7. TNM staging systems are also described for tumours of the oropharynx and tumours of the lips (Owen 1980).

Treatment

Surgery

Surgical resection is the single most effective means of treatment for oral tumours. For surgical treatment to be successful the entire tumour must be excised with adequate margins of surrounding normal tissue. Since a high proportion of oral tumours involve bone it is essential that the surgical margins are achieved in the bone as well as in the soft oral tissues. The techniques of mandibulectomy and maxillectomy have been well documented (Withrow & Holmberg 1983; White *et al.*

Table 7.6 Clinical stages (TNM) of canine/feline tumours of the oral cavity (Owen 1980).

T	*Primary tumour*
	Tis Pre-invasive carcinoma (carcinoma *in situ*)
	T0 No evidence of tumour
	T1 Tumour <2 cm maximum diameter
	T1a without bone invasion
	T1b with bone invasion
	T2 Tumour 2–4 cm maximum diameter
	T2a without bone invasion
	T2b with bone invasion
	T3 Tumour >4 cm maximum diameter
	T3a without bone invasion
	T3b with bone invasion
	The symbol (m) added to the appropriate T category indicates multiple tumours
N	*Regional lymph nodes (RLN)*
	N0 No evidence of RLN involvement
	N1 Movable ipsilateral nodes
	N1a nodes not considered to contain growth
	N1b nodes considered to contain growth
	N2 Movable contralateral or bilateral nodes
	N2a nodes not considered to contain growth
	N2b nodes considered to contain growth
	N3 Fixed nodes
	(−) histologically negative, (+) histologically positive.
M	*Distant metastases*
	M0 No evidence of distant metastasis
	M1 Distant metastasis detected (specify sites)

Table 7.7 Stage grouping for tumours of the oral cavity.

Stage Grouping	T	N	M
I	T1	N0 N1a N2a	M0
II	T2	N0 N1a N2a	M0
III	T3	N0 N1a N2a	M0
	Any T	N1b	
IV	Any T	Any N2b or N3	M0
	Any T	Any N	M1

1985). These techniques permit wide local excision of oral tumours with 1–2 cm margins of resection and have been used successfully in the management of basal cell carcinoma, squamous cell carcinoma and low grade fibrosarcoma. Such procedures are extremely well tolerated in dogs but may cause some degree of morbidity in cats.

The role of cryotherapy in the management of the malignant oral tumours is limited because it is difficult to achieve adequate treatment of the tumour margins, particularly those within the bone resulting in local tumour recurrence. Cryosurgery may be used in a palliative manner where more aggressive therapies are not feasible or appropriate.

Radiotherapy

Radiotherapy offers the advantage of treating larger areas of tissue surrounding the tumour than may be possible by surgery, and high energy megavoltage radiation has good penetration of bone.

Local lymph nodes can also be included in the treatment fields where necessary. The main indication for radiotherapy is in the treatment of oral tumours which, by virtue of their site or extent, are not amenable to surgical excision. Radiotherapy has been quite successful as a single agent in the management of gingival carcinomas in the dog and for palliation of oral malignant melanoma. The combination of surgery with post-operative radiotherapy is probably the most effective treatment for oral sarcomas in the dog.

Radiotherapy has been less successful in the management of malignant oral tumours in the cat.

Chemotherapy

Chemotherapy is not indicated treatment of most oral tumours in the cat or the dog, with the exception of mucocutaneous forms of lymphoma.

Benign/non-metastatic tumours of the oral cavity – The epulides

The 'epulides' are a group of common, non-metastatic oral tumours arising in association with the gingiva. As a group the epulides represent up to 40% of all oral tumours in the dog; they are relatively uncommon tumours in the cat. There is considerable confusion over the classification and nomenclature of these tumours. On the basis of clinical and radiographic behaviour the epulides can be considered to comprise two distinct tumour groups:

- Benign fibromatous/ossifying epulis (also termed peripheral odontogenic fibroma)
- Locally aggressive basal cell carcinoma (BCC) (also termed acanthomatous epulis and in some cases, incorrectly, adamantinoma).

Peripheral odontogenic fibroma (POF)

Epidemiology/aetiology

Fibromatous/ossifying epulis (POF) is the most common oral tumour in the dog, where it typically affects middle aged to older dogs of any breed. Brachycephalic dogs such as boxers may be prone to

developing multiple epuli (Fig. 7.14). These tumours are rare in the cat. The aetiology is not known.

Presentation

This tumour presents as a firm–hard mass usually with a smooth, non-ulcerated surface. It is firmly attached to the gingiva and periosteum of the dental arcade and grows outward, often from a relatively narrow base.

Pathology

Tumours show varying degrees of mineralisation, leading to the arbitrary distinction between the fibromatous and ossifying forms. The term peripheral odontogenic fibroma has been proposed to encompass both types on the basis that although

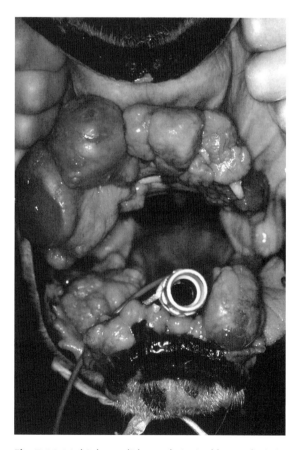

Fig. 7.14 Multiple epulides and gingival hyperplasia in a boxer dog. (Courtesy of Dr R.A.S. White, Department of Clinical Veterinary Medicine, University of Cambridge.)

they contain elements of odontogenic epithelium, they appear to be of mesenchymal origin (Bostock & White 1987).

Behaviour/treatment/prognosis

Clinically these tumours are benign, never invade into the adjacent bone and never metastasise. The treatment of choice is local surgical excision. Resection of alveolar bone at the base of the mass may be necessary to effect a complete removal but the prognosis is excellent.

Basal cell carcinoma (BCC)

Epidemiology/aetiology

Whilst less common than the fibromatous/ossifying epulis the BCC still represents a sizeable propor-

tion of all canine oral tumours. Tumours occur principally in middle-aged dogs (mean age 6.9 ± 2.4 years in one series (White & Gorman 1989)), although they are occasionally reported in younger animals. Medium to large breeds tend to be affected; there might be a male predilection. The aetiology is not known.

Presentation

The gross appearance of this tumour is variable. It may present as an irregular, fungating epithelial mass (Fig. 7.15) or may be more invasive with an ulcerated appearance and occasionally contains areas of necrosis. Radiographically there is usually lysis of adjacent alveolar bone, and displacement or loss of teeth is common (Fig. 7.16). Occasionally the soft tissue of the tumour becomes mineralised.

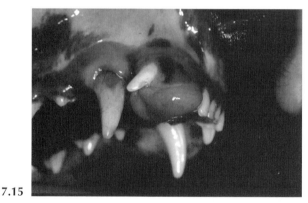

7.15

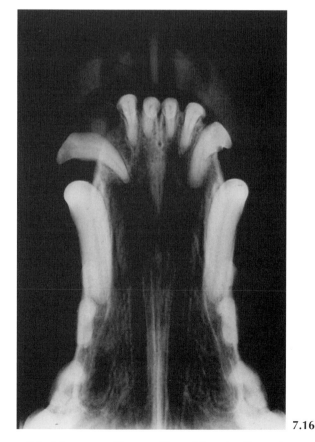

7.16

Figs 7.15 and 7.16 Basal cell carcinoma (acanthomatous epulis) of the premaxilla gross (Fig. 7.15) and radiograph (Fig. 7.16). These tumours invariably invade into the underlying bone causing lysis and dental displacement.

Pathology

The term basal cell carcinoma has been applied to this tumour on the basis that the lesion is predominantly composed of clumps of basal epithelium attached to and apparently originating from the stratum germanitivum of the overlying gum. The consistent infiltration into bone is characteristic of the behaviour of a carcinoma.

Tumour behaviour/treatment/prognosis

BCC is a locally aggressive tumour and invariably invades the adjacent alveolar bone. Although BCC does not metastasise, it does present a clinical problem by virtue of the invasive pattern of growth. Simple local excision with minimal tumour margins is rarely sufficient to prevent local recurrence. The treatment of choice is wide local excision including a margin of at least 1 cm of alveolar bone beyond the gross or radiographic limit of the tumour. This surgical approach has been shown to be effective in achieving a local cure (White & Gorman 1989). BCC are radio-sensitive and high cure rates can also be achieved by radiotherapy. However, surgery is the preferred treatment because there is a risk of the subsequent development of malignant tumours at the site of irradiated BCC (White *et al.* 1986).

Ameloblastoma

Epidemiology/aetiology

Ameloblastoma is a rare dental tumour which arises from odontogenic epithelium. Typically it occurs in young animals. In dogs the mandible is the usual site whereas a fibromatous form of ameloblastoma appears to be more frequent in the maxilla of young cats, especially the region of the upper canine.

Presentation

At either site the expansive growth of the tumour results in gross swelling and distortion of the bone. The tumour is composed of well-defined, large cystic cavities and thus has a characteristic multiloculate radiographic appearance (Figs 7.17, 7.18 and 7.19).

Tumour behaviour/treatment/prognosis

These tumours follow a benign course and can be cured by complete surgical resection. There is some evidence that curretage of the bony cavities is sufficient to achieve local control.

Squamous cell carcinoma (SCC)

Epidemiology

Squamous cell carcinoma (SCC) is the most common malignant oral tumour in the dog and cat. In the dog it accounts for approximately 20–30% of malignant oral tumours and tends to occur in older animals (average 8–10 years) of medium to larger breeds. There is no sex predilection. In the cat, SCC accounts for 70% of malignant oral tumours; it also occurs in older animals (average age 10 years) with no sex predilection.

For descriptive and prognostic purposes oropharyngeal SCC may be divided into:

- Gingival
- Labial
- Tonsillar
- Lingual (see tongue later in this chapter).

Gingival SCC – presentation

Gingival SCC may arise at any site in the upper and lower dental arcades. The tumour usually begins at the gingival margin and its invasive growth leads to destruction of the peridontal tissues and loosening of the teeth. The gross appearance is of an irregular, proliferative or ulcerative epithelial lesion (Fig. 7.20). The tumour is often friable and haemorrhagic and secondary bacterial infection is common. Invasion and lysis of adjacent bone occurs in over 70% of cases (Fig. 7.21).

Gingival SCC – tumour behaviour/treatment/prognosis

Gingival SCC has a low rate of metastasis, hence the major therapeutic priority is control of the primary tumour. In the dog, surgery is the treatment of choice for early stage lesions particularly those affecting rostral areas of the mouth. Wide local excision by maxillectomy or mandibulectomy

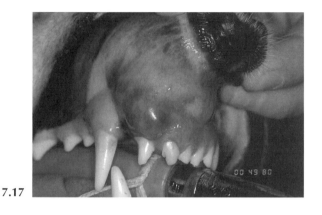

7.17

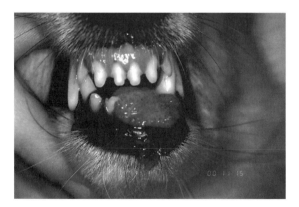

7.19

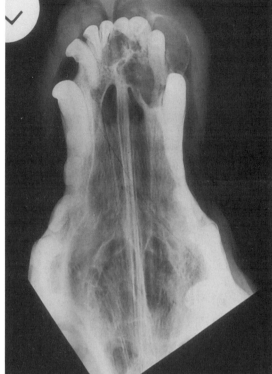

7.18

Figs 7.17, 7.18 and 7.19 Gross and radiographic appearance of ameloblastoma in the premaxilla of a dog (Figs 7.17 and 7.18) and in the rostral mandible of a young cat (Fig. 7.19).

Fig. 7.20 Gingival SCC, rostral mandible in a dog.

as appropriate is frequently curative, and one year survival rates are in the order of 84% (White 1991). Tumours sited more caudally in the mouth and particularly those involving the caudal maxilla, tend to be more invasive and carry a worse prognosis. SCC is radiosensitive and radiotherapy may provide palliation of more advanced tumours or those involving sites where surgery is not feasible.

Gingival SCC is a much more aggressive neoplasm in the cat and there is often severe, deep invasion of bone at the time of presentation (Fig. 7.22, and Chapter 6, Fig. 6.5). The extent of the tumour often precludes surgery and even those tumours deemed operable carry a poor prognosis. The outcome following radiotherapy is poor. As a result of the extensive invasion of bone by the tumour, radiation often results in large necrotic cavities within the bone, which fail to heal. One year survival rates rarely exceed 10%.

On occasion SCC arises in the epithelium of the mucosal surface of the lip or cheek. Tumours at this site are often more ulcerative than proliferative in nature and may initially be mistaken for oral ulceration. SCC of the lip is not generally as aggressive

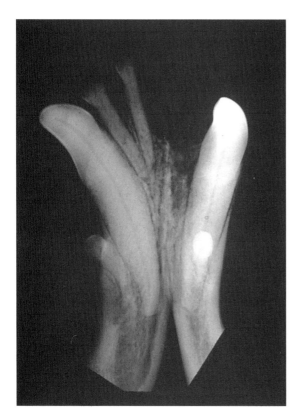

Fig. 7.21 Intraoral radiograph of case in Fig. 7.20.

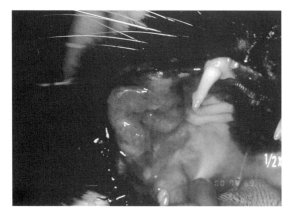

Fig. 7.22 Oral SCC in a cat, an extensive tumour of the maxilla invading into the soft tissue of the cheek.

as the lingual form but the lesion is often acutely painful to the animal. Wide local surgical resection is the treatment of choice; radiotherapy may also be appropriate in some cases.

Fibrosarcoma

Epidemiology

Fibrosarcoma is the third most common malignant tumour of the canine oral cavity, representing 10–20% of malignant tumours at this site. It tends to occur in younger dogs; the mean age of onset is 7.5 years but up to 25% occur in animals under five years of age. There is a 2:1 male:female ratio and in our experience the retriever breeds appear to suffer a particularly high incidence. Although fibrosarcoma is a common tumour in the cat, its incidence in the oral cavity is low (less than 20% of tumours at this site), sites of predeliction being the soft tissues of the head, trunk and limbs.

Presentation

In the dog, oral fibrosarcoma most commonly involves the upper dental arcade often extending dorsally and laterally into the paranasal region and medially onto the palate (Figs 7.23 and 7.24). Fibrosarcoma usually presents as a firm, smooth mass with a broad base and in its early stages may be difficult to distinguish on gross inspection from gingival hyperplasia or POF. Radiographic evidence of bone involvement is common in more advanced tumours but in general fibrosarcoma tends to cause less lysis than SCC or BCC and is more often associated with a proliferative periosteal reaction.

Tumour behaviour/treatment/prognosis

The histological appearance of fibrosarcoma of the oral cavity does not always correlate well with the biological behaviour of the tumour. Some tumours may appear histologically low grade and yet show a very aggressive and infiltrating behaviour. Local and distant metastasis occurs in around 25% of cases but the prognosis is always guarded due to the extensive infiltration of adjacent tissues. No single form of treatment has been found to be entirely effective in treatment of oral fibrosarcoma. Wide local surgical excision by mandibulectomy and maxillectomy may control early stage, low grade tumours but even such aggressive surgery does not achieve the compartment type of resection which is necessary to erradicate most oral fibrosarcomas.

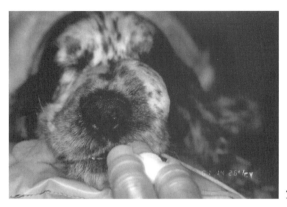

7.24

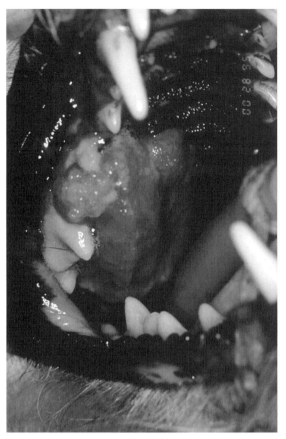

7.23

Figs 7.23 and 7.24 Canine maxillary fibrosarcomas – the lesion in Fig. 7.23 is invading across the hard palate whilst that shown in Fig. 7.24 has infiltrated the paranasal tissues.

One year survival rates with surgery alone are about 50% (White 1991). Fibrosarcoma is not particularly sensitive to radiation and radiotherapy alone does not appear to offer any significant improvement in local tumour control over surgery. However, the combination of surgery with radiation has been shown to improve the initial tumour response and extend patient survival, although local recurrence can still occur.

Undifferentiated sarcomas

Epidemiology

A number of less well differentiated sarcomas including haemangiosarcoma, spindle cell sarcomas and anaplastic sarcomas may also arise in the oral cavity of the dog. As a group these tumours respresent 10–20% of canine malignant oral tumours.

Presentation

In gross appearance they may resemble fibrosarcoma but in many cases they are more aggressive tumours and present as a rapidly growing mass which may be friable or haemorrhagic and contain areas of necrosis.

Behaviour/treatment/prognosis

As with fibrosarcoma these tumours are characterised by an infiltrative pattern of growth and are often locally advanced by the time of diagnosis.

A higher proportion of these tumours metasta-sise, usually via the haematogenous route to the lungs and other internal organs. The principles of management are essentially as for fibrosarcoma although the prognosis is often worse due to the rapid growth rate and higher risk of distant metas-tases. Small early stage tumours may be surgically resected and, although most soft tissue sarcomas are not very radioresponsive, cytoreductive sur-gery combined with radiation therapy can be ben-eficial in the management of the more advanced tumours.

Rarely, undifferentiated malignant tumours arise in young dogs under two years of age of large breeds. These highly malignant tumours are usually sited in the maxilla, involving the palate, upper molar teeth and often the orbit (Fig. 7.25). Most animals present with widespread metastases. No effective treatment has been described.

Melanoma

Epidemiology

Malignant melanomas represent about 30–40% of malignant tumours of the oral cavity in the dog. Oral melanoma is rare in the cat. In the dog oral melanomas characteristically develop in older animals; the average age is 9–12 years. There appears to be a sex predilection with male dogs affected four times more frequently than bitches. Certain breeds of dog, particularly those with pig-mented oral mucosa, e.g. poodle and pug, may be predisposed to this tumour.

Presentation

Common sites in order of prevalence are the gums (especially in the region of the molar teeth), the labial mucosa and the hard palate. The tumour usually presents as a rapidly growing friable and haemorrhagic soft tissue mass. The degree of pig-mentation varies considerably, some tumours being heavily pigmented whilst others contain little to no pigment (Figs 7.26 and 7.27). Secondary bacterial infection and necrosis may be present. Invasion of the bone is less common in oral melanoma than with SCC and fibrosarcoma.

Tumour behaviour/treatment/prognosis

Canine oral melanomas are among the most malignant neoplasms encountered in companion

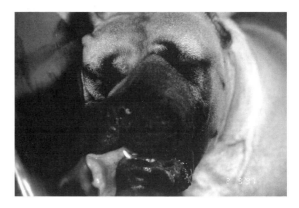

Fig. 7.25 An extensive anaplastic tumour of the maxilla and nasal cavity in a young bullmastiff.

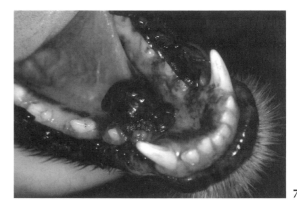

7.26   7.27

Figs 7.26 and 7.27 Gross appearance of canine oral melanomas. Figure 7.26 shows a partly pigmented lesion of the maxilla. Figure 7.27, a heavily pigmented and well circumscribed lesion in the floor of the mouth.

animals. Local control can be achieved by wide surgical resection where the site of the tumour is appropriate or by radiotherapy. The human cutaneous melanoma is generally regarded as being radioresistant but our experience in the treatment of canine oral melanoma suggests these tumours do respond to hypofractionated radiotherapy, with local response rates approaching 70% (Blackwood & Dobson 1996). Irrespective of local tumour control, the major problem presented by melanoma is the high incidence of both regional (nodal) and distant metastasis. In the absence of an effective method for the prevention or treatment of disseminated melanoma the prognosis for these tumours is poor and survival rates are in the order of three to six months.

SITE SPECIFIC TUMOURS OF THE OROPHARYNX

Tongue

Tumours of the tongue are not common in either the cat or the dog but squamous cell carcinoma is the most common histological type of tumour at this site in both species. Other tumour types reported to affect the tongue in the dog include:

- Granular cell myoblastoma (see below)
- Rhabdomyosarcoma
- Mast cell tumour
- Fibrosarcoma
- Lymphoma
- Malignant melanoma.

Presentation

Lingual tumours are often painful and interfere with the function of the tongue. Affected animals may present with:

- Difficulties in prehension, mastication and drinking
- Excessive salivation (often purulent or blood-tinged)
- Halitosis
- Lack of grooming in cats.

Some tumours may present as an obvious mass on the surface of the tongue but lingual squamous cell carcinoma often arises on the ventral surface of the tongue in the area of the frenulum (especially in cats) and may not be readily detected on brief visual inspection of the mouth.

Tumour behaviour/treatment/prognosis

SCC of the tongue is a particularly aggressive neoplasm which is characterised by rapid extension and invasion into the tongue such that the tumour often involves the full thickness of the tongue by the time of presentation (Fig. 7.28). Lymphatic invasion and metastasis are common. Surgery is the treatment of choice for tumours of the tongue. Dogs will tolerate partial glossectomy involving up to 50% of the tongue quite well but in the case of lingual SCC the extensive infiltration of the tongue at the time of presentation often precludes surgical resection. Although at other sites SCC is usually radiosensitive, the tongue is very sensitive to radiation toxicity and because normal tissue tolerance at this site is so poor, radiotherapy has not been a successful treatment for lingual tumours in cats and dogs. There have been some reports of chemotherapeutic treatment of lingual SCC in dogs and cats with drugs such as cisplatin (not cats), mitoxantrone and doxorubicin (Carpenter et al. 1993) but chemotherapy has not become established as an effective treatment for such tumours. Overall the prognosis for lingual SCC in both dogs and cats is poor. In dogs where complete surgical resection is possible, one year survival rates may exceed 50% but such

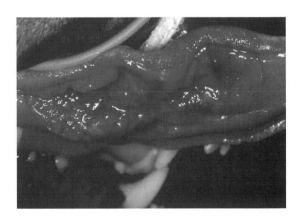

Fig. 7.28 Squamous cell carcinoma of the tongue – dog.

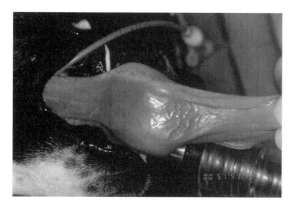

Fig. 7.29 Rhabdomyoma of tongue – dog.

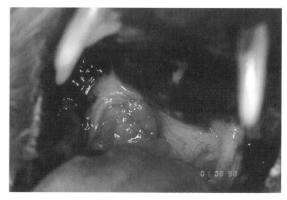

Fig. 7.30 SCC tonsil – dog.

cases are not common and one year survival rates are usually less than 25%.

Granular cell myoblastoma

Although rare, granular cell myoblastoma is reported to be the second most common tumour of the tongue in dogs. The origin of this tumour is unclear, although it has been suggested that it may arise from Schwann cells in the tongue. Morphologically, it is difficult to distinguish from other eosinophilic granular cell tumours such as rhabdomyoma, rhabdomysarcoma and oncocytoma. Ultrastructural and immunocytochemical studies are required to differentiate these entities (Liggett *et al.* 1985; Lascelles *et al.* 1998). Clinically these tumours present as a soft tissue mass within the tongue (Fig. 7.29). Although the lesions often appear large and invasive, their behaviour is usually benign. Local surgical removal is usually possible leading to a favourable prognosis with local control rates in excess of 80%.

Tonsil

Squamous cell carcinoma is the most common tumour to affect the tonsil in dogs and cats. Other tumours which may arise in the tonsil include:

- Lymphoma (usually as part of multicentric lymphoma – Chapter 15)
- Metastatic tumours from the oral cavity, especially malignant melanoma.

Tonsillar SCC is less common than the gingival form in the dog and cat but there is considerable regional variation in the reported incidence and it appears that this form of the disease may have been more common in the past (particularly in animals living in cities). Aetiologic associations with environmental pollutants have been implied (see earlier). In the dog the average age of onset of the disease is 9–10 years and males are affected three times more often than bitches. SCC of the tonsil is rare in the cat.

Presentation

Tonsillar SCC usually presents as a unilateral lesion although bilateral involvement has been reported. In early cases the tonsil is of relatively normal size but has a number of small papillomatous growths on its surface. Infiltration and destruction of the tonsil develops rapidly and the tumour progresses to involve the pharyngeal wall and soft palate (Fig. 7.30). This lesion is often acutely painful and affected animals present with signs of:

- Dysphagia
- Difficulty swallowing
- Gagging
- Hypersalivation
- Weight loss
- Temporal muscle atrophy.

Occasionally the first manifestation of the disease is an enlarged retropharyngeal lymph node which on histological/cytological examination reveals metastatic squamous cell carcinoma. In such cases the primary tonsillar mass may be small and asymptomatic.

Tumour behaviour/treatment/prognosis

SCC of the tonsil is a locally aggressive tumour with a high rate of metastasis to the retropharyngeal and cervical lymph nodes. Haematological dissemination may also occur. By virtue of its rapid local progression and high rate of metastasis, the prognosis for tonsillar SCC is poor. The results of therapy by surgical resection or radiotherapy or by combinations are usually disappointing and median survival times are in the region of two months; less than 10% of affected animals are alive at one year. There is no effective chemotherapeutic treatment for this condition.

Nasopharyngeal polyps

Nasopharyngeal polyps are not true neoplasms but inflammatory lesions originating from the middle ear or eustachian tube in young (usually <2 year old) cats. No breed or sex predilection is known. Polyps may grow into the external ear canal where they can be seen as a pink, fleshy mass but most grow via a pedicle into the pharynx where they may cause signs of:

- Stridor/stertor/difficulty breathing
- Change in voice
- Sneezing
- Swallowing problems
- Rhinitis
- Horner's syndrome (associated with otitis media).

Nasopharyngeal polyps may be seen as soft tissue masses on radiographs of the pharynx or visualised by retraction of the soft palate. Most nasopharyngeal polys can be removed by traction. If an underlying cause can be identified (e.g. middle ear disease) then this should be treated appropriately to prevent recurrence.

OSTEOSARCOMA OF THE SKULL

Osteosarcoma of the axial skeleton, particularly the skull, is less common than that of the long bones in dogs. There are two distinct variants of osteosarcoma which affect the bones of the canine skull:

- Multilobular osteoma/chondroma/ osteochondrosarcoma/chondroma rodens
- Mandibular osteosarcoma.

Multilobular osteochondrosarcoma

Multilobular oesteochondrosarcoma is an uncommon tumour which primarily occurs in older, medium to large breed dogs. It is a relatively slowly growing tumour which usually affects the bones of the calvarium. Animals present with an enlarging mass which is hard and fixed in nature. This is an osteoproductive tumour and gives rise to a characteristic radiographic appearance of dense bony mass of nodular or stippled density (Fig. 7.31). The tumour is locally invasive and may cause lysis of underlying bone. Surgical resection is the only effective treatment but complete surgical removal of the tumour may be difficult or impossible. These tumours were once considered to be benign as most animals were animals euthanased because of the primary mass without any evidence of metastases. However, with the advent of more aggressive surgical approaches to the management of these tumours, leading to prolonged survival, it has become apparent that metastasis will occur in 50% or more cases (Dernell et al. 1998).

Mandibular osteosarcoma

Osteosarcoma may arise in the ramus of the mandible; indeed it is one of the five most common tumours of the mandible in the dog. Osteosarcoma at this site is noteworthy as it is often possible to achieve primary tumour control by hemimandibulectomy (Fig. 7.32). By virtue of the fact that the tumour is contained within the deep periosteal fascia, such surgery actually achieves compartmental resection. Rapid metastasis is not a feature of tumours at this site and a one year survival rate of 71% was reported following mandibulectomy in one study (Straw et al. 1996).

Craniomandibular osteopathy (CMO) is an important differential diagnosis for a bony swelling of the mandible but in contrast to osteosarcoma:

- CMO usually occurs in juveniles, less than one year of age
- CMO usually affects both mandibles, although lesions are not necessarily bilaterally symmetrical

- CMO is strongly breed associated and occurs particularly in West Highland white and cairn terriers, although it can arise in other breeds, e.g. dobermann.

EARS

For anatomical, descriptive purposes, the ear is divided into three areas:

- The external ear, comprising the pinna and ear canal
- The middle ear, sited in the tympanic bulla of the temporal bone
- The inner ear, comprising the cochlea and semicircular canal system.

Primary tumours may arise at any of these sites in cats and dogs but the pinna and external ear are more common than the middle ear or inner ear, both of which are rare. The ear is an unusual site for secondary, metastatic tumour development but the external ear may be involved in widespread or diffuse cutaneous tumours such as cutaneous lymphoma. A variety of cutaneous tumours may arise on the pinna, as listed in Table 7.8; these tumours are discussed in Chapter 4. Most of the following discussion will concern tumours of the ear canal.

Epidemiology

Tumours of the ear canal are not common in either species, representing 1–2% of all feline tumours

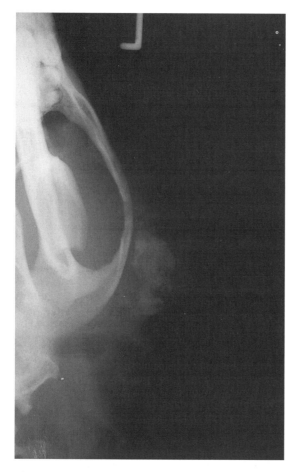

Fig. 7.31 Radiograph of skull showing typical radiographic appearance of a multilobular osteosarcoma of the caudal zygoma.

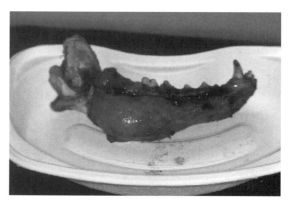

Fig. 7.32 Resected mandibular osteosarcoma.

Table 7.8 Tumours which commonly arise on the pinna.

Cats	Squamous cell carcinoma
	Basal cell tumour
	Mast cell tumour
	Cutaneous lymphoma
Dogs	Histiocytoma
	Plasmacytoma
	Mast cell tumour
	Basal cell tumour
	Cutaneous lymphoma

and 2–6% of all canine tumours. They tend to occur in older animals, mean age 7–11 years in cats and 9–10 years in dogs. (Inflammatory polyps may affect the ear canal in young cats – see above.) No sex predilection has been reported in either species, but in the dog the cocker spaniel appears to be at increased risk of developing tumours of the ear canal.

Aetiology

Chronic, long-standing inflammation may be a factor in the development of both benign and malignant ceruminous gland tumours (London *et al*. 1996; Moisan & Watson 1996) and this might explain the increased incidence of such tumours in the cocker spaniel, where otitis externa is a common problem.

Pathology

The epithelium of the ear canal is rich in sebaceous glands and ceruminous glands (modified apocrine glands). It is these glands that give rise to the most common tumours at this site. Benign ear canal tumours include ceruminous gland adenomas, inflammatory polyps, basal cell tumours and papillomas. In the cat, ceruminous gland cysts are tumour-like masses of the ear canal which often contain blue–black viscous fluid. Their heavily pigmented gross appearance may lead to confusion with melanoma and basal cell tumour.

Excluding inflammatory polyps, approximately 85% of all feline and 60% of all canine ear canal tumours are malignant (London *et al*. 1996). Ceruminous gland adenocarcinoma is the most common malignant tumour of the ear canal in both species; also reported at this site are squamous cell carcinoma and carcinoma of unknown origin.

Any cutaneous tumour may, on occasion, arise in the ear canal.

Tumour behaviour/paraneoplastic syndromes

Benign tumours of the ear canal may give rise to a number of clinical problems as discussed below but these tumours are not locally invasive and they do not metastasise. Ceruminous gland carcinomas and other carcinomas of the ear canal are locally invasive tumours and not only do they cause surface ulceration within the ear canal, but will invade into the deeper cartilagenous and bony structures associated with the ear. Up to 25% of malignant tumours show radiographic evidence of invasion of the tympanic bulla. The incidence of metastasis is not well documented but these tumours are capable of invasion of local lymphatics and metastasis to the regional (retropharyngeal) lymph nodes and, in a small percentage of cases, pulmonary metastases will be detected at the time of presentation. The behaviour of ceruminous gland and other carcinomas of the ear canal tends to be more aggressive in the cat than in the dog.

No paraneoplastic syndromes are commonly associated with tumours of the ear canal; the presenting signs tend to be associated with local, invasive growth of the primary mass.

Presentation/signs

Ear canal tumours may arise anywhere in the vertical or horizontal portion of the ear canal. On occasion there may be an obvious mass visible at the external auditory meatus but in most cases the presenting signs of an ear tumour will be similar to those of a chronic ear infection:

- Aural discharge
- Aural odour
- Aural irritation or discomfort
- Aural pain.

Otoscopic examination of the ear canal may be necessary to locate and visualise the tumour. Benign tumours tend to appear as a non-ulcerated, raised, sometimes pedunculated mass. Malignant tumours are more likely to be ulcerated and haemorrhagic.

Where the tumour is invasive and/or located in the middle or inner ear the animal may present with neurological signs:

- Vestibular signs: circling, head tilt, nystagmus
- Horner's syndrome.

These are reported in 10% of dogs with malignant tumours and in 25% of cats either as a result of benign polyps or as a result of invasive malignant tumours.

Investigations

Bloods

Routine haematological/biochemical analyses are not generally very helpful in the diagnosis of tumours of the ear.

Imaging techniques

Radiography of the skull is indicated in the investigation of tumours affecting the ear canal as up to 25% of malignant tumours at this site show radiographic evidence of bulla involvement. Inflammatory polyps and evidence of middle ear disease may be appreciated on skull radiography.

Radiography is also indicated for evaluation of retropharyngeal lymph nodes and thoracic metastasis.

Biopsy/FNA

In most cases the diagnosis will depend on a grab or incisional biopsy of the aural mass. Fine needle aspirate/cytology is of limited value in the diagnosis of most ear tumours but is useful for evaluation of local lymph node enlargement for metastasis.

Staging

A staging system for tumours of the ear canal has not been devised.

Treatment

Surgery

Surgery is the treatment of choice for most primary tumours of the ear canal in dogs and cats. The surgical approach depends on the nature, the site and the extent of the tumour. Options include:

- Excisional biopsy – only really indicated for inflammatory polyps
- Lateral ear canal resection – benign tumours affecting the vertical ear canal
- Total ear canal ablation and lateral bulla osteotomy – malignant tumours.

Whilst conservative surgery may be a tempting option for carcinomas involving the vertical ear canal, it has been shown that total ear canal ablation plus bulla osteotomy provide better surgical margins and hence a better prognosis (see below) (London *et al.* 1996). Possible complications of more aggressive surgery include damage to the facial nerve and the sympathetic trunk.

Radiotherapy

Radiotherapy is a possible alternative or adjunct to surgery although there are few reports documenting the efficacy of radiotherapy in either situation. The proximity of the tumour to the brain stem may complicate treatment planning and delivery.

Chemotherapy

Chemotherapy is indicated in the treatment of cutaneous forms of lymphoma with involvement of the pinna or ear canal, but little/no information exists on the efficacy of chemotherapy in the management of ceruminous gland or other carcinomas of the ear canal.

Prognosis

The prognosis for benign tumours of the ear following conservative surgical treatment is good. Occasionally inflammatory polyps may recur, especially if the underlying cause cannot be treated effectively.

In the case of malignant tumours of the ear canal, several factors have been shown to be of prognostic importance:

In cats:
- Histological type – ceruminous gland carcinomas carry a more favourable prognosis than squamous cell carcinoma or carcinoma of undetermined origin.

In both cats and dogs, negative prognostic factors include:
- Histological evidence of lymphatic or vascular invasion
- Presence of neurological signs
- Involvement of the tympanic bulla

Table 7.9 Surgical management of malignant tumours of the ear canal in dogs and cats.

Conservative Lateral ear canal resection	*Aggressive* Total ear canal ablation with lateral bulla osteotomy
Cats (ceruminous gland adenocarcinoma*) Median disease free survival = 10 months 1 year survival rate = 33% Recurrence rate = 66%	Median disease free survival = 42 months 1 year survival rate = 75% Recurrence rate = 25%
Dogs (ceruminous gland adenocarcinoma**) N = 4 Median follow up = 4 months (range 3–9 months) Recurrence rate = 75%	N = 11 Median survival = 36 months (range 8–72 months) No local recurrence

* Marino *et al.* 1994.
** Marino *et al.* 1993.

- Conservative treatment – surgical approach strongly influences the prognosis; those animals treated conservatively show considerably reduced survival times (Table 7.9).

SALIVARY GLANDS

Epidemiology

Tumours of the salivary glands are not common in the dog and are rare in the cat. In both species they are reported to occur in older animals; the mean age of affected animals is about 10 years in dogs and 12 years in cats. No breed or sex predilections have been reported.

Aetiology

The aetiology of tumours of salivary glands is undetermined.

Pathology

Tumours may arise in any of the major salivary glands or in the minor glands sited in the oral mucosa, gingiva and palate. Benign tumours of salivary glands are rare. Most tumours are malignant arising either from glandular tissue or from ductal epithelium, thus various types of salivary gland carcinoma/adenocarcinoma may be described (Table 7.10).

Tumour behaviour/paraneoplastic syndromes

Salivary carcinomas are usually locally invasive although the rate of growth and incidence of metastasis can vary considerably. Some tumours may grow slowly and be slow to metastasise but adenocarcinomas often display rapid growth and feature central tumour necrosis. The pattern of growth is invasive and such tumours frequently extend through the capsule of the gland to infiltrate adjacent tissues. Infiltration of local lymphatics may lead to local oedema. Metastasis is more common in the cat than in the dog and is to local and regional lymph nodes. Distant and widespread metastsis can occur.

No paraneoplastic syndromes are commonly associated with tumours of the salivary glands.

Presentation/signs

Most animals present with a firm, painless swelling of the affected salivary gland:

- Parotid – base of the ear
- Mandibular – upper neck (Fig. 7.33)

Table 7.10 Tumours of the salivary glands.

Histological type	Comment
Mixed tumour (pleomorphic adenoma)	Composed of a mixture of epithelium, myoepithelium, chondroid material and bone Rare tumour in cats and dogs, may be locally invasive and difficult to excise
Monomorphic adenoma	Predominantly glandular tumour with little stroma and no myxoid or chondroid areas Usually well encapsulated. Rare
Mucoepidermoid tumour	Composed of mucous filled spaces lined by secretory epithelium and strands of squamous epithelium Rare
Acinic cell tumour	Tumour of glandular epithelium which may be arranged in acini or solid sheets. Reported in both major and minor salivary glands in the dog. May show invasive growth but slow to metastasise
Adenocarcinoma	Malignant tumour of glandular tissue forming tubules or solid cords of epithelial cells Most common salivary gland tumour in the cat and moderately common in the dog
Undifferentiated carcinoma	Spindle shaped to round epithelial cells arranged in irregular masses. Rare tumour but metastasis reported
Non-neoplastic conditions (differential diagnoses)	Ductal hyperplasia Sialosis: bilateral enlargement of salivary glands due to hypertrophy of serous acinar cells Sialocoele (salivary mucocoele) Salivary gland infarction

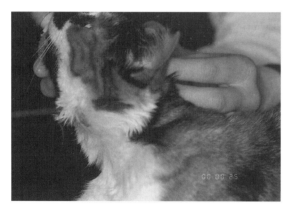

Fig. 7.33 Salivary carcinoma – firm, immobile mass in the mandibular salivary gland of a cat.

- Sublingual – upper neck/floor of the mouth
- Zygomatic – lip and maxilla; may also be associated with ocular signs including exophthalmos.

Excessive salivation and dysphagia may occasionally result from obstruction of the oropharynx.

Tumours of minor salivary glands may arise in the oral mucosa of the lip, palate and tongue; these tumours have a greater tendency to be ulcerated (Fig. 7.34).

Investigations

Bloods

Routine haematological/biochemical analyses are not generally very helpful in the diagnosis of tumours of salivary glands.

Imaging techniques

Radiography of the skull may be indicated in the investigation of tumours which are fixed, invasive and adjacent to bone, especially those affecting the orbit. Ultrasound of the orbit may also be indicated in cases with ocular involvement.

Radiography is indicated for evaluation of

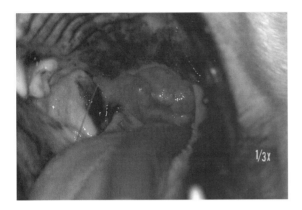

Fig. 7.34 Salivary carcinoma – forming an ulcerated lesion on the soft palate in a dog.

retropharyngeal lymph nodes and thoracic metastasis.

Biopsy/FNA

Fine needle aspirates may be helpful in the initial investigation to distinguish a salivary gland tumour from other salivary lesions (Table 7.9). Lymphoma would also be a differential diagnosis for a mass in the submandibular/parotid region.

In most cases the definitive diagnosis will depend on a needle or an incisional wedge biopsy of the mass.

Staging

A specific staging system for tumours of salivary glands has not been devised.

Treatment and prognosis

Surgical removal is the theoretical treatment of choice for tumours of salivary glands but in practice many tumours are too extensive at the time of presentation to permit an aggressive surgical resection in an area of the body containing many vital structures. Post-operative radiotherapy may prolong survival following incomplete tumour removal, but there is little information available on the success of radiotherapy alone or on the value of chemotherapy in the management of such tumours.

References

Adams, W.M., Withrow, S.J., Walshaw, R. *et al.* (1987) Radiotherapy of malignant nasal tumours in 67 dogs. *Journal of the American Veterinary Medical Association*, (191), 311–15.

Blackwood, L. & Dobson, J.M. (1996) Radiotherapy of oral malignant melanomas in dogs. *Journal of the American Veterinary Medical Association*, (209), 98–102.

Bostock, D.E. (1986) Neoplasms of the skin and subcutaneous tissues in dogs and cats. *British Veterinary Journal*, (142), 1–19.

Bostock, D.E. & White, R.A.S. (1987) Classification and behaviour after surgery of canine 'epulides'. *Journal of Comparative Pathology*, (97), 197–206.

Burk, R.L., (1992) Computed tomographic imaging of nasal disease in 100 dogs. *Veterinary Radiology & Ultrasound*, (33), 177–80.

Carlisle, C.H. & Gould, S. (1982) Response of squamous cell carcinoma of the nose of the cat to treatment with x-rays. *Veterinary Radiology*, (23), 186–92.

Carpenter, L.G., Withrow, S.J., Powers, B.E. *et al.* (1993) Squamous cell carcinoma of the tongue in 10 dogs. *Journal of the American Animal Hospital Association*, (29), 17–24.

Cox, N.R., Brawner, W.R. Jr, Powers, R.D. *et al.* (1991) Tumours of the nose and paranasal sinuses in cats: 32 cases with comparison to a national data base (1977–1987). *Journal of the American Animal Hospital Association*, (27), 339–47.

Dernell, W.S., Straw, R.C., Cooper, M.F., Powers, B.E., LaRue, S.M. & Withrow, S.J. (1998) Multilobularosetochondrosarcoma in 39 dogs: 1979–1993. *Journal of the American Animal Hospital Association*, (34), 11–18.

Head, K.W. (1990) Tumors of the alimentary tract. In: *Tumours of Domestic Animals*, 3rd edn, (ed. Jack E. Moulton), p.347. University of California Press.

LaDue, T.A., Dodge, R., Page, R.L., Price, G.S., Hauck, M.L. & Thrall, D.E. (1999) Factors influencing survival after radiotherapy of nasal tumours in 130 dogs. *Veterinary Radiology & Ultrasound*, (40), 312–17.

Lana, S.E., Oglivie, G.K., Withrow, S.J., Straw, R.C. & Rogers, K.S. (1997) Feline cutaneous squamous cell carcinoma of the nasal planum and the pinnae: 61 cases. *Journal of the American Animal Hospital Association*, (33), 329–32.

Lascelles, B.D.X., McInnes, E., Dobson, J.M. & White, R.A.S. (1998) Rhabdomyosarcoma of the tongue in a dog. *Journal of Small Animal Practice*, (39), 587–91.

Liggett, A.D., Weiss, R. & Thomas, K.L. (1985) Canine laryngopharyngeal rhabdomyoma resembling an oncocytoma: light microscopic, ultrastructural and comparative studies. *Veterinary Pathology*, (8), 256–9.

London, C.A., Dubilzeig, R.R. & Vail, D.M. *et al.* (1996) Evaluation of dogs and cats with tumours of the ear canal: 145 cases. *Journal of the American Veterinary Medical Association*, (208), 1413–18.

MacEwen, E.G., Withrow, S.J. & Patnaik, A.K. (1977) Nasal tumours in the dog: retrospective evaluation of diagnosis, prognosis and treatment. *Journal of the American Veterinary Medical Association*, (170), 45–8.

Madewell, B.R., Priester, W.A., Gillette, E.L. & Snyder, S.P. (1976) Neoplasms of the nasal passages and paranasal sinuses in domestic animals as reported by 13 veterinary colleges. *American Journal of Veterinary Research*, (37), 851–6.

Marino, D.J., MacDonald, J.M., Matthiesen, D.T. *et al.* (1993) Results of surgery and long term follow up in dogs with ceruminous gland adenocarcinoma. *Journal of the American Animal Hospital Association*, (29), 560–63.

Marino, D.J., MacDonald, J.M., Matthiesen, D.T. & Patnaik, A.K. (1994) Results of surgery in cats with ceruminous gland adenocarcinoma. *Journal of the American Animal Hospital Association*, (30), 54–8.

Moisan, P.G. & Watson, G.L. (1996) Ceruminous gland tumours in dogs and cats: a review of 124 cases. *Journal of the American Animal Hospital Association*, (32), 448–52.

Morris, J.S., Blackwood, L., Dobson, J.M. & Villiers, E.J. (1996a) Association between nasal and renal lymphoma in cats. *Clinical Research Abstracts*, British Small Animal Veterinary Association Congress, p.241.

Morris, J.S., Dunn, K.J., Dobson, J.M. & White, R.A.S. (1996b) Radiological assessment of severity of canine nasal tumours and relationship with survival. *Journal of Small Animal Practice*, (37), 1–6.

Owen, L.N. (1980) *TNM Classification of Tumours in Domestic Animals*. World Health Organization, Genera.

Peaston, A.E., Leach, M.W. & Higgins, R.J. (1993) Photodynamic therapy for nasal and aural squamous cell carcinoma in cats. *Journal of the American Veterinary Medicial Association*, (202), 1261–5.

Straw, R.C., Powers, B.E., Klausner, J. *et al.* (1996) Canine mandibular osteosarcoma: 51 cases (1980–1992). *Journal of the American Animal Hospital Association*, (32), 257–62.

Theon, A.P., Madewell, B.R., Harb, M.F. & Dungworth, D.L. (1993) Megavoltage irradiation of neoplasms of the nasal and paranasal cavities in 77 dogs. *Journal of the American Veterinary Medical Association*, (202), 1469–75.

Theon, A.P., Peaston, A.E., Madewell, B.R. & Dungworth, D.L. (1994) Irradiation of non-lymphoproliferative neoplasms of the nasal cavity and paranasal sinuses in 16 cats. *Journal of the American Veterinary Medical Association*, (204), 78–83.

Thrall, D.E. & Adams, W.M. (1982) Radiotherapy of squamous cell carcinomas of the canine nasal plane. *Veterinary Radiology*, (23), 193–5.

Thrall, D.E., Robertson, I.D., McLeod, D.A., Heidner, G.L., Hoopes, J. & Page, R.L. (1989) A comparison of radiographic and computed tomographic findings in 31 dogs with malignant nasal cavity tumors. *Veterinary Radiology*, (30), 59–66.

White, R.A.S., Gorman, N.T., Watkins, S.B. & Brearely, M.J. (1985) The surgical management of bone involved oral tumours in the dog. *Journal of Small Animal Practice*, (26), 693–708.

White, R.A.S., Jefferies, A.R. & Gorman, N.T. (1986) Sarcoma development following irradiation of acanthomatous epulis in two dogs. *Veterinary Record*, (118), 668.

White, R.A.S. & Gorman, N.T. (1989) Wide local excision of acanthomatous epulides in the dog. *Veterinary Surgery*, (18), 12–14.

White, R.A.S. (1991) Mandibulectomy and maxillectomy in the dog: long term survival in 100 cases. *Journal of Small Animal Practice*, (32), 69–74.

Withrow, S.J. (1996) Tumours of the respiratory system. In: *Small Animal Clinical Oncology*, 2nd edn, (S.J. Withrow & E.G. MacEwen) pp.268–86. JB Lippincott Company, Philadelphia.

Withrow, S.J. & Holmberg, D.L. (1983) Mandibulectomy in the treatment of oral cancer. *Journal of the American Animal Hospital Association*, (19), 273–86.

Withrow, S.J. & Straw, R.C. (1990) Resection of the nasal planum in nine cats and five dogs. *Journal of the American Animal Hosptial Association*, (26), 219–22.

8
Gastro-intestinal Tract

Gastro-intestinal tract tumours of the dog occur most often in the stomach but even at this site they are still uncommon. In the cat, they affect the intestines more frequently, with lym-phoma predominating. Primary tumours of the liver, spleen and pancreas are also rare, although the liver is a common site for metastatic tumours.

OESOPHAGUS

Epidemiology

Oesophageal cancer is extremely rare in dogs and cats (0.5% of all cancer) except in areas where the parasite *Spirocerca lupi* is endemic and causes secondary sarcomas (Ridgeway & Suter 1979). Most animals are old and no sex or breed predisposition is reported.

Aetiology

In Africa and south-eastern USA oesophageal fibrosarcomas and osteosarcomas are caused by the parasitic worm *Spirocerca lupi*, probably by secreting a carcinogen (Chapter 1). No aetiology is known for carcinomas which usually predominate in other regions, although ingestion of carcinogens may play a role.

Pathology

Malignant tumours such as squamous cell carcinoma, leiomyosarcoma, fibrosarcoma and osteosarcoma occur most commonly (Table 8.1). Squamous cell carcinoma often occurs in the middle third of the oesophagus, anterior to the heart as an annular thickening. Benign tumours are rarely reported but are usually located in the caudal oesophagus and cardia. Primary tumours may arise from tissues adjacent to the oesophagus and invade it by direct extension.

Tumour behaviour

Malignant tumours are usually aggressive and locally invasive with lymphatic metastasis to draining lymph nodes or haematogenous spread.

Table 8.1 Tumours of the oesophagus.

Benign	Malignant
Leiomyoma	Squamous cell carcinoma
	Leiomyosarcoma
	Fibrosarcoma
	Osteosarcoma
	Plasmacytoma

Tumours spread within the oesophagus longitudinally and circumferentially and may result in complete obstruction.

Paraneoplastic syndromes

Hypertrophic osteopathy (Chapter 2, Table 2.7) has been reported with oesophageal tumours, particularly with sarcomas caused by *Spirocerca lupi*.

Presentation/signs

Animals may present with vague signs such as weight loss or anorexia, but usually pain or difficulty in swallowing, dysphagia or regurgitation is also noted. Secondary aspiration pneumonia may occur with persistent regurgitation resulting in respiratory signs.

Investigations

A presumptive diagnosis of an oesophageal tumour is usually made on history and clinical signs but some further investigations may be necessary.

Bloods

No specific haematological or biochemical changes are associated with oesophageal tumours.

Imaging techniques

Plain radiography of the neck and thoracic cavity may reveal a mass, gas retention or oesophageal dilation cranial to a stricture but contrast studies (barium swallow) may be needed to confirm the diagnosis by demonstrating irregularities of the oesophageal mucosa, filling defects

Table 8.2 Clinical stages (TNM) of the oesophagus. Owen (1980).

T   *Primary tumour*
(add 'm' to the appropriate T category for multiple tumours)
T0   No evidence of tumour
T1   Tumour confined to the oesophagus
T2   Tumour invading neighbouring structures

N   *Regional lymph nodes (RLN)*
N0   No evidence of RLN involvement
N1   RLN involved

M   *Distant metastasis*
M0   No evidence of metastasis
M1   Distant metastasis detected

or a stricture with or without megaoesophagus. Fluoroscopy may also be useful to assess swallowing or regurgitation.

Biopsy/FNA

Endoscopy should allow visualisation and biopsy of the lesion.

Staging

The TNM system is applicable to oesophageal tumours but no stage grouping is recommended (Table 8.2). Clinical and surgical examination is required for primary tumour, regional lymph nodes and metastatic sites although endoscopy of the primary tumour may be sufficient. Regional lymph nodes are the cervical and prescapular (cervical oesophagus) or mediastinal (thoracic oesophagus) nodes. Radiography of the thorax is required to screen for pulmonary metastases.

Treatment

Surgery

Although surgical resection of oesophageal tumours is the treatment of choice, complete excision of the tumour and anastomosis of the oesophagus are difficult to achieve unless the mass is very small and non-invasive. The majority of tumours remain untreatable because of their size and the difficulties of reconstruction if adequate surgical margins are to be obtained. The oesophagus is prone to wound healing complications due to a segmental blood supply, lack of omentum and absence of serosa. Full thickness resections have the added complication of tension on the surgical repair and those greater than 2 cm may require sophisticated reconstruction techniques (Fingeroth 1993).

Radiotherapy

Radiotherapy is not used for oesophageal tumours in small animals because of the potentially harmful side-effects to surrounding structures and the risk of oesophageal stricture.

Chemotherapy

Chemotherapy has not been shown to be effective in the treatment of oesophageal tumours. Although drugs such as doxorubicin have a potential role

for the post-operative treatment of sarcomas, trials have not been established to demonstrate a response.

Other

For oesophageal tumours causing strictures, palliation of signs such as regurgitation may be achieved by serial bouginage of the oesophagus. Alternatively, a gastrostomy tube could be used as a short-term measure to feed an animal which was otherwise not in pain.

Prognosis

The prognosis for most oesophageal tumours is poor because they are usually advanced at the time of diagnosis and the treatment options are therefore limited.

STOMACH

Epidemiology

Tumours of the stomach are more common than those of the oesophagus, but are still relatively uncommon. Male dogs are more frequently affected than females and benign tumours such as leiomyomas tend to occur in much older animals (mean age 15 years) than do carcinomas (mean age 8 years) (Patnaik et al. 1977). Cats affected with gastric carcinoma are generally over 10 years old.

Aetiology

Long term ingestion of dietary carcinogens may play a role in the aetiology of gastric cancers. The bacterium Helicobacter pylori is associated with gastric carcinoma and lymphoma in humans but although it causes gastritis and ulceration in dogs and cats, its relationship to gastric tumours is uncertain (Marks 1997). In the Belgian shepherd dog, a genetic predisposition to gastric carcinoma has been suggested (Scanzianzi et al. 1991). Although lymphoma occurs commonly in the stomach of the cat, few cases appear FeLV positive.

Pathology

Gastric tumours often involve the cardia, lesser curvature or pyloric antrum of the stomach. In the dog, two thirds of gastric tumours are adenocarcinomas although a variety of tumour types and benign polyps also occur (Table 8.3). In the cat, the predominant tumour type is lymphoma (usually FeLV negative) with adenocarcinoma occurring less frequently and mast cell tumour more rarely.

Adenocarcinoma usually occurs in the pyloric antrum extending into the body of the stomach. Grossly it often appears as an ulcerated, plaque-like thickening, a diffuse non-ulcerated thickening or less commonly as a raised sessile polyp (Fig. 8.1). The plaque-like ulcers can be up to 5 cm in diame-

Table 8.3 Tumours of the stomach.

Benign	Malignant
Polyps	Adenocarcinoma
Leiomyoma	Squamous cell carcinoma
	Lymphoma
	Leiomyosarcoma
	Fibrosarcoma
	Plasmacytoma

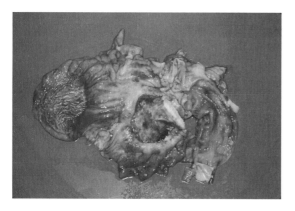

Fig. 8.1 Gastric carcinoma, gross specimen showing ulcerated tumour at pylorus. (Courtesy of Mr A. Jefferies, Department of Clinical Veterinary Medicine, University of Cambridge.)

ter with a depressed base and overhanging margins. Mucosal rugae around the crater are thickened and lost and a very fibrous or scirrhous appearance is common.

Leiomyosarcoma arises in the inner smooth muscle layer producing an extensive, plaque-like bulge into the lumen, usually without surface ulceration. Leiomyoma has a similar appearance and is frequently multiple.

Lymphoma produces diffuse non-ulcerated thickening similar to adenocarcinoma but not scirrhous in nature and with less ulceration and crater formation. Multiple plaques may be noted on the gastric lumen, and tumour may be present in the intestines and abdominal organs as well as the stomach.

Tumour behaviour

Gastric adenocarcinoma is usually locally aggressive and may lead to perforation of the stomach wall and peritonitis if ulceration is deep. Obstruction to pyloric outflow may occur in some cases. Tumour plugs often develop in surrounding blood vessels causing ischaemic necrosis, and local metastasis to gastroduodenal and splenic lymph nodes may occur. Distant metastasis to abdominal organs is common, often by the time of diagnosis, although the lungs are rarely involved. In contrast to gastric carcinoma, leiomyosarcoma rarely metastasises. Lymphoma may be restricted to the stomach, may involve other abdominal organs and lymph nodes, or may be multicentric. Plasmacy-

toma of the stomach often metastasises to local lymph nodes, unlike cutaneous plasmacytoma which is benign.

Paraneoplastic syndromes

Gastric lymphoma may be accompanied by paraneoplastic syndromes, particularly hypercalcaemia (Chapter 2).

Presentation/signs

Although mild or vague signs may occur early in the disease, animals with gastric neoplasia often present with persistent vomiting or haematemesis, with partially digested blood producing a 'coffee grounds' appearance. Anorexia and weight loss are common and overt melaena or occult faecal blood may be present. Some animals show anterior abdominal pain.

Investigations

Bloods

Regenerative anaemia may be detected on haematological analysis due to gastric haemorrhage but dehydration and haemoconcentration due to vomiting may mask the anaemia. Electrolyte imbalances may be obvious on biochemical assessment because of vomiting, and renal parameters such as BUN and creatinine may be elevated due to dehydration.

Imaging techniques

Plain radiography of the abdomen rarely reveals gastric neoplasia and so positive contrast with barium or fluoroscopic examination is usually required (Fig. 8.2). Changes may include:

- Gastric thickening or ulceration
- Filling defects
- Loss of rugal folds
- Delayed gastric emptying
- Reduced or abnormal gastric motility in particular areas.

Ultrasonography can be used to diagnose gastric neoplasia, detect enlarged lymph nodes and assess other abdominal organs for metastasis. A thickened

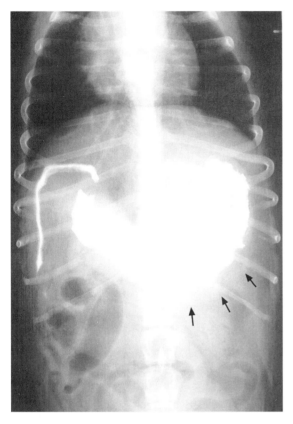

Fig. 8.2 Radiograph of abdomen following oral administration of barium. Gross thickening along the greater curvature of the stomach is evident (see arrows). The histological diagnosis was gastric carcinoma. (Courtesy of Radiology Department, Department of Clinical Veterinary Medicine, University of Cambridge.)

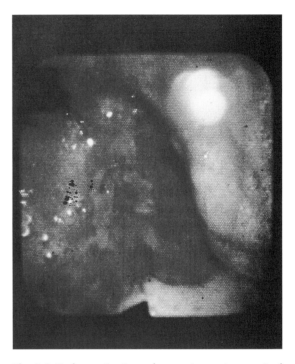

Fig. 8.3 Endoscopic view of a gastric carcinoma sited near the pylorus in a rough collie. (See also Colour plate 26, facing p. 162.) (Courtesy of Mr M. Herrtage, Department of Clinical Veterinary Medicine, University of Cambridge.)

gastric wall with disruption of the wall layers is characteristic of neoplasia and ulceration may be recognised as a focal outpouching of the luminal surface that contains trapped gas bubbles. Endoscopy will usually allow visualisation of any gastric lesion and enable a grab biopsy to be taken (Fig. 8.3).

Biopsy/FNA

A definitive diagnosis can be achieved by histological analysis of a representative biopsy. Endoscopic biopsy is least invasive but can produce false-negative results. Gastrotomy should produce a more representative biopsy of the lesion which may have to be combined with surgical treatment.

Staging

TNM staging is applicable to gastric tumours but no stage grouping is recommended at present (Table 8.4). Surgical exploration of the abdominal cavity is required to examine primary tumour, regional (gastrosplenic) nodes and other possible metastatic sites, although endoscopy may be sufficient for the primary tumour. Radiography of the thorax is necessary to screen for distant metastasis.

Treatment

Surgery

Surgical resection is the treatment of choice for tumours which have not metastasised but wide local excision is often hard to achieve while allowing satisfactory reconstruction of the stomach and adequate post-operative function. Tumours on the lesser curvature are generally considered unresectable, whereas those on the fundus or

Table 8.4 Clinical stages (TNM) of tumours of the stomach. Owen (1980).

T *Primary tumour*
(add 'm' to the appropriate T category for multiple
  tumours)
T0   No evidence of tumour
T1   Tumour not invading serosa
T2   Tumour invading serosa
T3   Tumour invading neighbouring structures

N *Regional lymph nodes (RLN)*
N0   No evidence of RLN involvement
N1   RLN involved
N2   Distant LN involved

M *Distant metastasis*
M0   No evidence of distant metastasis
M1   Distant metastasis detected

body can be resected successfully. Post-operative complications are much higher with pyloric resections.

Pylorectomy and gastroduodenostomy or gastro-jejunostomy have been described for wide local excision of antral tumours but these procedures are technically difficult and there is a significant risk of iatrogenic injury to the pancreas, extrahepatic biliary system and local blood supply.

Radiotherapy

Radiotherapy is not usually used for gastric tumours in animals.

Chemotherapy

Lymphoma is the only gastric tumour that may respond to systemic chemotherapy. If restricted to the stomach and easily resectable, surgery may remain the treatment of choice since chemotherapy carries a potential risk of gastric perforation if tumour cells are present across the full thickness of the stomach wall and they are lysed by drug treatment. For non-resectable or widespread disease, chemotherapy remains an option (see Chapter 15 for protocols).

Adenocarcinomas and other tumours do not usually respond well to chemotherapy and so it is not recommended.

Other

Medical management of clinical signs such as vomiting may improve quality of life in non-resectable tumours. Anti-emetics, e.g. metoclopramide, and H_2 antagonists, e.g. cimetidine and ranitidine, may be tried although any response will be of short-term benefit only.

Prognosis

Highly variable survival times are reported for gastric neoplasms. Even with surgical resection the prognosis for most malignant gastric tumours is poor with survival times of six months or less because of recurrent or metastatic disease. Survival rates for gastric lymphoma are also low because it does not usually respond well to chemotherapy. In contrast, benign gastric tumours have a good prognosis and are often cured by surgical resection.

INTESTINES

Epidemiology

The intestines are not a common site for neoplasia in either the cat or the dog. Tumours tend to occur in older animals (cats often older than dogs) although colorectal polyps may occur in middle-aged dogs. More male than female cats may be affected and the Siamese may have an increased risk of adenocarcinoma.

Aetiology

The cause of intestinal tumours is not known although it is possible that diet may play a role. A history of chronic colitis or dietary sensitivity may predispose to polyps. Cases of lymphoma in the cat are usually not FeLV positive.

Pathology

In the dog, most tumours occur in the large intestine, particularly the distal third of the colon and the rectum. Adenocarcinoma/carcinoma is the most common malignant tumour, and leiomyosarcoma is the most common sarcoma (Figs 8.4 and 8.5). Other tumour types, inflammatory and benign lymphoid lesions, and non-neoplastic adenomatous polyps may also be found, particularly in the rectum (Table 8.5). In the cat, most tumours arise in the small intestine, with the ileocaecocolic junction, jejunum and ileum being most commonly affected.

Lymphoma (Fig. 8.6) predominates here followed by mast cell tumour and adenocarcinoma. In the feline large intestine, adenocarcinoma may be more common than lymphoma.

Adenomas are usually plaque-like sessile masses or pedunculated polyps with broad or narrow stalks. Most rectal adenomatous polyps occur within 2 cm of the anus and are usually solitary (Fig. 8.7).

Intestinal carcinomas also usually occur as single, discrete lesions and may be either intramural, intraluminal or annular in nature (Fig. 8.4). The latter are usually scirrhous and may stenose the lumen, causing partial or total obstruction of the gut, or leave it unaffected. Smooth muscle atrophy may occur with non-scirrhous tumours, causing ballooning and perforation of the intestine. Intramural or intraluminal carcinomas may be nodular or plaque-like. Nodular tumours mimic polyps and tend to grow into the lumen, occasionally occluding it.

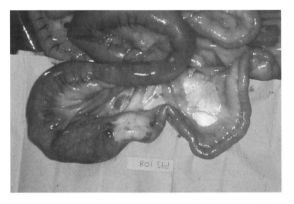

Fig. 8.4 Post mortem picture of adenocarcinoma of the intestine in a dog. (Courtesy of Dr P. Nicholls.)

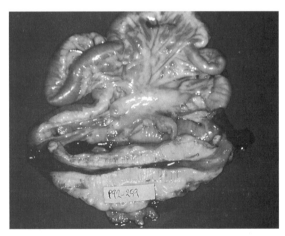

Fig. 8.6 Post mortem picture of intestinal lymphosarcoma in a cat. (Courtesy of Dr P. Nicholls.)

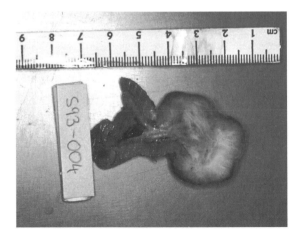

Fig. 8.5 Post mortem picture of leiomyoma of the intestine in a dog. (Courtesy of Dr P. Nicholls.)

Table 8.5 Tumours of the intestines.

Benign	Malignant
Polyps	Adenocarcinoma/carcinoma
Adenoma	Lymphoma
Leiomyoma	Leiomyosarcoma
	Mast cell tumour
	Carcinoid tumour
	Plasmacytoma

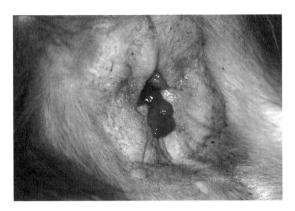

Fig. 8.7 Rectal polyp.

Carcinoid tumours are derived from the enterochromaffin cells of the intestinal mucosa and are only rarely reported in the ileum, jejunum and rectum of dogs and cats. They are often expansile and infiltrative.

Intestinal lymphoma may be diffuse or local. Local infiltrates may be single or multiple and may appear plaque-like, fusiform or nodular. Intramural tumours are most common although intraluminal forms do occur. Lymphocytes invade the intestinal wall and produce muscle atrophy and ballooning of a segment which may then rupture if it becomes thin enough. Mesenteric lymph nodes, liver and spleen are often involved.

In the cat mast cell tumours can occur as primary tumours in the gut and metastasise widely elsewhere. This type of visceral mast cell disease is distinct from systemic mastocytosis which primarily affects spleen (Chapter 4.)

Tumour behaviour

Most malignant intestinal tumours are locally invasive and have metastasised by the time of diagnosis to draining lymph nodes and liver. Tumours may cause partial or total intestinal obstruction or lead to gut perforation and peritonitis. Abdominal effusion may result from widespread carcinomatosis. Benign adenomatous polyps have been demonstrated to progress to carcinoma *in situ* and then invasive carcinoma if left alone. Plasmacytomas of the intestine often metastasise to local lymph nodes, unlike those of the skin which are benign.

Paraneoplastic syndromes

In general, paraneoplastic syndromes are rarely associated with gastro-intestinal tumours. Those that are reported include:

- Hyperhistaminaemia with mast cell tumours – produces gastric irritation and vomiting (Chapter 2)
- Hypercalcaemia with intestinal lymphoma
- Hypoglycaemia with jejunal leiomyoma.

Intestinal carcinoids in man may release serotonin or other amines which produce signs of chronic diarrhoea and weight loss but this has not been documented in animals.

Presentation/signs

Most animals with small intestinal neoplasia present with vague signs such as anorexia, weight loss, vomiting, diarrhoea or melaena. Those with large intestinal neoplasia usually present with constipation, tenesmus or haematochezia. The onset is usually insidious although an acute crisis caused by gut perforation and peritonitis may sometimes occur. An abdominal mass may be palpable, especially in cats. Alimentary lymphoma in the dog may present with a malabsorption type syndrome.

Investigations

The history and clinical signs are very important for making a diagnosis of intestinal neoplasia and often help locate the disease to the small or large intestine. Lesions close to the anus may be detected by rectal examination.

Bloods

A regenerative anaemia may be detected on routine haematological analysis due to intestinal haemorrhage. Electrolyte disturbances detected on biochemical screening may suggest intestinal obstruction, and low serum proteins may result from infiltrating tumours, especially in the dog.

Imaging techniques

Plain abdominal radiography may detect an abdominal mass, dystrophic calcification, or 'gravel signs' suggestive of an obstruction, but it may not reveal any abnormalities. A barium series or enema is usually necessary to see thickening of the intestinal wall, luminal narrowing, ulceration or mucosal irregularities, outlining of a polypoid mass, or to detect an abnormal transit time.

Ultrasonography can be helpful in localising an abdominal mass to the intestines and in assessing local lymph nodes and abdominal organs for metastasis. The different layers of intestine can be assessed, making it useful in diagnosis too.

Endoscopy may be useful to diagnose intestinal neoplasia, particularly for tumours in the proximal small intestine. Proctoscopy is more helpful for visualising colorectal lesions.

Biopsy/FNA

A suitable biopsy may be obtained by endoscopy or proctoscopy, although in some cases a histological diagnosis may have to wait for an incisional or excisional biopsy at celiotomy.

Staging

The TNM system is applicable to intestinal tumours although no group staging is recommended at present (Table 8.6). Clinical examination, surgical exploration of the abdomen and thoracic radiography are needed for complete assessment of the three categories. Regional lymph nodes are the mesenteric, caecal, colic and rectal nodes.

Treatment

Surgery

Wide local excision is the treatment of choice for intestinal tumours which show no evidence of metastasis. At celiotomy, the liver, spleen and kidneys should be carefully examined first for evidence of metastasis and then the entire gastrointestinal tract for evidence of diffuse disease or multiple tumours. Finally regional lymph nodes should be examined and aspirated to check for

Table 8.6 Clinical stages (TNM) of tumours of the intestines. Owen (1980).

T *Primary tumour*
(add 'm' to the appropriate T category for multiple tumours)
T0   No evidence of tumour
T1   Tumour not invading serosa
T2   Tumour invading serosa
T3   Tumour invading neighbouring structures
N *Regional lymph nodes (RLN)*
N0   No evidence of RLN involvement
N1   RLN involved
N2   Distant LN involved
M *Distant metastasis*
M0   No evidence of distant metastasis
M1   Distant metastasis detected

metastasis prior to resection of the tumour, or removed if grossly enlarged. Any mesenteric or omental adhesions should also be removed en bloc.

In the small intestine, enterectomy and anastomosis with surgical margins of at least 5 cm is usually possible without compromising intestinal function. Proximal duodenal tumours, however, may be difficult to resect without damage to the pancreatic blood supply or duodenal papilla.

Large intestinal tumours may be resected with a subtotal colectomy and this is the recommended procedure for unidentified colonic masses or colonic adenocarcinoma in cats. Dogs tend to tolerate colonic resection less well than cats and it should be considered a major procedure. Tumours at the colorectal junction or in the rectum are more difficult to resect owing to reduced mobility of the rectum and therefore increased tension on the anastomosis (Fig. 8.8). Rectal resections have a high rate of post-operative complications due to the lack of omentum and poor surgical access. Major resections can be accomplished via an osteotomy of the pubis ('pelvic split') or a rectal pull-through procedure has been described which combines celiotomy with a per-rectal approach. These are fraught with difficulties at the reconstruction stage and the poor healing and high bacterial load in the large bowel significantly increase the risk of dehiscence.

Colorectal polyps should be excised with a wide

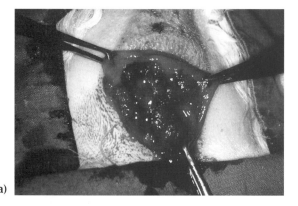

(a)

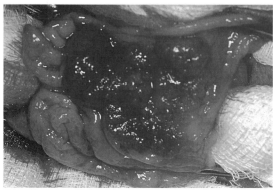

(b)

Fig. 8.8 Carcinoma of the rectum (a) exposed at surgery (b) resected. (Courtesy of Dr R.A.S. White, Department of Clinical Veterinary Medicine, University of Cambridge.)

surgical margin because of the potential for malignant transformation. They are accessed by a rectal pull-out approach and can be excised using a partial thickness dissection, not perforating the serosa. Wide full thickness resections of rectal tumours that are not annular can also be achieved using this approach. Post-operatively these patients should receive stool softeners (isogel) for life. For extensive or inaccessible benign rectal tumours, transanal endoscopic resection and cautery has also been proposed (Holt & Durdley 1999).

Post-operatively, all intestinal tumour resections should be closely monitored for 48–72 hours as the risk of dehiscence is high, particularly if diffuse tumour tissue is present at the anastomosis site. Hypoproteinaemic patients with a serum albumin of less than 20g/l are also at increased risk of dehiscence.

Radiotherapy

Radiotherapy is not generally used for intestinal or rectal tumours in animals because of the problems associated with accurate delivery of the dose and side-effects on the normal sections of gut which are extremely radiosensitive and easily damaged.

Chemotherapy

Intestinal lymphoma is the only tumour suitable for chemotherapy but this is not without complications as perforation of the intestinal wall may occur, with a dramatic response of tumour cells to the cytotoxic agents. Focal lesions may therefore be more safely treated by surgical resection, with careful monitoring for the development of disease at new sites or a short (six month) course of post-operative chemotherapy. In one study (Slawienski *et al.* 1997), cats treated with combination chemotherapy after resection of colonic lymphoma did not survive longer than those without chemotherapy. However, cats receiving post-operative doxorubicin therapy after resection of colonic adenocarcinoma did survive significantly longer than those which only had surgery.

Other

Medical management with stool softeners (isogel) may provide some palliation for inoperable cases.

Prognosis

Benign tumours of the small intestine carry an excellent prognosis if surgically resected. Adenocarcinoma of the small intestine also carries a good prognosis if adequately excised and there are no gross signs of metastatic disease. Cats with resected small intestinal adenocarcinoma have been reported to survive for over a year (Kosovsky *et al.* 1988).

The prognosis for colorectal polyps is also good although recurrence is possible with large or sessile lesions and with carcinoma *in situ*. Malignant tumours of the large intestine, however, carry a worse prognosis because of the difficulties with surgical access, making local recurrence and distant metastasis more likely after resection. Subtotal colectomy may be necessary in some cases to achieve prolonged survival times. Colorectal adenocarcinoma which presents as an annular stricture often has a shorter survival time than nodular or pedunculated masses (Church *et al.* 1987).

Diffuse canine lymphoma does not respond well to chemotherapy but solitary or nodular disease has a better response. Mean survival times for cats with alimentary lymphoma treated with combination chemotherapy are approximately six months.

PERIANAL TUMOURS

Three types of tumour occur commonly around the anus of the dog and since their behaviour is quite different it is important to distinguish them:

• Perianal/circumanal gland (hepatoid) tumour
• Apocrine gland tumour of anal sac
• Apocrine gland tumour around anus.

Cats may occasionally develop apocrine gland tumours but they have no sebaceous glands analogous to the perianal/hepatoid glands of the dog. The apocrine tumours of the anal sacs and around the anus are discussed here as part of the gastrointestinal tract, but hepatoid gland tumours of the dog are discussed along with other skin tumours in Chapter 4.

Epidemiology

Apocrine gland tumours of the anal sac tend to occur in old female dogs whereas the other apocrine gland tumours, which are much less common, have no breed or sex predisposition.

Aetiology

There is no obvious cause for the apocrine gland tumours of either type.

Pathology

Apocrine tumours of the anal sac

These tumours are derived from apocrine sweat glands around the anal sac and are therefore modified sweat gland tumours, usually adenocarcinomas. They can be quite small grossly and easily missed unless a rectal examination is performed. Bilateral tumours occur infrequently.

Apocrine tumours around the anus

These are derived from apocrine sweat glands in the skin and are usually solitary adenomas.

Tumour behaviour

Apocrine adenocarcinomas of the anal sac are malignant despite their small size and may metastasise to the regional lymph nodes, abdominal organs or lungs. Apocrine gland tumours around the anus are usually benign.

Paraneoplastic syndromes

Only the apocrine gland adenocarcinomas of the anal sac are associated with a paraneoplastic syndrome. Hypercalcaemia is frequently present and is often noted clinically before the tumour is detected (Chapter 2).

Presentation/signs

Apocrine adenomas around the anus present as solitary, discrete, skin masses which may become ulcerated or secondarily infected if licked. Apocrine adenocarcinomas of the anal sac usually present with signs of hypercalcaemia such as polyuria, polydipsia, muscle tremors, weakness and lethargy. A large, subcutaneous, infiltrating or discrete mass may be noted ventro-lateral to the anus (Fig. 8.9) but often only a small mass, invisible externally but palpable per rectum, is present. Occasionally, animals may present with constipation or caudal abdominal pain if the primary tumour is not obvious, but the sublumbar lymph nodes are sufficiently enlarged to obstruct the rectum.

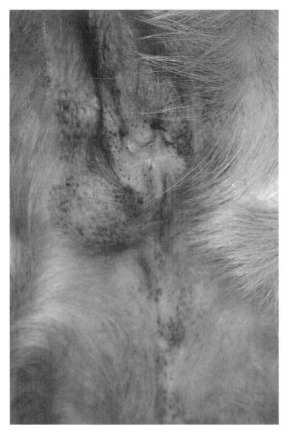

Fig. 8.9 Apocrine adenocarcinoma of the anal sac, in this case a relatively discrete mass associated with the left anal sac.

Investigations

Palpation

Gross inspection and physical palpation of the mass including a rectal examination should indicate whether it is discrete, superficial and likely to be benign or whether it is extensive, infiltrative and likely to be an adenocarcinoma. Abdominal or rectal palpation may reveal enlarged sublumbar lymph nodes.

Bloods

Blood samples are extremely important for apocrine tumours of the anal sac which present with hypercalcaemia. Routine biochemical analysis will show the severity of the hypercalcaemia and may show secondary azotemia. The degree of dehydration can be assessed using PCV and total protein. Haematological assessment is necessary to rule out other causes of hypercalcaemia such as lymphoma and leukaemia.

Imaging techniques

Abdominal and thoracic radiographs are essential for suspected adenocarcinomas to search for metastatic disease in the regional lymph nodes, abdominal organs or lungs. Ultrasonography may be helpful to look for metastases in sublumbar lymph nodes and abdominal organs and to guide fine needle aspirates or biopsies.

Biopsy/FNA

A fine needle aspirate for cytological examination may give an indication of whether the tumour is benign or malignant and whether metastasis to the sublumbar lymph nodes has occurred. A definitive diagnosis, however, can only be made on histological examination of a biopsy sample. A punch or grab biopsy is best for superficial apocrine tumours, whereas a tru-cut technique may be needed for anal gland adenocarcinoma.

Staging

Both tumour types are staged using the TNM system as for skin tumours (Chapter 4). There is no group staging at present.

Treatment

Surgery

Surgical excision is the treatment of choice for both types of tumour. Care should be taken, however, since extensive resection of peri-anal tumours can result in faecal incontinence if more than 40–50% of the external anal sphincter is removed. Anal sac adenocarcinomas are often difficult to excise completely, unless they present as very small nodules, and local recurrence is a frequent problem. The rapid rate at which they metastasise often means that excision of the primary tumour is not appropriate unless it is causing local problems such as dyschezia.

Radiotherapy

Inadequately excised adenocarcinomas, both around the anus and of the anal sac, may benefit from a course of post-operative radiotherapy but care must be taken to avoid damaging the anal sphincter and causing excessive radiation side-effects in the distal rectum. Local recurrence is often delayed but not always prevented by post-operative radiotherapy. Irradiation of the sublumbar nodes is technically difficult and so radiotherapy of cases with nodal spread is not usually attempted.

Chemotherapy

Since most adenocarcinomas respond poorly to cytotoxic drugs, chemotherapy is not usually recommended for their treatment. Some protocols have been tried but their efficacy is unproven.

Other

Hypercalcaemia associated with anal sac adenocarcinomas may require special treatment. The severity of the hypercalcaemia is often less than that associated with lymphoma and saline diuresis may not be necessary prior to surgical excision of the tumour. If excision is complete, the hypercalcaemia should resolve. However, the hypercalcaemia often persists after treatment of the primary tumour because of its inadequate resection or because of metastatic disease. Since the response of residual tumour to chemotherapy is often poor, symptomatic treatment of the hypercalcaemia with drugs such as bisphonates may be tried although it is often unrewarding. (Chapter 2).

Prognosis

The prognosis for perianal apocrine adenomas is excellent if surgically excised, although their malignant counterpart carries a worse prognosis because of problems with local recurrence and possible metastasis. Apocrine adenocarcinomas of the anal sac have the worst prognosis since complete local excision may be difficult to achieve; they have often metastasised by the time of diagnosis and persistent hypercalcaemia may remain a long term problem.

LIVER

Epidemiology

Although primary liver tumours are rare in small animals, the liver is a very common site for metastatic tumours because of the rich blood supply provided by the hepatic portal vein and hepatic artery (Fig. 8.10). Hepatic carcinoma is seen in older dogs (over 10 years of age) and is reported to be more common in the male than the female. Cholangiocellular carcinoma is more frequent in the cat and may be more common in females.

Aetiology

Exposure to carcinogens and toxins such as nitrosamines has been shown to induce hepatic tumours experimentally.

Pathology

Metastatic tumours are the most common tumours occurring in the liver. These must be distinguished

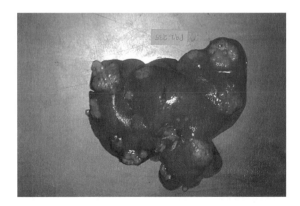

Fig. 8.10 Post mortem picture of metastases in cat liver, from a small intestinal carcinoma. (Courtesy of Dr P. Nicholls.)

from benign nodular hyperplasia which is very common in dogs.

Primary tumours may be described in three ways:

- Massive – affecting one liver lobe with smaller metastatic nodules throughout
- Nodular – discrete nodules in several lobes
- Diffuse – large areas of the liver infiltrated by non-encapsulated tumour.

The primary tumours affecting the liver are listed in Table 8.7. The most important primary tumours of the dog are hepatocellular adenoma (hepatoma), hepatocellular carcinoma, cholangiocarcinoma and hepatic carcinoids. In cats, hepatocellular carcinoma and cholangiocarcinoma are most important.

Hepatocellular adenoma/carcinoma

Hepatocellular carcinoma is the most common of the malignant primary liver tumours in the dog

and is also important in the cat. It usually occurs in the massive form (Fig. 8.11) and histologically cells may vary from well differentiated to anaplastic (Fig. 8.12). Its benign equivalent, the hepatocellular adenoma, is more common than hepatocellular carcinoma in dogs and can occur as single or multiple masses which are often spherical but not necessarily encapsulated. It may be difficult to distinguish from well-differentiated hepatocellular carcinoma in some cases.

Cholangiocellular adenoma/carcinoma

Cholangiocellular (bile duct) adenoma is rare but cholangiocellular carcinoma (Fig. 8.13) is more common, particularly in the cat. Intrahepatic forms usually occur in dogs and cats, although extrahepatic bile ducts may be affected. Carcinomas may be diffuse, nodular or massive and although usually solid, cystic forms which secrete mucous may occur (cystadenocarcinomas). Adenomas may be solitary or multiple and may also be cystic.

Gall bladder adenoma/carcinoma

These are very rare in the dog and cat. Adenomas may appear as papillary masses protruding into the gall bladder.

Other primary tumours

Neuro-endocrine carcinoid tumours are occasionally reported in the dog, and sarcomas such as haemangiosarcoma, leiomyosarcoma, fibrosarcoma

Table 8.7 Tumours of the liver.

Benign	Malignant
Hepatocellular adenoma (hepatoma)	Hepatocellular carcinoma
Bile duct/cholangiocellular adenoma	Bile duct/cholangiocellular carcinoma
Gall bladder adenoma	Gall bladder carcinoma
	Hepatic carcinoids
	Haemangiosarcoma
	Other sarcomas
	Mast cell tumour

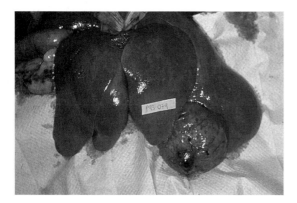

Fig. 8.11 Post mortem picture of hepatocellular carcinoma in dog. (Courtesy of Dr P. Nicholls.)

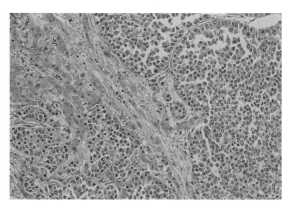

Fig. 8.12 Histological section of a hepatocellular carcinoma from a dog.

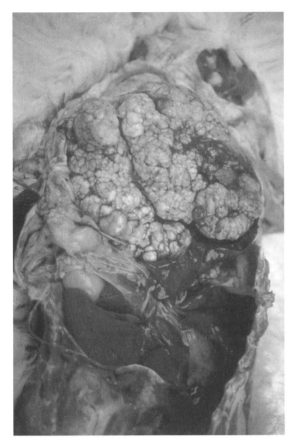

Fig. 8.13 Gross appearance of a cholangiocellular carcinoma in a dog. (Courtesy of Dr P. Nicholls.)

or osteosarcoma may occur as primary tumours. The latter should be differentiated from metastases.

Tumour behaviour

Both hepatocellular and cholangiocellular carcinomas are locally invasive and highly metastatic tumours, spreading within the liver and to local lymph nodes, lungs, abdominal organs and peritoneum. The corresponding adenomas grow expansively within the liver parenchyma.

Paraneoplastic syndromes

Hypoglycaemia is reported with some liver neoplasms and is attributed to increased use of glucose or production of hormones with insulin-like activity (Chapter 2, Table 2.5).

Presentation/signs

Liver tumours usually present with vague clinical signs such as anorexia, weight loss, vomiting, polydipsia, ascites or hepatic encephalopathy (CNS signs). Icterus is uncommon in dogs (less than 20% of cases) and is usually associated with liver disease other than neoplasia. Many hepatic tumours, particularly hepatomas, may be palpable as a mass in the anterior abdomen.

Investigations

Bloods

The most consistent finding for hepatic tumours on biochemical analysis of blood is increased activity of ALT and SAP, although AST and LDH are also frequently elevated. Serum bilirubin is increased in a minority of dogs but is more common in cats with hepatocellular carcinoma. Serum proteins may be low because of interference with their production and since clotting factors may be affected, clotting tests should be performed before major surgery. Hypoglycaemia may be detected.

Imaging techniques

Diffuse or focal hepatomegaly, rounding of liver margins or irregularity of liver outline with displacement of adjacent abdominal organs may be visible on plain radiographs of the abdomen. Occasionally localised calcification or loss of abdominal detail associated with ascites may be seen. A normal size and shape to the liver does not preclude neoplasia, however, and ultrasonography is more helpful in defining a mass or assessing a neoplastic infiltrate in the liver.

Abdominocentesis

If abdominal fluid is present, neoplastic cells may be detected on cytological examination of sediment. Most effusions are modified transudates but haemorrhage may occur with tumour rupture.

Table 8.8 Clinical stages (TNM) of tumours of the liver. Owen (1980).

T   *Primary tumour*
(add 'm' to the appropriate T category for multiple
  tumours)
T0   No evidence of tumour
T1   Tumour involving one lobe
T2   Tumour involving more than one lobe
T3   Tumour invading neighbouring structures

N   *Regional lymph nodes (RLN)*
N0   No evidence of RLN involvement
N1   RLN involved
N2   Distant LN involved

M   *Distant metastasis*
M0   No evidence of metastasis
M1   Distant metastasis detected

Biopsy/FNA

Ultrasound guided aspirates often reveal neoplastic cells and may distinguish between benign and malignant tumours although hepatoma and well differentiated carcinomas can be difficult. A definitive diagnosis is dependent on biopsy. Needle core biopsies will give more information if suffcent tissue is obtained but if a larger sample is required, a celiotomy will be necessary.

Staging

The TNM staging system can be applied to liver tumours (Table 8.8) but no group staging is recommended at present. All three categories require surgical examination (celiotomy or laparoscopy) for complete assessment, the regional lymph nodes being the hepatic and diaphragmatic nodes. Radiography of the thorax is also indicated to look for pulmonary metastases.

Treatment

Surgery

Surgical excision has the best chance of cure for hepatic adenoma, massive hepatocellular carcinoma and hepatobiliary cystadenocarcinoma. For discrete tumours affecting one or more lobe, surgical excision may be possible either by nodulectomy or lobectomy. Large portions of the liver may be removed without its loss of function since its powers of regeneration are good. Diffuse tumours and widespread nodular disease are more difficult to deal with, however.

Radiotherapy

Radiotherapy is not usually used to treat liver tumours in animals because of the potential side-effects on other abdominal organs.

Chemotherapy

No chemotherapy regimes are recommended for the treatment of primary liver tumours. Some metastatic sarcomas, e.g. haemangiosarcoma, may respond to cytotoxic drugs but treatment for such tumours is better administered before metastatic disease is detected clinically (see Chapters 3 and 5).

Prognosis

The prognosis for benign liver tumours is good if they can be adequately excised. Malignant tumours and metastatic tumours have a poor prognosis because treatment options are restricted, although mean survival times of approximately a year have been reported for massive hepatocellular carcinoma following surgery (Kosovsky *et al.* 1989).

PANCREAS (EXOCRINE)

Epidemiology

Primary tumours of the pancreas are relatively rare but the pancreas is also a site for metastatic tumours, particularly from the gastro-intestinal tract. Older female dogs (mean age 10 years) and the Airedale terrier breed may be predisposed to pancreatic carcinoma. Affected cats are also old (mean age 12 years).

Aetiology

The cause of pancreatic neoplasms is unknown in both the dog and cat.

Pathology

It is important to distinguish primary pancreatic tumours from metastatic tumours and from nodular hyperplasia which is common in older animals. Primary tumours are derived from the acinar cells or the pancreatic ducts and are therefore adenomas, adenocarcinomas, or carcinomas, the latter being much more common in both the dog and cat. Most are located in the middle portion of the pancreas and may occur as single discrete masses or multiple dispersed masses. Mineralisation and fat necrosis may be noted. Histologically, tubular structures, acini or solid sheets of cells may be seen and these need to be distinguished from carcinomas of the pancreatic islet cells (see Chapter 14).

Tumour behaviour

Pancreatic adenomas are often small, solitary tumours which have functional effects because they compress the surrounding pancreas but they do not metastasise. Carcinomas, however, are relatively aggressive (Fig. 8.14), invading the stomach or duodenum locally and metastasising most commonly to the liver, but also to the lymph nodes, other abdominal organs, peritoneal surface and lungs. Metastases to vertebrae and the femur have also been reported. Tumours may block the common bile duct and cause an obstruction to biliary flow or, in extreme cases, exocrine pancreatic insufficiency if

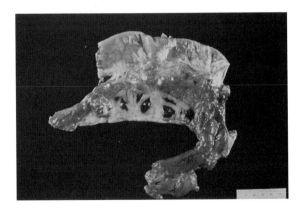

Fig. 8.14 Post mortem picture of pancreatic carcinoma in dog. (Courtesy of Dr P. Nicholls.)

pancreatic atrophy occurs. Tumour necrosis may arise if the vascular supply is inadequate and this may produce an inflammatory response that can lead to pancreatitis.

Paraneoplastic syndromes

Paraneoplastic alopecia affecting the ventrum, limbs, face or diffuse zones has been reported in cats with pancreatic adenocarcinoma (Brooks *et al.* 1994; Tasker *et al.* 1999).

Presentation/signs

Clinical signs are usually non-specific and include weight loss, anorexia, lethargy, vomiting, diarrhoea, constipation, abdominal pain or distension. Clinical signs may be related more to hepatic metastases than to pancreatic disease. Animals with biliary obstruction may present with jaundice or other signs of liver disease. Pancreatic tumours are not easily palpable in dogs, but in cats they are often larger and more easily felt in the abdomen.

Investigations

Bloods

Haematological and biochemical parameters are often within normal limits but elevated liver enzymes or bilirubinaemia may indicate cholestasis or biliary obstruction. Hyperglycaemia associated with concurrent beta cell destruction, neutrophilia, anaemia and hypokalaemia have been reported. Amylase and lipase serum activities are rarely elevated.

Imaging techniques

An ill-defined mass or a mottled appearance due to local peritonitis may be identifiable on plain abdominal films. The descending duodenum and pylorus may appear displaced but the proximal duodenum often appears fixed in a 'c-shape' on the ventrodorsal view due to spasticity and dilation. Generalised loss of abdominal detail and increased radiodensity may be noted with peritoneal metastasis and effusion.

Ultrasonography can be more helpful, especially in cases where radiographic detail in the cranial abdomen is lost. It should give an indication of tumour size and invasiveness.

Biopsy/FNA

Ultrasound guided fine needle aspiration is possible if a suspicious mass is identifiable but often the pancreatic tumour cells do not exfoliate well and a cytological diagnosis is difficult to obtain. Even cytological examination of peritoneal effusions rarely reveals tumour cells. A histological diagnosis is usually made at exploratory celiotomy, either by excising the whole tumour or if inoperable, by taking a small sample. Pancreatic biopsy can be carried out by a shave of the abnormal tissue with a scalpel blade or crush ligation of a small portion with a ligature. Normal pancreatic tissue should be left undisturbed if possible. In some cases, the diagnosis is not made until post mortem examination.

Staging

A TNM staging scheme is available for pancreatic tumours (Table 8.9) but requires surgical exploration (celiotomy or laparoscopy) to evaluate the primary tumour, regional (splenic and hepatic) nodes and metastatic disease. Radiography of the thorax is also indicated to look for pulmonary metastases.

Table 8.9 Clinical stages (TNM) of tumours of the pancreas. Owen (1980).

T	*Primary tumour*
T0	No evidence of tumour
T1	Tumour present
N	*Regional lymph nodes (RLN)*
N0	No evidence of RLN involvement
N1	RLN involved
N2	Distant LN involved
M	*Distant metastasis*
M0	No evidence of metastasis
M1	Distant metastasis detected

Treatment

Surgery

Partial pancreatectomy is the treatment of choice for small pancreatic adenomas identified at celiotomy. Adenocarcinomas, however, are often identified at a late stage when metastasis or considerable local invasion has often occurred. For those rare cases without metastasis, surgical resection can be attempted but complete excision is not easy to achieve. A sound understanding of the regional anatomy is essential in order to prevent post-operative morbidity due to obstruction of the main pancreatic duct or damage to the vascular supply of the proximal duodenum. Tumours in the body or base of the pancreas are usually considered inoperable. Total pancreatectomy is associated with high morbidity and mortality and should not be attempted.

Radiotherapy

Radiotherapy is of limited value for tumours of the pancreas and is not recommended.

Chemotherapy

Chemotherapy is of limited value for tumours of the pancreas and is not recommended.

Prognosis

The prognosis for pancreatic adenocarcinomas is poor because of their invasive nature and early metastasis. Survival times do not exceed a year.

References

Brooks, D.G., Campbell, K.L., Dennis, J.S. & Dunstan, R.W. (1994) Pancreatic paraneoplastic alopecia in three cats. *Journal of the American Animal Hospital Association*, (30), 557–63.

Church, E.M., Mahlhaff, C.J. & Patnaik, A.K (1987) Colorectal adenocarcinoma in dogs: 78 cases (1973–1984). *Journal of the American Veterinary Medical Association*, (191), 727–30.

Fingeroth, J.M. (1993) Surgical techniques for oesophageal disease. In: *Textbook of Small Animal Surgery* (ed. D. Slatter), 2nd edn, pp. 549–53. W.B. Saunders, Philadelphia.

Holt, P.E. & Durdley, P. (1999) Transanal endoscopic treatment of benign canine rectal tumours: preliminary results in six cases (1992–1996). *Journal of Small Animal Practice*, (40), 423–7.

Kosovsky, J.E., Matthiesen, D.T. & Patnaik, A.K. (1988) Small intestinal adenocarcinoma in cats: 32 cases (1978–1985). *Journal of the American Veterinary Medical Association*, (192), 233–5.

Kosovsky, J.E., Manfara-Marretta, S., Matthiesen, D.T. *et al.* (1989) Results of partial hepatectomy in 18 dogs with hepatocellular carcinoma. *Journal of the American Animal Hospital Association*, (25), 203–206.

Marks, S.L. (1997) Bacterial gastroenteritis in dogs and cats: more common than you think. *Proceedings of the American College of Veterinary Internal Medicine*, (15), 237–9.

Owen, L.N. (1980) TNM Classification of Tumours in Domestic Animals. World Health Organisation, Geneva.

Patnaik, A.K., Hurvitz, A.I. & Johnson, G.F. (1977) Gastrointestinal neoplasms. *Veterinary Pathology*, (14), 547–55.

Ridgeway, R.L. & Suter, P.F. (1979) Clinical and radiographic signs in primary and metastatic oesophageal neoplasms of the dog. *Journal of the American Veterinary Medical Association*, (174), 700–704.

Scanzianzi, E., Giusti, A.M., Gualtieri, M. & Fonda, D. (1991) Gastric carcinoma in the Belgian shepherd dog. *Journal of Small Animal Practice*, 32, 465–9.

Slawienski, M.J., Mauldin, G.E., Mauldin, G.N. & Patnaik, A.K. (1997) Malignant colonic neoplasia in cats: 46 cases (1990–1996). *Journal of the American Veterinary Medical Association*, (211), 878–81.

Tasker, S., Griffon, D.J., Nuttall, T.J. & Hill, P.B. (1999) Resolution of paraneoplastic alopecia following surgical removal of a pancreatic carcinoma in a cat. *Journal of Small Animal Practice*, (40), 16–19.

Further reading

Birchard, S.J., Couto, C.G. & Johnson, S. (1986) Nonlymphoid intestinal neoplasia in 32 dogs and 14 cats. *Journal of the American Veterinary Medical Association*, (22), 533–7.

Couto, C.G., Rutgers, H.C., Sherding, R.G. & Rojko, J. (1989) Gastrointestinal lymphoma in 20 dogs. *Journal of Veterinary Internal Medicine*, (3), 73–8.

Fonda, D., Gualtieri, M. & Scanziani, E. (1989) Gastric carcinoma in the dog: a clinicopathological study of 11 cases. *Journal of Small Animal Practice*, (30), 353–60.

Gibbs, C. & Pearson, H. (1986) Localised tumours of the canine small intestine: a report of 20 cases. *Journal of Small Animal Practice*, (27), 507–19.

Holt, P.E. & Lucke, V.M. (1985) Rectal neoplasia in the dog: a clinicopathologic review of 31 cases. *Veterinary Record*, (116), 400–405.

Kapatkin, A.S., Mullen, H.S., Matthiesen, D.T. & Patnaik, A.K. (1992) Leiomyosarcoma in dogs: 44 cases (1983–1988). *Journal of the American Veterinary Medical Association*, (201), 1077–79.

Lamb, C.R. & Grierson, J. (1999) Ultrasonographic appearance of primary gastric neoplasia in 21 dogs. *Journal of Small Animal Practice*, (40), 211–15.

Patnaik, A.K. (1992) A morphologic and immunocytochemical study of hepatic neoplasms in cats. *Veterinary Pathology*, (29), 405–15.

Patnaik, A.K., Liu, S.K. & Johnson, G.F. (1976) Feline intestinal adenocarcinoma in cats: 32 cases (1978–1985). *Veterinary Pathology*, (13), 1–10.

Patnaik, A.K., Hurvitz, A.I. & Lieberman, P.H. (1980) Canine hepatic neoplasms: a clinicopathologic study. *Veterinary Pathology*, (17), 553–64.

Penninck, D.G., Moore, A.S. & Gliatto, J. (1998) Ultrasonography of canine gastric epithelial neoplasia. *Veterinary Radiology and Ultrasound*, (39), 342–8.

Steiner, J.M. & Williams, D.A. (1997) Feline exocrine pancreatic disorders: insufficiency, neoplasia and uncommon conditions. *Compendium of Continuing Education for the Practising Veterinarian*, (19), 836–48.

Sullivan, M., Lee, R., Fisher, E.W., Nash, A.S. & McCandlish, I.A.P. (1987) A study of 31 cases of gastric carcinoma in dogs. *Veterinary Record*, (120), 79–83.

White, R.A.S. & Gorman, N.T. (1987) The clinical diagnosis and management of rectal and pararectal tumours in the dog. *Journal of Small Animal Practice*, (28), 87–107.

9
Respiratory Tract

The lung is the commonest site for tumours of the respiratory system (excluding the nasal cavity), although primary lung tumours occur infrequently compared to metastatic tumours. Most primary lung tumours are malignant with adenocarcinoma predominating. Laryngeal and tracheal tumours are rare.

LARYNX

Epidemiology

Cancer of the larynx is rare in the dog and cat. Although most tumour types are likely to occur in middle-aged or older animals, the laryngeal specific tumour, the oncocytoma, occurs in young mature dogs.

Aetiology

There are no known aetiological factors for primary lung tumours in animals but smoking and alcohol consumption predispose to laryngeal cancer in man.

Pathology

A variety of laryngeal tumours have been reported in the dog (Table 9.1). Of these, squamous cell carcinoma is the most common, but all are rare. Benign tumours include lipoma, leiomyoma, rhabdomy-oma and oncocytoma, the latter being unique to the larynx. Occasionally, thyroid carcinomas may invade locally to involve the larynx.

In the cat, lymphoma is the most common laryngeal tumour but squamous cell carcinoma and more rarely, adenocarcinoma, have been reported.

Canine oncocytoma

Grossly, the oncocytoma usually develops as a well circumscribed mass (Fig. 9.1) although it can become very large and protrude from the laryngeal ventricle. Histologically, sheets of large, epithelioid cells with granular, acidophilic cytoplasm are seen in the submucosa. These are divided into lobules by fibrovascular stroma. Areas of haemorrhage and necrosis are common, making haemangiosarcoma an important differential, but the overlying mucosa is usually intact. The histogenesis of the oncocytes is not known although in man they are derived from glandular epithelia of the head and neck.

Table 9.1 Tumours of the larynx.

Benign	Malignant
Rhabdomyoma	Squamous cell carcinoma
Oncocytoma	Adenocarcinoma
Leiomyoma	Fibrosarcoma
Lipoma	Osteosarcoma
Osteochondroma	Chondrosarcoma
	Rhabdomyosarcoma
	Lymphoma
	Mast cell tumour
	Malignant melanoma

Tumour behaviour

Oncocytomas in the dog are benign and minimally invasive but can grow quite large, whereas all malignant tumours of the larynx are very locally invasive and metastatic.

Paraneoplastic syndromes

No paraneoplastic syndromes are commonly associated with laryngeal tumours.

Presentation/signs

Animals with laryngeal tumours usually present with insidious signs such as a progressive change in vocalisation, stertorous breathing, coughing, exercise intolerance, dysphagia or dyspnoea. Advanced cases with respiratory obstruction or animals with acute laryngeal spasm due to inflammation and pain may present with syncope or cyanosis.

Investigations

Direct visualisation

Most laryngeal tumours can be visualised under general anaesthesia although care should be taken to ensure a narrow endotracheal tube can be passed to maintain the airway. A tracheostomy should be performed if a large laryngeal mass is suspected. The larynx often appears very inflamed and oedematous secondary to air turbulence caused by the tumour.

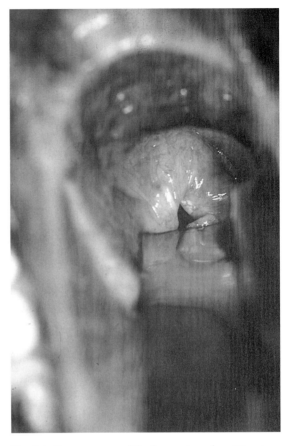

Fig. 9.1 Oncocytoma of the larynx in a dog. (Courtesy of Dr R.A.S. White, Department of Clinical Veterinary Medicine, University of Cambridge.)

Bloods

No haematological or biochemical changes are commonly associated with laryngeal tumours.

Imaging techniques

Radiography of the larynx is not usually necessary but may reveal a soft tissue swelling displacing adjacent structures in the neck and pharyngeal region (Fig. 9.2). Radiography of the thorax is essential for all malignant tumours to screen for pulmonary metastases. Ultrasonography and MRI can also be used to image the larynx and cartilages.

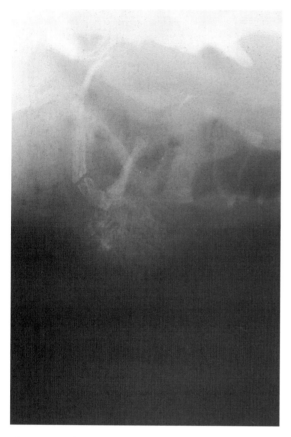

Fig. 9.2 Radiograph of chondrosarcoma associated with hyoid apparatus. (Courtesy of Radiology Department, Department of Clinical Veterinary Medicine, University of Cambridge.)

Biopsy/FNA

Ulcerating neoplasia needs to be differentiated from granulomatous laryngitis which responds to medical management. A definitive diagnosis of neoplasia can only be obtained by histological examination of a biopsy taken from the laryngeal mass. This is best obtained via the oropharynx under general anaesthesia. Care should be taken to minimise haemorrhage or post-operative inflammation and swelling. After a biopsy procedure, dexamethasone may be helpful.

Staging

A combined TNM staging system is available for the larynx, trachea and lungs (see Table 9.4,

lungs). Regional lymph nodes for the larynx are the anterior cervical and pharyngeal nodes.

Treatment

Surgery

The oncocytoma is usually the best candidate for surgical excision and preservation of laryngeal function although it may also be possible for other benign tumours such as rhabdomyoma. Excision of malignant tumours is usually impossible due to their invasive nature.

Before laryngeal surgery, care should be taken to assess the larynx for other obstructive airway disease such as laryngeal paralysis or laryngeal collapse which may compromise airflow in the recovery period. During surgery, the airway should be maintained with a suitable endotracheal tube or temporary tracheostomy while the oncocytoma is dissected from its submucosal location. Tumours are best approached intra-orally to minimise disruption to the larynx. Haemostasis and gentle handling of the tissues are essential to prevent airway obstruction in the recovery period although this risk is also avoided with a temporary tracheostomy.

Although partial, hemi and total laryngectomy are reported for resection of laryngeal tumours, post-operative management is difficult and they should only be undertaken with extreme caution.

Radiotherapy

External beam radiotherapy is not usually applied to laryngeal tumours in small animals because of potential radiation side-effects to the normal cartilage and other radio-sensitive structures in the pharynx and neck. It may, however, be of palliative value in selected cases or in laryngeal lymphoma.

Chemotherapy

Chemotherapy may be of use for laryngeal lymphoma (see Lymphoma in Chapter 15) but most other tumours are not chemosensitive.

Prognosis

Benign tumours of the larynx carry a good prognosis if they can be surgically resected.

Oncocytomas are generally slow growing and local recurrence, if they are inadequately excised, may take months or years. Malignant tumours carry a very poor prognosis since wide resection is too difficult and respiratory obstruction is inevitable.

TRACHEA

Epidemiology

Tumours of the trachea occur even more rarely than laryngeal tumours in dogs and cats. They are likely to occur in middle-aged or older animals but osteochondromas have been recorded in young growing dogs with active osteochondral ossification sites.

Aetiology

There are no known aetiological factors.

Pathology

Malignant tumours reported in the trachea are listed in Table 9.2. Benign tumours include leiomyoma and osteochondroma. The latter grow from the cartilagenous tracheal rings in immature dogs and may not be truly neoplastic.

Tumour behaviour

Tumours of the trachea may extend into the lumen or invade local tissues. Metastasis to local lymph nodes and lungs is common.

Paraneoplastic syndromes

No paraneoplastic syndromes are commonly associated with tracheal tumours.

Table 9.2 Tumours of the trachea.

Benign	Malignant
Leiomyoma	Squamous cell carcinoma
Polyps	Adenocarcinoma
Osteochondroma	Chondrosarcoma
Chondroma	Rhabdomyosarcoma
	Osteosarcoma
	Lymphoma
	Plasmacytoma

Presentation/signs

The presenting signs of tracheal tumours are often insidious but usually include coughing, respiratory obstruction or exercise intolerance.

Investigations

Bloods

No haematological or biochemical changes are expected with tracheal tumours.

Imaging techniques

A tracheal mass may be visible on plain radiographs of the neck or cranial thorax. Narrowing of the tracheal lumen is often noted and metastasis to the bronchial lymph nodes may be seen. The whole thorax should be radiographed to screen for pulmonary metastases if a malignant tumour is suspected.

Biopsy/FNA

A suitable biopsy can usually be obtained using a rigid bronchoscope or an endoscope if the mass protrudes into the lumen of the trachea. Alternatively, an excisional biopsy may have to be performed when the mass is explored surgically as part of the treatment procedure.

Staging

A combined TNM staging system is available for the larynx, trachea and lungs (see Table 9.4, lungs). Regional lymph nodes for the anterior trachea are the anterior cervical and pharyngeal nodes and for the rest of the trachea, the intrathoracic nodes.

Treatment

Surgery

Benign osteochondromas can be surgically excised relatively easily and the trachea joined by end-to-end anastomosis. Some malignant tumours may be amenable to surgery if small and minimally invasive. Great care must be taken not to damage the caudal thyroid artery that supplies the trachea. Up to a third of the trachea can be removed in adults provided the remainder can be sufficiently mobilised to allow anastomosis. Puppies and kittens can only tolerate 25% removal as the tracheal rings are unable to tolerate the tension in the stay sutures. Tension on the anastomosis increases the likelihood of granulation tissue forming and thus stenosis at the surgical site. It may be reduced by using tension sutures, providing lateral and ventral support to the anastomosis or by keeping the animal's head in flexion for two weeks post-operatively.

Radiotherapy

Radiotherapy is not usually used for tracheal tumours because of potential radiation side-effects to the cartilage of the normal tracheal rings and other structures of the neck and thorax.

Chemotherapy

Few malignant tracheal tumours except lymphoma are amenable to chemotherapy. Even post-operative therapy for highly metastatic tumours is rarely attempted because so few tumours are amenable to surgical excision.

Prognosis

Benign tumours carry a reasonable prognosis if surgically excised, but malignant tumours are rarely treated successfully.

LUNG

Epidemiology

Primary lung tumours are relatively uncommon in small animals, accounting for approximately 1% of all tumours in the dog and less than 0.5% in the cat. In contrast, the lungs are one of the most common sites for metastatic tumours in small animals.

An annual incidence of 4.17 cases per 100000 dogs and 2.2 cases per 100000 cats has been reported for primary lung tumours (Dorn *et al.* 1968). Older dogs (mean 9–11 years) and aged cats (mean 11–12 years) tend to be affected. Tumours may occur more frequently in the right lung, particularly the caudal lobe in the dog or the left lobes of the cat, although others agree that left and right lungs are equally affected.

Aetiology

There is experimental evidence of an association between cigarette smoke exposure and development of lung tumours in beagle dogs mimicking the effect of similar carcinogen exposure in man. Ionising radiation, atmospheric pollutants and aromatic amines also cause lung tumours in experimental animals.

Pathology

The most common type of primary lung tumour in dogs and cats is adenocarcinoma (Table 9.3). Squa-

Table 9.3 Primary lung tumours in the dog and cat.

Histological types (Moulton 1990)
Adenocarcinoma/carcinoma
  bronchial gland
  bronchogenic
  bronchiolar-alveolar
Squamous cell (epidermoid) carcinoma
Anaplastic carcinoma
  small cell
  large cell
Sarcomas
Benign tumours
Lymphomatoid granulomatosis (rare)

mous cell carcinoma and anaplastic carcinoma (small and large cell) are less common and sarcomas and benign tumours are rare.

Carcinoma or adenocarcinoma of the lung may be classified as differentiated or undifferentiated and although the site of origin may be difficult to determine for a large, advanced tumour, it may also be classified by its location as:

- Bronchial gland
- Bronchogenic
- Bronchiolar-alveolar.

Bronchiolar-alveolar carcinoma accounts for over 70% of lung tumours in the dog and cat and is usually peripheral and multifocal in nature. Differentiated tumours are characterised by well-formed glands of bronchiolar/alveolar derivation which may have a papillary appearance. Metaplasia of the stroma to bone or cartilage may be noted and some tumours may produce mucinous material. Undifferentiated tumours are more common in the cat and are characterised by irregular, poorly formed glands resembling immature bronchioles or alveoli, and squamous metaplasia.

Bronchial carcinomas, in contrast, are derived from the serous or mucous bronchial glands in the wall of the major airways around the hilus and are therefore located in this region. Squamous metaplasia may be noted, or hyperplastic thickening of the bronchial epithelium overlying the neoplastic tissue.

Bronchogenic carcinoma which is common in man, is very rare in animals. It arises from the pseudostratified columnar surface epithelium of a bronchus and shows papillary or glandular morphology.

Squamous cell carcinoma represents about 15% of lung tumours in the dog and cat, which is much less than in man. It develops where the bronchial mucosa has undergone squamous metaplasia, usually in the major bronchi. Solid branching cords of epithelial cells without a glandular pattern and varying degrees of keratinisation are characteristic. Tumours are very invasive and there is always much fibrosis of the stroma.

Anaplastic small cell and large cell carcinomas are also much less common than in man and are derived from alveolar epithelium, either type I or type II pneumocytes. The virtue of dividing them into small and large cell types is debatable in dogs and cats.

Tumour behaviour

The behaviour of primary lung tumours depends to some extent on their degree of differentiation, undifferentiated bronchiolar-alveolar carcinoma, which is common in cats, being highly invasive and metastatic. Squamous cell carcinoma and anaplastic carcinoma generally have a higher metastatic rate than adenocarcinoma. Primary lung tumours may spread in a limited way via the alveoli and airways or by pleural invasion and adhesions, but more commonly via the lymphatics or blood. Metastatic spread may be detected within the lungs, the bronchial lymph nodes, distant sites within the pleural cavity or, if haematogenous spread occurs, extrathoracic sites such as skeletal muscle, skin, abdominal organs, bone or brain. Metastasis to the digits has also been reported as a syndrome associated with primary lung cancer (usually squamous cell carcinoma) in cats (May & Newsholme 1989; Scott Moncrieff *et al.* 1989).

Paraneoplastic syndromes

Hypertrophic osteopathy (Maries' disease) is the commonest paraneoplastic syndrome associated with a lung mass, occurring in up to 15% of canine cases but more rarely in the cat (Figs 9.3–9.5) (see Chapter 2, Table 2.7 for details). Hypercalcaemia has also been reported in some dogs with lung tumours, as has adrenocorticotrophic hormone (ACTH) secretion and generalised neuropathy. Both adenocarcinoma and small cell lung carcinoma can secrete neuropeptides in man but this has not been reported in animals.

Presentation/signs

Most dogs have clinical signs associated with a primary tumour although 30% may be asymptomatic (McNiel *et al.* 1997). Asymptomatic presentation is less common in the cat, although the clinical signs detected in a third of cases may not be associated with respiratory disease (Hahn & McEntee 1997). The most common presenting signs include non-productive or productive cough, lethargy, haemoptysis and dyspnoea. Pleural effusion or regurgitation may occur (particularly in the cat) and non-specific signs such as anorexia, pyrexia, weight

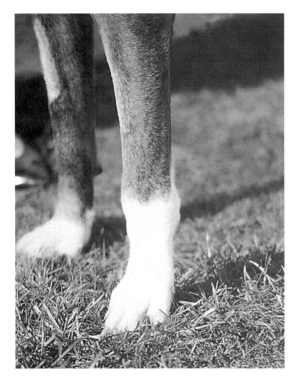

Fig. 9.3 Four year old boxer bitch presented with painful swelling of the distal limbs.

loss (common in the cat), lameness (either as a paraneoplastic syndrome or due to skeletal and bone metastases) and exercise intolerance may be reported.

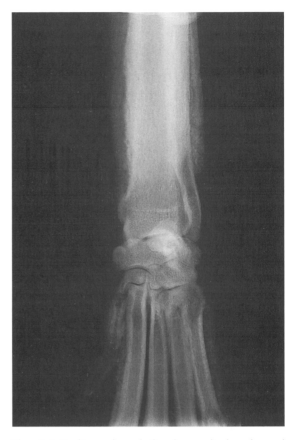

Fig. 9.4 Radiographs of the lower limbs showed periosteal new bone characteristic of hypertrophic osteopathy.

Investigations

Bloods

No haematological or biochemical changes are commonly expected with lung tumours.

Imaging techniques

Thoracic radiography is the most important diagnostic tool and will reveal a primary lung neoplasm in most cases (Fig. 9.6). This may present as:

- A solitary mass
- Multiple nodules
- A diffuse reticulonodular pattern of all lobes
- Consolidation of one or more lobes.

Both lateral views and dorso-ventral views may be needed to ensure small masses are detected and to

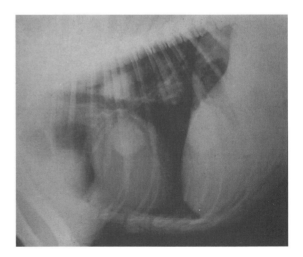

Fig. 9.5 Radiograph of the thorax showed several large pulmonary masses, the cause of the hypertrophic osteopathy. On histopathology these were anaplastic soft tissue sarcomas, possibly rhabdomyosarcoma.

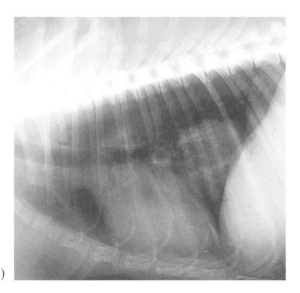

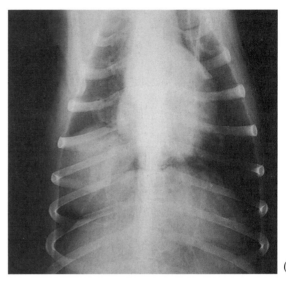

(a)   (b)

Fig. 9.6 Lateral (a) and dorsoventral (b) radiographs of the thorax of a dog with a solitary soft tissue mass in the right dorsal lung. This was a primary bronchial carcinoma.

locate the lung lobe affected. Pleural fluid, hilar or mediastinal lymphadenopathy or calcification of the lesion may also be present. Radiography of the abdomen and skeleton should be performed to look for distant metastases and hypertrophic osteopathy.

To detect metastatic lung tumours, both left and right lateral thoracic views are essential to view each lung fully aerated but dorso-ventral views are not always necessary. Metastases are usually noted as:

- Well defined 'cannon-balls'
- Multiple, small miliary nodules
- A diffuse interstitial – more common for lymphoma or mast cell tumours.

Ultrasonography may be useful to image a lung tumour in cases where the mass is large and there is no overlying air-filled lung, i.e. if it contacts the thoracic wall or diaphragm or if pleural fluid is present.

Bronchoscopy/tracheo-bronchial washes

Bronchoscopy may be useful in viewing a hilar mass and accessing it for grab biopsy, but for more peripheral cases, endoscopy may not be appropriate. Similarly, cytological examination of tracheo-bronchial washes may or may not detect neoplastic cells.

Thoracocentesis

For cases with pleural effusion, a modified transudate is usually obtained at thoracocentesis. Neoplastic cells may be visible on cytological examination.

Biopsy/FNA

In some cases, a diagnosis may be made on cytological examination of tracheobronchial washes or percutaneous ultrasound-guided fine needle aspirates (Fig. 9.7). In some samples, however, inflammation, haemorrhage and necrotic debris may obscure any neoplastic cells. Alternatively, a bronchoscopic grab biopsy or a percutaneous needle biopsy may be used to obtain a sample for histopathology. More reliable results may be obtained with cats than dogs, but if non-diagnostic samples are consistently obtained, a thoracotomy may be needed for a definitive biopsy. Some argue that the risks of tumour seeding, pneumothorax and haemorrhage, along with the poor diagnostic assistance often obtained from aspirate or biopsy procedures, suggest that surgical exploration should be the first approach to a solitary lung mass detected radiographically.

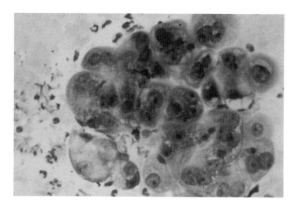

Fig. 9.7 Fine needle aspirate of pulmonary carcinoma.

Staging

A combined TNM staging system is available for laryngeal, tracheal and lung tumours (Table 9.4). All three categories should be assessed clinically and surgically in addition to endoscopy, bronchoscopy and radiography of the primary tumour. Radiography of the thorax is necessary to screen for distant metastases, if not already performed for the primary tumour. No stage grouping is recommended at present.

Treatment

Surgery

Surgical resection of the mass or lung lobe is the treatment of choice for a primary lung tumour. This necessitates a thoracotomy using a lateral intercostal approach or sternal split. A sternal split gains better access to both sides of the thoracic cavity but makes dissection and ligation of the hilar vessels and bronchus very difficult. An intercostal incision should be made further caudally if there is any doubt as to which lung lobe is affected since ribs are more easily retracted cranially.

Partial lobectomy may be used for peripheral lung masses but, without surgical stapling equipment, may prove lengthier and technically more difficult than lobectomy. Lobectomy is easier to perform via an intercostal approach, and involves ligation of the pulmonary artery and vein before transection and oversew of the bronchus. The artery should be ligated first in order to minimise lobe

Table 9.4 Clinical stages (TNM) of tumours of the larynx, trachea and lungs. Owen (1980).

T   *Primary tumour*
(multiple tumours should be classified independently)
T0   No evidence of tumour
TX   Tumour proven by presence of malignant cells in bronchopulmonary secretions but not seen by radiography or bronchoscopy
T1   Solitary tumour surrounded by lung or visceral pleura
T2   Multiple tumours of any size
T3   Tumour invading neighbouring tissues

N   *Regional lymph nodes (RLN)*
N0   No evidence of RLN involvement
N1   Bronchial LN involved
N2   Distant LN involved

M   *Distant metastasis*
M0   No evidence of metastasis
M1   Distant metastasis detected

congestion and haemorrhage during dissection. There is little chance of seeding of neoplastic cells through the venous outflow as the lung lobe collapses after arterial ligation. With multiple masses or affected lymph nodes it may not be possible to excise all tumour. Pneumonectomy can be performed if lesions have extended to all the lung lobes unilaterally and the contralateral lung is unaffected. However, a right sided pneumonectomy removes more than 50% of lung tissue and is thus fatal. Although nodes should be inspected for staging of the disease, and metastatic enlargement carries a worse prognosis, it is not necessarily recommended to remove affected nodes.

The post-operative care involves placement of a thoracostomy tube to allow drainage of air and early detection of haemorrhage if ligatures were insufficient or there is bronchial leakage. Post-operative monitoring of ventilation and oxygenation are important as the animal's dependent lungs will be collapsed on recovery and oxygen supplementation via a mask or nasogastric tube is strongly recommended until the animal has completely recovered from general anaesthesia.

Metastatic tumours are usually multiple and not amenable to surgery, although excision of solitary, slow-growing metastases has been attempted, particularly if in the caudo-dorsal lung fields and easily accessible via a caudal intercostal approach.

Radiotherapy

The lungs are particularly radiosensitive tissues and susceptible to radiation side-effects. It is not usually recommended to treat dog and cat primary or metastatic lung tumours with radiation.

Chemotherapy

Since most primary lung tumours in the dog and cat are carcinomas they are not particularly sensitive to chemotherapy. However, treatment with combinations of cisplatin, doxorubicin or mitoxantrone, cyclophosphamide and 5-fluorouracil have been reported anecdotally with limited success. Intra-cavitory cisplatin or sclerosing agents such as tetracycline have been tried for malignant pleural effusion.

Treatment of metastatic tumours is most successful in the micrometastatic stage, i.e. before radiographic detection. To prolong survival times with tumours known to have a high risk of lung metastasis, such as osteosarcoma and haemangiosarcoma, chemotherapy should be employed routinely after surgery (see Chapters 3, 5, and 6).

Prognosis

Survival times for many small primary lung tumours with no evidence of metastasis can extend to over 12 months. Factors associated with a poorer prognosis (shorter survival and disease free interval) in dogs are:

- Large tumour size (>5 cm diameter)
- Detection of clinical signs
- Metastasis to regional lymph nodes (TNM staging).

Adenocarcinoma of the lung tends to have a slightly better prognosis (mean survival time of 19 months) than squamous cell carcinoma (mean survival time 8 months) and anaplastic carcinoma (Mehlaff *et al.* 1983). Histological grading of tumours is important in that dogs and cats with well differentiated tumours have a better survival time and disease free interval than those with moderately or poorly differentiated tumours.

References

Dorn, C.R., Taylor, P.O., Frye, F.L. *et al.* (1968) Survey of animal neoplasms in Alameda and Contra Costa Counties, California. I. Methodology and description of cases. *Journal of the National Cancer Institute*, (40), 295–305.

Hahn, K.A. & McEntee, M.F. (1997) Primary lung tumours in cats: 86 cases (1979–1994). *Journal of the American Veterinary Medical Association*, (211), 1257–60.

May, C. & Newsholme, S.J. (1989) Metastasis of feline pulmonary carcinoma presenting as multiple digital swelling. *Journal of Small Animal Practice*, (30), 302–10.

McNeil, E.A., Ogilvie, G.K., Powers, B.E., Hutchison, J.M., Salman, M.D. & Withrow, S.J. (1997) Evaluation of prognostic factors for dogs with primary lung tumours: 67 cases (1985–1992). *Journal of the American Veterinary Medical Association*, (211), 1422–7.

Mehlaff, C.J., Leifer, C.E., Patnaik, A.K. & Schwarz, P.D. (1983) Surgical treatment of primary pulmonary neoplasia in 15 dogs. *Journal of the American Animal Hospital Association*, (20), 799–803.

Moulton, J.E. (1990) Tumours of the respiratory system. In: *Tumours in Domestic Animals*, 3rd edn., pp. 309–346. *University of California Press*, Los Angeles.

Owen, L.N. (1980) TNM Classification of Tumours in Domestic Animals. World Health Organisation, Geneva.

Scott-Moncrieff, J.C., Elliot, G.S., Radovsky, A. & Blevins, W.E. (1989) Pulmonary squamous cell carcinoma with multiple digital metastases in a cat. *Journal of Small Animal Practice*, (30), 696–9.

Further reading

Barr, F.J., Gibbs, C. & Brown, P.J. (1986) The radiological features of primary lung tumours in the dog: a review of 36 cases. *Journal of Small Animal Practice*, (27), 493–505.

Barr, F.J., Gruffydd-Jones, T.J., Brown, P.J. & Gibbs, C. (1986) Primary lung tumours in the cat. *Journal of Small Animal Practice*, (28), 1115–25.

Hahn, K.A. & McEntee, M.F. (1998) Prognostic factors for survival in cats after removal of a primary lung tumour: 21 cases (1979–1994). *Veterinary Surgery*, (27), 307–11.

O'Brien, M.G., Straw, R.C., Withrow, S.J. *et al.* (1993) Resection of pulmonary metastases in canine osteosarcoma: 36 cases (1983–1992). *Veterinary Surgery*, (22), 105–109.

Ogilvie, G.K., Haschek, W.M, Withrow, S.J. *et al.* (1989) Classification of primary lung tumours in dogs: 210 cases (1975–1985). *Journal of the American Veterinary Medical Association*, (195), 106–108.

Ogilvie, G.K., Weigel, R.M., Haschek, W.M. *et al.* (1989) Prognostic factors for tumour remission and survival in dogs after surgery for primary lung tumour: 76 cases (1975–1985). *Journal of the American Veterinary Medical Association*, (195), 109–12.

10
Urinary Tract

The bladder is the commonest site for urinary tract tumours in the dog; in the cat, it is the kidney. Most bladder and renal tumours are malignant and carry a poor prognosis.

KIDNEY

Epidemiology

Primary renal neoplasia is uncommon, accounting for less than 1.7% and 2.5% of all canine and feline tumours respectively (Crow 1985). Affected dogs are usually old (mean age nine years) except for those with embryonal tumours which are often less than a year old (mean age four years). Males are affected more than females. The mean age of cats with renal lymphoma is six or seven years but no sex predisposition has been reported. In contrast to primary renal neoplasia in small animals, secondary (metastatic) cancer is common because of the high blood flow and rich capillary network within the kidney.

Aetiology

For most primary renal tumours, there is no known aetiology. Bilateral renal cystadenocarcinoma, however, is seen almost exclusively in the German shepherd dog as part of a syndrome involving nodular dermal fibrosis and uterine polyps and may be familial (Atlee *et al.* 1991; Moe & Lium 1997). FeLV may be responsible for renal lymphoma in the cat but only 50% of cases are FeLV positive.

Pathology

Primary renal tumours are usually solitary and unilateral in contrast to metastatic tumours which are often multiple and bilateral. Ninety per cent of primary renal neoplasms in the dog and cat are malignant and more than half of these are epithelial. The various histological types are listed in Table 10.1.

Renal adenocarcinoma/carcinoma is derived from tubular epithelium and can be described histologically as tubular, solid, acinar or papillary. It usually grows from one pole and can become quite large, with areas of haemorrhage and necrosis (Fig. 10.1). Some may appear well demarcated and resemble renal adenoma while others are more invasive.

Transitional cell tumours are derived from renal pelvis epithelium and are rarer than renal carcinoma. Small cauliflower-like lesions without invasion are usually papillomas but larger, more invasive lesions are usually carcinomas.

Table 10.1 Tumours of the kidney.

Benign	Malignant
Adenoma	Adenocarcinoma/carcinoma
Transitional cell papilloma	Transitional cell carcinoma
Leiomyoma	Leiomyosarcoma
Haemangioma	Haemangiosarcoma
Fibroma	Fibrosarcoma
Interstitial cell tumour	Lymphoma
	Nephroblastoma

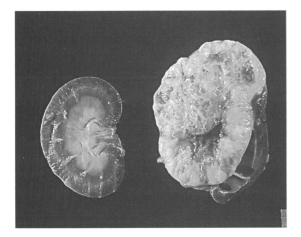

Fig. 10.1 Gross appearance of renal carcinoma, post mortem. (Courtesy of Dr P. Nicholls.)

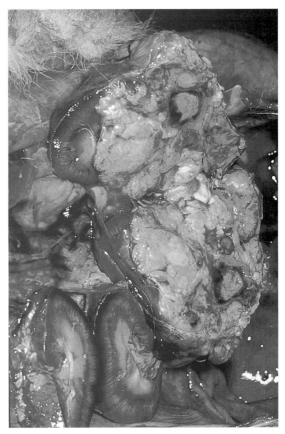

Fig. 10.2 Gross appearance of a nephroblastoma (post mortem). (Courtesy of Mr A. Jefferies, Department of Clinical Veterinary Medicine, University of Cambridge.)

Twenty per cent of primary renal tumours are mesenchymal and these include haemangiosarcoma, and fibrosarcoma in dogs. Lymphoma is the most common feline renal tumour. It is usually bilateral and often progresses to generalised form or spreads to the CNS. There may be an association between nasal and renal lymphoma since many cases presenting with nasal lymphoma subsequently develop the renal form.

Ten per cent of renal tumours are derived from primitive tissues. Nephroblastoma which is also called embryonal nephroma or Wilm's tumour is less common in dogs than other species. Grossly, one pole of the kidney may be affected by a solitary mass originating from the renal cortex, but multiple or bilateral tumours can occur (Fig. 10.2). Primitive epithelial and mesenchymal tissues such as vestigial tubules, muscle, cartilage and bone are seen histologically.

Benign tumours are rare but include fibroma, haemangioma, adenoma, transitional cell papilloma, leiomyoma and interstitial cell tumour.

Tumour behaviour

Renal carcinoma may be very small and confined to the cortex or it may extend into the peri-renal tissues and form adhesions. Invasion of the renal arteries and veins, vena cava and aorta may occur as well as metastasis to regional lymph nodes, lung, liver, bone or skin (the latter may often be mistaken for apocrine sweat gland adenocarcinoma). Tumours are usually fast growing and prone to metastasis by the time of diagnosis. Transitional cell carcinomas may obstruct urine flow and cause hydronephrosis but are less metastatic than renal adenocarcinoma.

Nephroblastoma may also extend beyond the renal cortex, and invade the medulla and pelvis. Approximately half of canine nephroblastomas metastasise, but nephrectomy is sometimes curative.

Paraneoplastic syndromes

Polycythaemia may result if a renal carcinoma autonomously produces erythropoietin (see Chapter 2, Table 2.4). Other paraneoplastic syndromes occasionally reported are hypertrophic osteopathy, hypercalcaemia and nodular dermatofibrosis.

Presentation/signs

Many renal tumours present with vague signs of illness such as anorexia, depression, weight loss, lethargy, or sub-lumbar pain. More specific signs may include:

- An abdominal mass may be palpated and bilateral renomegaly is often palpable in the cat with renal lymphoma.
- Abdominal distension may occur with nephroblastoma or bilateral cystadenoma bullet haematuria may be associated with tumours of the renal pelvis or haemangiosarcoma.
- Hind limb oedema can occasionally be seen if lymphatic drainage is obstructed.

Signs of renal failure such as polyuria, polydipsia, vomiting or diarrhoea are not noted unless there is bilateral involvement. Some tumours, however, may be asymptomatic and discovered as an incidental finding on radiography, at celiotomy or at post mortem examination.

Investigations

Bloods

Regenerative anaemia may be noted if haematuria is present, or polycythaemia if erythropoietin production is increased. Serum biochemistry is often normal unless renal function is compromised.

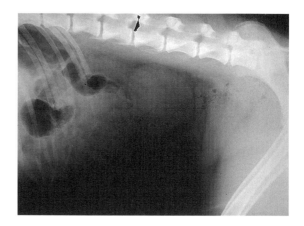

Fig. 10.3 Lateral abdominal radiograph showing a large circumscribed renal mass in the caudal–dorsal abdomen. (Courtesy of Radiology Department, Department of Clinical Veterinary Medicine, University of Cambridge.)

Imaging techniques

Renomegaly, a change in renal shape, or undefined dorsal abdominal mass(es) and displacement of other abdominal organs may be detected on plain abdominal films (Fig. 10.3) but contrast (intravenous urography or renal angiography) will be necessary to demonstrate a change in renal architecture and to help visualise the renal pelvis, cortex and ureters. Dystrophic calcification may be noted in some cases. Thoracic radiography should also be performed to screen for pulmonary metastasis.

Ultrasonography is often useful to confirm an abdominal mass as renal and to assess renal architecture. It may also be used to guide an aspirate or biopsy needle. MRI is becoming increasingly used to assess abdominal organs in animals. Although scintigraphy is used in humans to assess renal blood flow and function, as yet it is not much used in the veterinary field for this purpose.

Urinalysis

Proteinuria is a common finding but haematuria is only seen with haemangiosarcoma or transitional cell carcinoma of the renal pelvis. Tumour cells may occasionally be detected on cytological examination of urinary sediment but this is not a reliable finding on which to make a diagnosis.

Biopsy/FNA

Ultrasound-guided biopsy or fine needle aspirate is fairly non-invasive and easily performed by experienced operators. An incisional biopsy can be taken at exploratory celiotomy if surgical excision is not possible.

Staging

A TNM staging system is available for renal tumours (Table 10.2) and requires clinical and surgical (celiotomy or laparoscopy) examination to view primary tumour, regional (lumbar) nodes and distant metastatic sites as well as radiography of the chest. No group staging is recommended.

Table 10.2 Clinical stages (TNM) of canine tumours of the kidney. Owen (1980).

T	*Primary tumour*
T0	No evidence of tumour
T1	Small tumour without deformation of the kidney
T2	Solitary tumour with deformation and/or enlargement of the kidney
T3	Tumour invading perinephric structures (peritoneum) and/or pelvis, ureter and/or renal blood vessels
T4	Tumour invading neighbouring structures
N	*Regional lymph nodes (RLN)*
N0	No evidence of RLN involvement
N1	Ipsilateral RLN involved
N2	Bilateral RLN involved
N3	Other LN involved (abdominal and pelvic LN)
M	*Distant metastasis*
M0	No evidence of metastasis
M1	Distant metastasis detected
M1a	Single metastasis in one organ
M1b	Multiple metastases in one organ
M1c	Multiple metastases in various organs

Treatment

Surgery

Ureteronephrectomy is the treatment of choice for unilateral renal tumours without evidence of metastatic disease. Ideally, the function of the opposite kidney should be checked by excretion urography or scintigraphy before surgery. At celiotomy, the tumour should be handled as little as possible to reduce the risk of peritoneal seeding and the renal vessels ligated as soon as possible to prevent embolic spread. The renal capsule should be left intact if the tumour is contained within it.

Radiotherapy

Radiotherapy is not generally used for the treatment of renal tumours in small animals.

Chemotherapy

Combination chemotherapy is more appropriate than surgery for treating renal lymphoma because it is often bilateral or generalised. Standard protocols may be used (Chapter 15). Adjuvant therapy with 5 fluorouracil, actinomycin-D, doxorubicin and cyclophosphamide has been used following surgical removal of renal carcinoma but objective evidence for a response is lacking. Although cisplatin is effective in treating human urogenital tumours, this is not the case in dogs (Klein *et al.* 1988).

Prognosis

The prognosis for most renal tumours is poor because of their invasive nature and tendency to metastasise. Even after surgical removal, survival times are generally short (6–12 months) although occasional animals survive for a few years. Nephroblastoma carries a better prognosis with many more cases cured by surgery. Cases of renal lymphoma respond less well to chemotherapy than other forms of the disease and long-term remission and survival are difficult to achieve.

URETER

Pathology

Neoplasia of the ureters is extremely rare but transitional cell carcinoma, leiomyoma, or leiomyosarcoma can develop. Direct extension of renal pelvis tumours or of bladder tumours into the distal ureter can also occur.

Tumour behaviour

Most tumours will protrude into the ureteral lumen, eventually causing urinary obstruction, hydroureter and hydronephrosis. Local invasion of surrounding tissues may occur as well as distant metastasis to other abdominal organs.

Presentation/signs

Clinical signs for ureteral tumours are generally non-specific and may include lower back pain or stiffness. Most will be detected in the late stages when hydorureter or hydronephrosis have occurred.

Investigations

Bloods

No specific haematological or biochemical changes are expected with ureteral tumours.

Imaging techniques

Normal ureters are rarely visible on radiographs, but plain abdominal radiography may show a soft tissue sublumbar mass or a change in renal size or shape due to hydronephrosis. Contrast radiography (IVU) is essential for a more precise diagnosis and will reveal a filling defect, irregularity or stricture in the ureter. With complete obstruction, proximal dilation of the ureter may be present or if hydronephrosis has been present for some time and all nephrons destroyed, no excretion of contrast may be visible on the affected side. Thoracic radiographs should be performed to screen for pulmonary metastases.

Ultrasonography can be helpful in locating an abdominal mass to the ureter and in assessing associated changes in renal architecture.

Biopsy/FNA

Ultrasound-guided needle biopsy or fine needle aspirate may be possible with a large mass, but often a histological diagnosis may only be achieved by a laparoscopic biopsy or at exploratory celiotomy.

Staging

A TNM system is not available for ureteral tumours.

Treatment

Surgery

Ureteral tumours which have not invaded locally or metastasised can often be treated successfully by ureteronephrectomy. The function of the opposite kidney and ureter should be assessed prior to surgery.

Prognosis

Since most malignant ureteral tumours invade locally and metastasise, surgical resection is not always an option, making the prognosis generally poor. Benign tumours carry a much better prognosis.

BLADDER

Epidemiology

The bladder is the most common site in the canine urinary tract for neoplasia but fewer than 1% of all tumours in the dog occur here. Aged female animals (mean 10 years) are usually affected although embryonal rhabdomyosarcoma occurs in young dogs, particularly those of large breeds. Bladder cancer is much rarer in the cat than the

Table 10.3 Tumours of the bladder.

Benign	Malignant
Leiomyoma	Transitional cell carcinoma
Haemangioma	Adenocarcinoma
Fibroma	Squamous cell carcinoma
	Undifferentiated carcinoma
	Embryonal rhabdomyosarcoma
	Leiomyosarcoma
	Haemangiosarcoma
	Fibrosarcoma
	Lymphoma

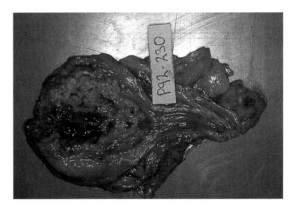

Fig. 10.4 Post mortem picture of bladder carcinoma. (Courtesy of Dr P. Nicholls.)

dog, accounting for less than 0.5% of all tumours. Aged male cats (mean 9–10 years) are most at risk.

Aetiology

Prolonged contact time between carcinogenic chemicals in stored urine and uropeithelial cells is thought to cause bladder cancer. In man, cigarette smoking, certain industrial chemicals (nitrosamines), tryptophan metabolites, cyclophosphamide and environmental pollutants are considered bladder carcinogens. Some of these chemicals may also predispose to tumour formation in dogs but it has been proposed that cats metabolise them differently and excrete lower quantities of the carcinogenic compounds.

Pathology

Malignant bladder tumours are more common than benign ones (Table 10.3). The majority of tumours in both the dog (97% of cases) and cat (80% of cases) are epithelial, the most common being transitional cell carcinoma. Squamous cell carcinoma and adenocarcinoma may arise due to metaplasia of the bladder epithelium but are much less common and appear to behave similarly to transitional cell carcinoma. Undifferentiated carcinoma is also reported.

All epithelial tumours may be solitary or multiple and appear as papillary or non-papillary, infiltrating or non-infiltrating growths. Transitional cell carcinoma is usually papillary, protruding into the lumen from a broad base, although an infiltrating, thickened plaque or ulcerated nodule may occur

(Fig. 10.4). Tumours most often arise at the trigone region of the bladder.

Mesenchymal bladder tumours are mainly derived from fibrous tissue or smooth muscle and these include leiomyoma, haemangioma and fibroma along with their malignant counterparts. Rhabdomyosarcoma (botryoid or embryonal sarcoma) is a rare embryonal myoblast tumour which sometimes occurs in the bladder wall. It arises in the trigonal region, is often multi-lobulated and may occlude the ureteric orifices. Lymphoma has also been occasionally reported.

Tumour behaviour

Transitional cell carcinoma is usually locally invasive. After infiltrating through the bladder wall, it extends into adjacent tissues and regional organs such as the pelvic fat, prostate or uterus, vagina or rectum. Peritoneal seeding may also occur as well as metastases to internal iliac and sublumbar lymph nodes, lungs, liver, spleen and pelvic bones.

Whereas most mesenchymal bladder tumours are locally invasive and less likely to metastasise than transitional cell carcinoma, embryonal rhabdomyosarcoma has a tendency for both local recurrence after surgery and distant metastasis.

Paraneoplastic syndromes

Hypertrophic osteopathy may be associated with embryonal rhabdomyosarcoma of the bladder (see Chapter 2).

Presentation/signs

Bladder tumours often present with signs similar to those of chronic cystitis including haematuria, dysuria and pollakiuria. Any elderly bitch presenting with recurrent cystitis should be considered for investigating the presence of an underlying bladder tumour.

Investigations

Bloods

No specific haematological or biochemical changes are expected with bladder tumours.

Imaging techniques

Plain abdominal radiographs are often unremarkable although a change in bladder shape or possibly just a distinct bladder may be visible. Negative (air) contrast is necessary to visualise most tumours (Fig. 10.5) but double contrast cystography is preferable. This allows coating of the bladder mucosa with a small amount of positive contrast prior to inflation with air. Multiple, discrete masses or a solitary mass often located at the bladder neck are easily visible, as well as diffuse tumours which cause thickening of the bladder wall or changes

in the mucosal surface. Epithelial tumours often appear ulcerated whereas mesenchymal ones have a smoother mucosal appearance. Hydronephrosis or hydroureter may also be noted (IVU may be needed) or metastases to sublumbar lymph nodes, lungs, spine or pelvis. Radiography of the skeletal long bones may reveal hypertrophic osteopathy. Thoracic radiographs should be taken to screen for pulmonary metastases.

Ultrasonography of the bladder is often more useful to visualise a mass or localised, irregular, bladder thickening, but it requires the bladder to be moderately distended with urine and should therefore be carried out before contrast radiography. Saline can be used to distend the bladder if necessary. Ultrasonography also gives information on the depth of invasion of the bladder wall and thus assists clinical staging (Fig. 10.6).

Urinalysis

Full urinalysis and cytological examination is necessary to distinguish between cystitis and neoplasia. Haematuria and proteinuria are common findings for both but the presence of pleomorphic tumour cells (Fig. 10.7) on cytological examination should differentiate the two conditions. These are not always noted, however, since some tumours, particularly sarcomas, do not exfoliate well. Conversely, atypical epithelial cells may sometimes be noted with cystitis since inflammation can induce changes which mimic malignancy. Bacterial culture

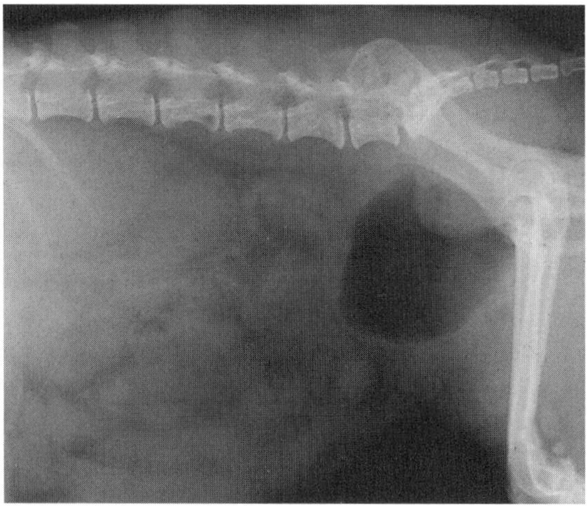

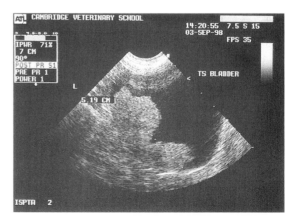

Fig. 10.5 Pneumocystogram – the air contrast assists visualisation of the mass in the caudal bladder.

Fig. 10.6 Ultrasound picture of transitional cell carcinoma of the bladder.

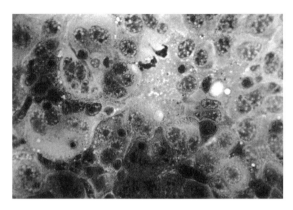

Fig. 10.7 Cytology of urine sediment showing neoplastic cells, leading to diagnosis of a transitional cell carcinoma. (See also Colour plate 27, facing p. 162.) (Courtesy of Ms K. Tennant, Department of Clinical Veterinary Medicine, University of Cambridge.)

Table 10.4 Clinical stages (TNM) of canine tumours of the urinary bladder. Owen (1980).

T	*Primary tumour*
	(add 'm' to appropriate T category for multiple tumours)
Tis	Carcinoma *in situ*
T0	No evidence of primary tumour
T1	Superficial papillary tumour
T2	Tumour invading the bladder wall with induration
T3	Tumour invading neighbouring organs (prostate, uterus, vagina, anal canal)
N	*Regional lymph nodes (RLN)*
N0	No evidence of RLN involvement
N1	RLN involved
N2	RLN and juxta RLN (lumbar) involved
M	*Distant metastasis*
M0	No evidence of metastasis
M1	Distant metastasis detected

may also be helpful although infection secondary to neoplasia is common.

Cystoscopy

Using a small diameter flexible endoscope, the bladder lumen can be examined for multiple, pedunculated masses or localised thickenings, the extent of any tumour determined and a biopsy obtained. The technique is easier for bitches than for dogs because of the length of the urethra.

Biopsy/FNA

Since some bladder lesions visible on radiography or ultrasonography may be inflammatory polyps or nodular hyperplasia, cytological or histological examination is required to differentiate these from neoplasia. Ultrasound-guided fine needle aspiration is easily performed for a large, discrete, bladder mass but other tumours may require biopsy. Biopsy may be performed using cystoscopy, or by applying negative pressure with a syringe to a catheter inserted into the bladder to suck in some tissue which can then be flushed into fixative. This does not require expensive endoscopic equipment but is relatively non-specific since it is performed blind and can produce false negatives. In many cases, an incisional biopsy may have to be taken at exploratory cystotomy, when surgical excision of any tumour may also be attempted.

Staging

A TNM system is available for bladder tumours (Table 10.4) but no group staging is recommended at present. For complete staging of primary tumour, regional (internal and external iliac) nodes and distant metastatic sites, clinical examination, cystography, radiography of the thorax and celiotomy or laparoscopy are required.

Treatment

Surgery

Early lesions or localised tumours may be resected by a partial cystectomy. However, this is often not possible because of the multiple or diffuse nature of many epithelial tumours which makes visualisation of the margins difficult and local recurrence is common. The ureters and trigone are often affected in dogs making resection of the tumour and reconstruction of a functional lower urinary tract difficult or impossible. Mesenchymal tumours may be completely excised more easily since the general recommendation is that two thirds of the bladder may be resected without interfering significantly with its function. In cats, tumours are often located at the bladder apex making surgical excision more likely to be effective.

Total cystectomy with diversion of the ureters to the distal ileum or proximal colon has been described but gives poor survival times and a very unsatisfactory quality of life due to reabsorption of toxic renal metabolites in the colon and the risk of ascending pyelonephritis.

Radiotherapy

External beam radiotherapy is not usually attempted for bladder tumours in dogs and cats because of the problems of radiation side-effects on other abdominal organs. Intra-operative radio-therapy delivered as one large fraction after surgical debulking of a bladder mass has produced variable survival times. It avoids side-effects to other abdominal organs since abdominal organs can be shielded and the radiation beam can be delivered to a more precise area, but there are often long term complications such as bladder fibrosis which may cause urinary dyssynergia or incontinence. Some of these cases respond to oxybutynin which encourages bladder filling. Orthovoltage radiation is generally recommended in the literature but we have used megavoltage radiation with suitable build-up to deliver the required dose to the bladder wall, while protecting the rest of the abdomen with lead shielding.

Chemotherapy

Various cytotoxic agents have been tried for the treatment of bladder tumours, intravesically or systemically, as a sole treatment or combined with surgery, but the results have proved inconsistent and the efficacy of such protocols has not been demonstrated. Direct application within the bladder of drugs such as 5-fluorouracil, cisplatin or thiotepa is only of use with very superficial tumours since penetration of the bladder wall is limited. Most canine tumours are deep and invasive, making this method of therapy rarely effective. Triethylenethiophosphoramide (thiotepa) is extremely toxic, requires special protective measures to the administrators and is therefore not recommended for use in general practice.

Systemic administration of 5-fluorouracil, doxorubicin, cyclophosphamide or cisplatin may have some effect, but often the tumour mass is too great to be significantly reduced in size. Cisplatin has proved variably effective depending on the dose used but carries a significant risk of renal toxicity. Carboplatin, which is less nephrotoxic, has minimal effect on survival time (Chun *et al.* 1997). Paradoxically, cyclophosphamide, a drug which may cause bladder cancer, has also been used in its treatment. A combination of doxorubicin and cyclophosphamide extended survival time in dogs with transitional cell carcinoma in one study (Helfand *et al.* 1994).

Other

The non-steroidal anti-inflammatory drug piroxicam (0.3 mg/kg po SID) has been used with partial success to treat transitional cell carcinoma of the bladder or at least obtain several months of palliation (Knapp *et al.* 1994). It may also be used postoperatively after surgical debulking of a tumour.

In some cases, palliative treatment in the form of repeated courses of antibiotics to control secondary infection may relieve the clinical signs and improve quality of life without addressing the primary problem. Particularly for old animals, some owners may prefer this approach.

Prognosis

The prognosis for most bladder carcinomas is poor because of their diffuse or multiple nature and the failure to control them satisfactorily by surgery or other means. Survival time following surgical excision is usually less than six months. Mesenchymal tumours may have a slightly better prognosis if diagnosed early and amenable to surgical excision.

URETHRA

Epidemiology

Tumours of the urethra are less common than those of the bladder in dogs and extremely rare in cats.

Aetiology

The same aetiological factors that induce bladder tumours probably affect the urethra too.

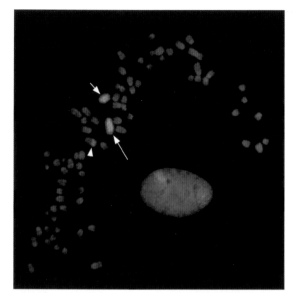

Plate 1

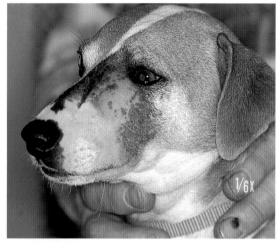

Plate 3

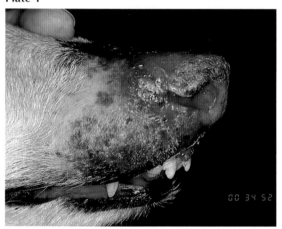

Plate 4

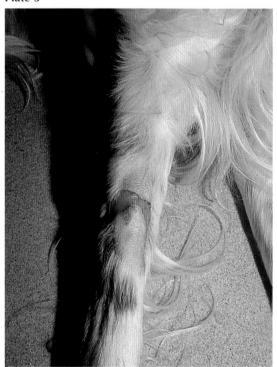

Plate 2

Plate 1 Hybridisation of dog chromosome 1 paint to a metaphase from a canine sarcoma. Chromosome 1 paint is labelled with the fluorescent dye Cy3 (pink) and the other chromosomes are counterstained with DAPI (blue). One normal copy of chromosome 1 (large arrow) is present in the metaphase, but the other copy (small arrow) has split and translocated to a third chromosome (arrow head). This shows that there is a translocation involving chromosome 1 and another as yet unidentified chromosome in this sarcoma. (Chromosome paint as from Yang *et al.* 1999.)

Plate 2 Acute radiation skin reaction – erythema of the skin and moist desquamation of the nasal planum following treatment of a SCC of the nasal planum.

Plate 3 Post radiation alopecia.

Plate 4 Local tissue damage following perivascular leakage of vincristine.

Plate 5 Red light source being used to treat superficial SCC on cat's nose.

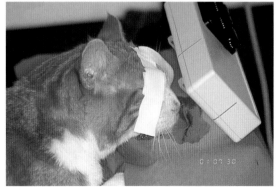

Plate 5

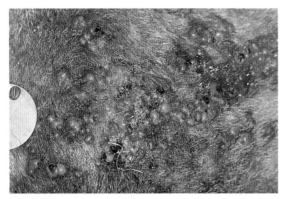

Plate 6

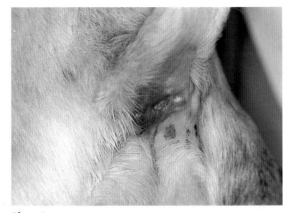

Plate 8

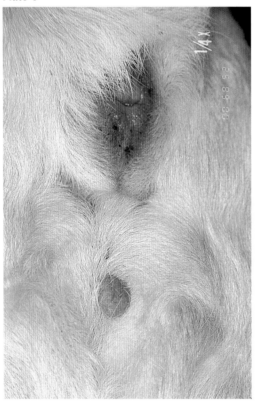

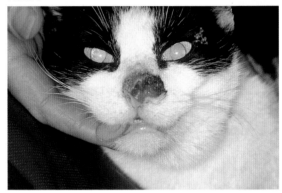

Plate 9

Plate 8 Perianal gland adenocarcinoma. (Courtesy of Dr R.A.S. White, Department of Clinical Veterinary Medicine, Cambridge.)
Plate 9 SCC nasal planum – cat.

Plate 7

Plate 6 Sweat gland adenocarcinoma, infiltrating widely throughout the skin.
Plate 7 Perianal gland adenoma.

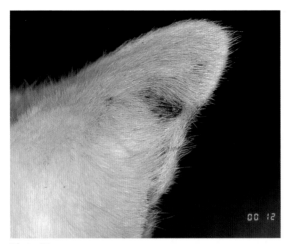

Plate 10

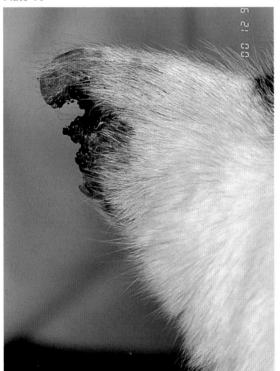

Plate 11

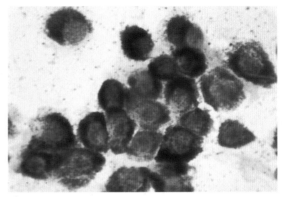

Plate 12

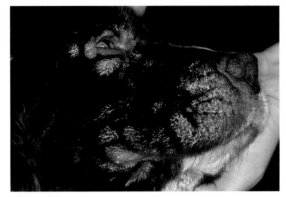

Plate 13

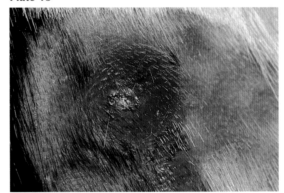

Plate 14

Plates 10 and 11 SCC of the pinna in a cat. **Plate 10** Early stage lesion with erythema and crusting is seen on the right ear. **Plate 11** A more advanced, ulcerated and invasive tumour is affecting the left pinna of the same cat.

Plate 12 Cytological appearance of a mast cell tumour. Mast cells may be recognised by the characteristic heavily staining cytoplasmic granules. (Neat Stain – Haematology and Gram – Guest Medical.)

Plate 13 Primary cutaneous T cell lymphoma, generalised erythematous plaques and nodules.

Plate 14 Primary cutaneous T cell lymphoma. Close up of erythematous nodule from a different dog. Note infiltration of surrounding skin.

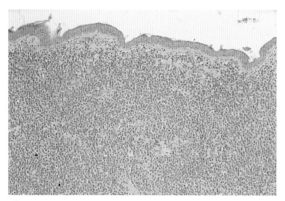

Plate 15

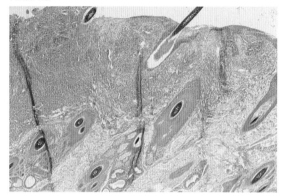

Plate 16

Plate 15 Histological appearance of primary cutanenous lymphoma. The tumour infiltrate affects the dermis, the epidermis is intact.
Plate 16 Histological appearance of epitheliotropic lymphoma. In contrast to Plate 15, the tumour cell infiltrate is in the epidermis.

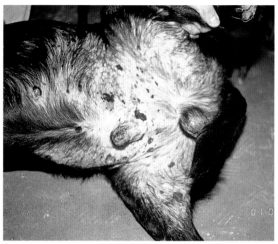

Plate 17

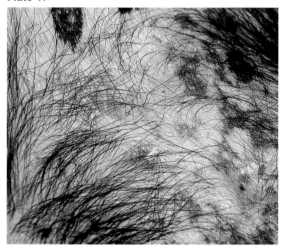

Plate 18

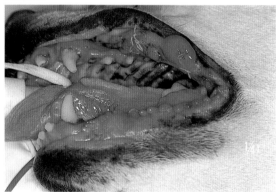

Plate 19

Plates 17 and 18 Epitheliotropic lymphoma (Plate 17) shows generalised nature of skin lesions (Plate 18) close up showing erythematous crusting nature of lesions.
Plate 19 Epitheliotropic lymphoma affecting oral mucocutaneous junctions and mucosae.

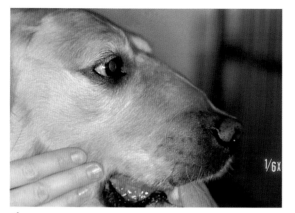

Plate 20

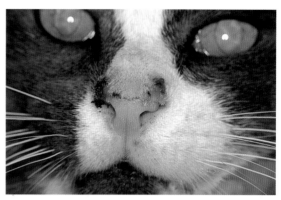

Plate 23

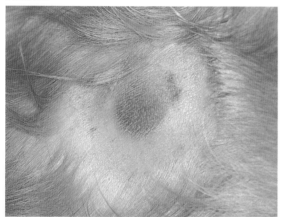

Plate 21

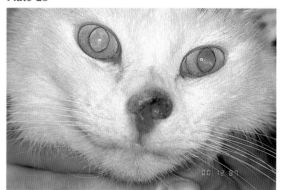

Plate 24

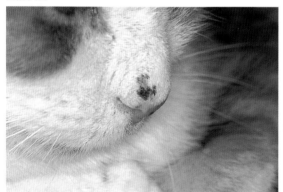

Plate 22

Plates 20 and 21 Cutaneous histiocytosis/pyogranulo-matous skin condition in a retriever. **Plate 20** The dog presented with a soft tissue swelling over the bridge of the nose. **Plate 21** Several other dermal masses were noted.

Plate 22 Early crusting lesion of carcinoma on cat's nose.

Plate 23 Minimally invasive, early SCC of nasal planum.

Plate 24 Invasive SCC of nasal planum in cat.

Plate 25 Invasive and destructive SCC of nasal planum in a dog.

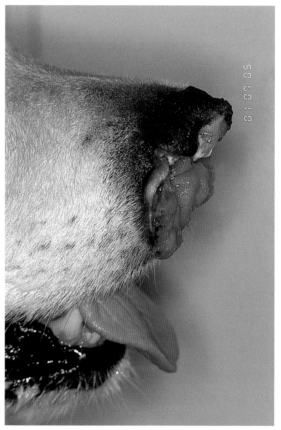

Plate 25

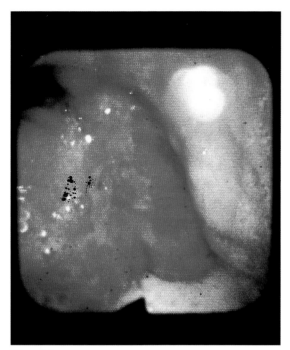

Plate 26

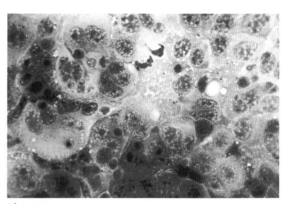

Plate 27

Plate 26 Endoscopic view of a gastric carcinoma sited near the pylorus in a rough collie.

Plate 27 Cytology of urine sediment showing neoplastic cells, leading to diagnosis of a transitional cell carcinoma. (Courtesy of Ms K. Tennant, Department of Clinical Veterinary Medicine, University of Cambridge.)

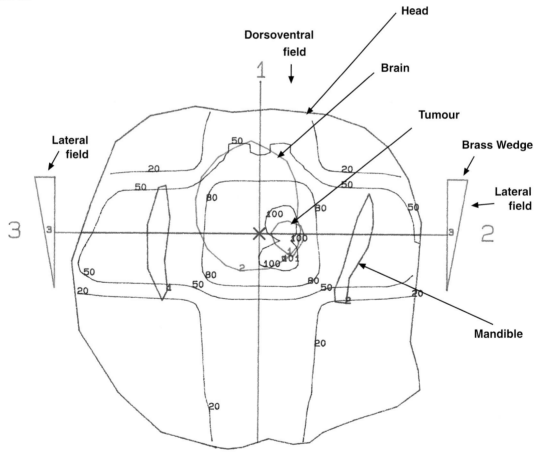

Plate 28 Computer generated treatment plan for a dog with a brain tumour. An MRI scan is digitised into the computer to provide a scaled line drawing of the outline of the dog's head (blue line) and mandibles (blue), the brain (outer red) and the tumour (inner red). The computer predicts the radiation dose deposition, shown as isodose contours (black lines; figures indicate percentage applied radiation dose) based on an isocentric treatment using three portals: dorsoventral and right and left lateral, with brass wedges (green triangles) used to attenuate the lateral beams.

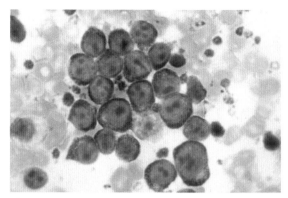

Plate 29

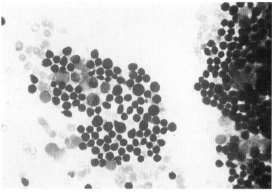

Plate 32

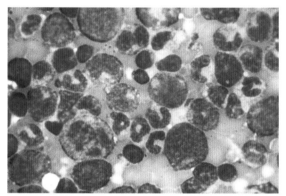

Plate 30

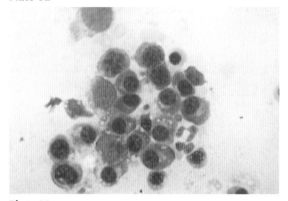

Plate 33

Plate 32 Bone marrow aspirate from dog with CLL. The marrow contains unusually high numbers of small lymphoid cells but normal erythroid and myeloid precursors are also present.

Plate 33 Bone marrow aspirate from dog with multiple myeloma, showing a cluster of plasma cells, some with secretory vacuoles in their cytoplasm.

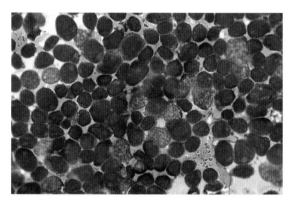

Plate 31

Plate 29 Fine needle aspirate of lymph node from dog with multicentric lymphoma. Cytology reveals a population of large, neoplastic lymphoblasts.

Plate 30 Bone marrow aspirate from dog with AML. Showing large undifferentiated myeloblasts.

Plate 31 Bone marrow aspirate from dog with ALL. The smear is dominated by medium to large lymphoblasts with very little normal erythroid or myeloid activity.

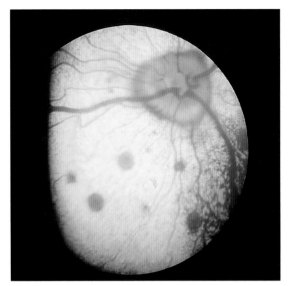

Plate 34

Plate 34 Retinal haemorrhages may be a feature of myeloma as a result of hyperviscosity or thrombocytopenia.

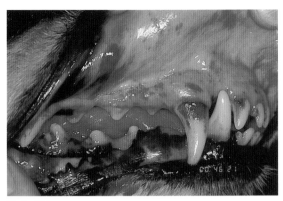

Plate 35

Plate 35 Petechiation of mucous membranes due to thrombocytopenia associated with multiple myeloma.

Pathology

Transitional cell carcinoma is the most common tumour in the proximal third of the urethra whereas squamous cell carcinoma often predominates in the distal two thirds. Often, however, carcinomas affect the whole length of the urethra and it may also be affected by direct extension of tumours from the bladder neck region.

Tumour behaviour

Urethral tumours may invade locally through the wall of the urethra or protrude into the lumen and cause urinary obstruction as they progress. Metastasis to local lymph nodes, other pelvic and abdominal organs or pelvic bones is frequently found.

Paraneoplastic syndromes

No paraneoplastic tumours are commonly associated with urethral tumours.

Presentation/signs

The clinical signs associated with urethral tumours are those of cystitis and urethritis and are often difficult to distinguish from those of bladder carcinoma. Haematuria, dysuria and pollakiuria are common although incontinence or urinary obstruction may develop later. Cases presenting with obstruction may require urinary diversion (cystostomy) while awaiting imaging and biopsy results.

Investigations

Some urethral tumours will be palpable per rectum or per vagina as a discrete, solitary mass or more diffuse swelling along the length of the urethra.

Bloods

No haematological or biochemical changes are expected with urethral tumours.

Urinalysis

Urinalysis will usually reveal haematuria and proteinuria as for bladder carcinoma and cytological examination of sediment may occasionally reveal neoplastic cells. These abnormalities will not determine whether the tumour is in the bladder or urethra, however.

Imaging techniques

Plain radiographs of the caudal abdomen may reveal some changes such as an elevated rectum, distended bladder due to urinary retention or a soft tissue mass in the region of the urethra. Retrograde urethrography or retrograde vaginourethrography, however, are necessary for a more precise diagnosis and to distinguish urethral tumours from bladder tumours. Irregularity of the urethral lumen or stricture are suggestive of neoplasia. Enlarged sublumbar lymph nodes and spinal or pelvic metastases may be noted. Chest radiographs should be performed to screen for pulmonary metastases.

Biopsy/FNA

It is important to distinguish urethral neoplasia from granulomatous urethritis which responds well to steroid therapy. Urethral tumours can often be sampled by passing a urinary catheter to the approximate location (measured on radiographs) and applying negative pressure via a syringe. Cytological examination of the aspirate should be possible or if a large piece of tissue is obtained, it can be fixed for histological examination. Alternatively, for more precise sampling, a narrow diameter endoscope can be used to visualise the tumour and biopsy it. In the bitch or queen, a Volkmann spoon can be passed into the urethral papilla and used to scrape tissue off the mucosal surface of the tumour.

Staging

There is no TNM system specifically for urethral tumours.

Treatment

Surgery

It may be possible to resect small, localised urethral tumours and anastomose the urethra but most tumours are too extensive for suitable surgical margins to be obtained. Access to the pelvic urethra is a problem and requires pubic symphysectomy. Tumours confined to the distal urethra may be managed by resection and pre-pubic urethrostomy if there is sufficient urethral length. In the male dog, distal urethral tumours may be managed by wide resection and scrotal urethrostomy. Radical resection of up to 50% of the urethra and urethral tubercle has been described, using the overlying proximal vagina to construct the urinary outflow tract. However, this only works well for benign tumours (White *et al.* 1996).

Radiotherapy

Radiotherapy of urethral tumours is not generally attempted in cats and dogs because of poor tumour response, radiation side-effects to local tissues and pelvic organs and the risk of urethral stricture.

Chemotherapy

Urethral tumours are not considered very chemosensitive and cytotoxic therapy has not been shown to be effective.

Other

Some animals may be managed on palliative antibiotic therapy to control secondary infection until urinary obstruction occurs. The anti-inflammatory drug piroxicam which has been recommended for treatment of transitional cell carcinoma of the bladder may also be of benefit for urethral tumours.

Prognosis

The prognosis for urethral tumours is poor because of their progressive nature and the difficulties associated with surgical treatment. Most animals are euthanased because of progressive symptoms and obstruction of the urethra.

References

Atlee, B.A., DeBoer, D.J., Ihrke, P.J., Stannard, A.A. & Willemse, T. (1991) Nodular dermatofibrosis in German shepherd dogs as a marker for renal cystadeno-carcinoma. *Journal of the American Animal Hospital Association*, (27), 481–7.

Chun, R., Knapp, D.W., Widmer, W.R., DeNicola, D.B. *et al.* (1997) Phase II clinical trial of carboplatin in canine transitional cell carcinoma of the urinary bladder. *Journal of Veterinary Internal Medicine*, (11), 279–83.

Crow, S.E. (1985) Urinary tract neoplasms in dogs and cats. *Compendium of Continuing Education for the Practising Veterinarian*, (7), 607–18.

Helfand, S.C., Hamilton, T.A., Hungerford, L.L., Jeglum, K.A. & Goldschmidt, M.A. (1994) Comparison of three treatments for transitional cell carcinoma of the bladder in the dog. *Journal of the American Animal Hospital Association*, (30), 270–5.

Klein, M.K., Cockerell, G.L., Harris, C.K., Withrow, S.J. *et al.* (1988) Canine primary renal neoplasms: a retrospective review of 54 cases. *Journal of the American Animal Hospital Association*, (24), 443–52.

Knapp, D.W., Richardson, R.C., Chan, T.C.K. *et al.* (1994) Piroxicam therapy in 34 dogs with transitional cell carcinoma of the urinary bladder. *Journal of Veterinary Internal Medicine*, (8), 273–8.

Moe, L. & Lium, B. (1997) Hereditary multifocal cystadenocarcinomas and nodular dermatofibrosis in 51 German shepherd dogs. *Journal of Small Animal Practice*, (38), 498–505.

Owen, L.N. (1980) TNM Classification of Tumours in Domestic Animals. World Health Organisation, Geneva.

White, R.N., Davies, J.V. & Gregory, S. (1996) Vaginourethroplasty for treatment of urethral obstruction in the bitch. *Veterinary Surgery*, (25), 503–10.

Further reading

Burnie, A.G. & Weaver, A.D. (1983) Urinary bladder neoplasia in the dog: a review of 70 cases. *Journal of Small Animal Practice*, (24), 129–43.

Cuypers, M.D., Grooters, A.M., Williams, J. & Partington, B.P. (1997) Renomegaly in dogs and cats. Part I. Differential diagnoses. *Compendium of Continuing Education for the Practising Veterinarian*, (19), 1019–32.

Lucke, V.M. & Kelly, D.F. (1976) Renal carcinoma in the dog. *Veterinary Pathology*, (13), 264–76.

Macy, D.W., Withrow, S.J. & Hoopes, J. (1983) Transitional cell carcinoma of the bladder associated with cyclophosphamide administration. *Journal of the American Animal Hospital Association*, (19), 965–9.

Magne, M.L., Hoopes, P.J., Kainer, R.A. *et al.* (1985) Urinary tract carcinomas involving the canine vagina and vestibule. *Journal of the American Animal Hospital Association*, (21), 767–72.

Mooney, S.C., Hayes, A.A., Matus, R.E. & MacEwen, E.G. (1987) Renal lymphoma in cats: 28 cases (1977–1984). *Journal of the American Veterinary Medical Association*, (191), 1473–77.

Norris, A.M., Laing, E.J., Valli, V.E.O., Withrow, S.J. *et al.* (1992) Canine bladder and urethral tumours: a retrospective study of 115 cases (1980–1985). *Journal of Veterinary Internal Medicine*, (6), 145–53.

Patnaik, A.K., Schwarz, P.D. & Greene, R.W. (1986) A histopathologic study of 20 urinary bladder neoplasms in the cat. *Journal of Small Animal Practice*, (27), 433–45.

Stone, E.A. (1985) Urogenital tumors. *Veterinary Clinics of North America*, (15), 597–608.

Tarvin, G., Patnaik, A. & Greene, R. (1978) Primary urethral tumors in dogs. *Journal of the American Veterinary Medical Association*, (172), 931–3.

Weller, R.E. & Stann, S.E. (1983) Renal lymphosarcoma in the cat. *Journal of the American Animal Hospital Association*, (19), 363–7.

11
Genital Tract

In the female dog, genital tract tumours occur most frequently in the vagina and vulva and rarely in the uterus or ovary. Vaginal and vulval tumours are usually benign and carry a good prognosis. In the cat, tumours at all sites of the female genital tract have a low incidence.

In the male dog, testicular tumours are relatively common in contrast to those of the penis, prepuce and prostate which occur more rarely. Only a minority of testicular tumours metastasise and the prognosis is therefore good. In the cat, tumours at all sites of the male genital tract are rare.

OVARY

Epidemiology

Ovarian neoplasia is uncommon in small animals due to ovariohysterectomy at an early age. It accounts for less than 1.2% and 3.6% of all neoplasms in the dog and cat respectively. Most animals are usually middle aged to old when affected but teratoma may occur in slightly younger dogs.

Aetiology

No aetiological factors are reported.

Pathology

Tumours of the ovary may arise from the surface epithelium, gonadostromal tissue (sex cord) or germ cells (Table 11.1).

Surface epithelium

Cystadenoma/adenocarcinoma, papillary adenoma/adenocarcinoma
Tumours arising from the surface cuboidal epithelium of the ovary account for 40–50% of canine ovarian tumours but are very rare in the cat. They may be unilateral or bilateral and can vary considerably in size. Both adenomas and adenocarcinomas can occur as papillary or cystic forms and transitional and undifferentiated carcinomas are also reported. Papillary adenocarcinoma gives the ovary a shaggy surface and histologically appears as multiple, branched papillae that arise multicentrically. Cystadenoma has a cystic appearance, with a variably-sized lumen containing a clear, watery, fluid.

Table 11.1 Tumours of the ovary.

Benign	Malignant
Surface epithelium	
Cystadenoma	Cystadenocarcinoma
Papillary adenoma	Papillary adenocarcinoma
Gonadostromal tissue	
Thecoma	Granulosa cell tumour
Luteoma	
Germ cell tumours	
	Dysgerminoma
Teratoma	Teratoma

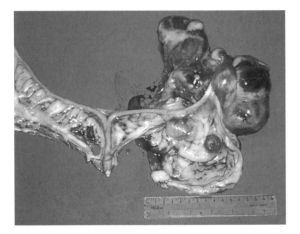

Fig. 11.1 Granulosa cell tumour of the ovary, post mortem. (Courtesy of Mr A. Jefferies Department of Clinical Veterinary Medicine, University of Cambridge.)

Gonadostromal tissue

Granulosa cell tumour

This gonadostromal tumour is derived from the outer layer of cells (granulosa cells) around the tertiary follicle. It accounts for approximately 50% of canine ovarian tumours and is the most common ovarian tumour in the cat. It is usually unilateral, spherical, firm and smooth surfaced, and can have solid and polycystic areas (Fig. 11.1). Some may reach considerable diameter. Histologically, the tumour appearance can be variable but the most common appearance in the dog and cat is of a well differentiated, uniform population of small cells around a pink or clear fluid.

Other gonadostromal tumours

Thecomas are derived from the fibrous collagen theca around the tertiary follicle and luteomas are derived from granulosa cells which have become luteal cells. Both are extremely rare, benign tumours which grow by expansion and do not metastasise.

Germ cell tumours

Dysgerminoma

This tumour arises from undifferentiated germ cells and is uncommon in the dog and cat. It is analogous to the seminoma and resembles it histologically as cords or sheets of undifferentiated cells, scattered with giant cells and histiocytes. Tumours are often large, soft masses with a smooth, lobulated surface.

Teratoma

This is rare in the dog and cat. It is often well differentiated and benign although malignant teratomas have been described in both species.

Tumour behaviour

Cystadenocarcinoma/papillary adenocarcinoma

Surface epithelial carcinomas often metastasise to renal or para-aortic lymph nodes, omentum, liver or lungs and can seed throughout the peritoneal cavity. They may cause peritoneal effusion due to lymphatic obstruction in the diaphragm or by fluid production from the tumour tissue. Pleural effusion may also occur.

Granulosa cell tumour

Although most granulosa cell tumours are considered benign, approximately 20% in the dog and up to 50% in the cat are malignant. Metastases are detected in the sublumbar lymph nodes, abdominal organs and lungs although peritoneal seeding is also possible.

Dysgerminoma

Growth of dysgerminomas is by expansion but up to 30% of cases metastasise to regional lymph nodes and abdominal organs in the dog and cat.

Paraneoplastic syndromes

Granulosa cell tumours in the dog and cat often produce oestrogen which may cause prolonged oestrus, mammary hyperplasia, swollen vulva, bilateral alopecia, cystic endometrial hyperplasia (CEH) or pyometra. Persistently elevated oestrogen levels may potentially cause myelosuppression although this is not widely reported.

Presentation/signs

Many ovarian tumours are asymptomatic and discovered as an incidental finding at celiotomy for ovariohysterectomy, or for another reason. In other cases, animals may present with:

- Ascites (peritoneal carcinomatosis)
- Lumbar pain
- A palpable abdominal mass.

An ovarian mass is often more mobile and may be relatively low in the abdomen compared to a renal mass. Advanced tumour cases may have cachexia or general weakness and lethargy. Abnormal oestrus cycles, vaginal discharge or clinical signs associated with pyometra/cystic endometrial hyperplasia may also be noted.

Investigations

Bloods

No haematological or biochemical abnormalities are commonly reported with ovarian tumours although myelosuppression (anaemia, thrombocytopenia, neutropenia) is a potential problem if a granulosa cell tumour produces persistently elevated oestrogen levels.

Imaging techniques

A soft tissue mass adjacent to the kidney may be obvious on plain radiography although it may be obscured by peritoneal effusion. Calcification of the mass may be noted with teratomas. Thoracic radiographs of the chest should be taken to

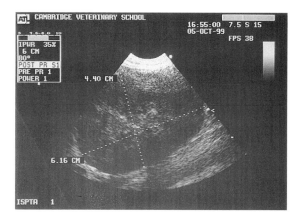

Fig. 11.2 Ultrasonogram of granulosa cell tumour of the ovary in a bitch.

screen for pulmonary metastases and to stage the tumour.

Ultrasonography may be useful to differentiate an ovarian from a renal mass and to assess its architecture (Fig. 11.2).

Abdominocentesis

If ascites is present, paracentesis usually reveals a modified transudate. Tumour cells may be detected on cytological examination of an ultra-spin sediment.

Biopsy/FNA

Ultrasound-guided fine needle aspirate or biopsy is often possible with large ovarian tumours but carries a theoretical risk of seeding malignant cells through the peritoneum. A definitive diagnosis is usually obtained by excisional biopsy (ovariectomy) at celiotomy when the rest of the abdomen can also be assessed.

Staging

A TNM staging system exists for ovarian tumours (Table 11.2) and requires clinical and surgical examination (celiotomy/laparoscopy) of the primary tumour, regional (lumbar) lymph nodes and distant sites of possible metastasis as well as radiography of the thorax.

Table 11.2 Clinical stages (TNM) of canine tumours of the ovary. Owen (1980).

T	*Primary tumour*
T0	No evidence of tumour
T1	Tumour limited to one ovary
T2	Tumours limited to both ovaries
T3	Tumour invading the ovarian bursa
T4	Tumour invading neighbouring structures
N	*Regional lymph nodes (RLN)*
N0	No evidence of RLN involvement
N1	RLN involved
M	*Distant metastasis*
M0	No evidence of distant metastasis
M1	Evidence of implantation(s) or other metastases:
M1a	In the peritoneal cavity
M1b	Beyond the peritoneal cavity
M1c	Both peritoneal cavity and beyond

Treatment

Surgery

Ovariectomy is the treatment of choice for ovarian tumours. In most cases, a complete ovariohysterectomy should be performed, particularly if there is any evidence of cystic endometrial hyperplasia or pyometra. Care should be taken in a myelosuppressed patient since there is often poor haemostasis, slow wound healing and decreased resistance to infection.

Radiotherapy

Radiotherapy is not usually used for ovarian tumours since those confined to the ovary are best treated surgically.

Chemotherapy

The role of systemic chemotherapy in the treatment of malignant ovarian tumours has not been established in animals since, in most cases, surgery alone is adequate. Peritoneal lavage or systemic therapy with chemotherapeutic agents such as cisplatin is theoretically possible where seeding has occurred, but is not widely reported.

Prognosis

The prognosis for benign ovarian tumours is extremely good after ovariohysterectomy. Since most tumours in the dog are benign, the prognosis for canine ovarian tumours is better than that for feline ones. Malignant tumours carry a more guarded prognosis especially if peritoneal seeding or other distant metastasis has occurred.

UTERUS AND CERVIX

Epidemiology

Uterine tumours are rare in the dog and cat. They occur mostly in older animals.

Aetiology

There is no known aetiology for tumours of the cervix and uterus.

Pathology

Benign mesenchymal tumours such as leiomyoma, fibroma or fibroleiomyoma are most common in the dog and may affect uterus, cervix or vagina. They often develop as multiple nodules in the uterine wall and may be associated with cystic endometrial hyperplasia, follicular cysts or mammary neoplasia. In the German shepherd dog, a syndrome associating these tumours with bilateral renal cystadenocarcinomas and nodular dermatofibrosis has been reported (Atlee *et al.* 1991; Moe & Liam 1997). Malignant mesenchymal tumours of the uterus are very rare (Table 11.3) but leiomyosarcoma, fibrosarcoma and lymphoma in cats have been reported occasionally.

Endometrial carcinoma/adenocarcinoma is more common in the cat than the dog. Tumours arise from the endometrial glands, often filling the uterine lumen and expanding outwards through the uterine wall (Fig. 11.3). Histologically, cells may be multinucleated and invade the myometrium singly,

Table 11.3 Tumours of the uterus and cervix.

Benign	Malignant
Leiomyoma	Leiomyosarcoma
Fibroma	Fibrosarcoma
Fibroleiomyoma	Lymphoma
	Adenocarcinoma

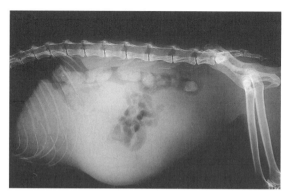

Fig. 11.4 Lateral abdominal radiograph of cat, showing grossly distended, fluid-filled loops of uterus. The animal had pyometra secondary to a uterine adenocarcinoma.

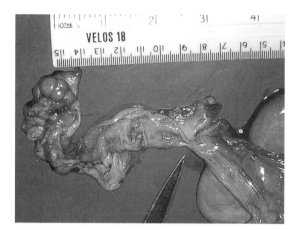

Fig. 11.3 Uterine adenocarcinoma, post mortem. (Courtesy of Mr A. Jefferies Department of Clinical Veterinary Medicine, University of Cambridge.)

in cords or in glandular formation. Squamous metaplasia may occur.

Tumour behaviour

Leiomyoma and other benign mesenchymal tumours are non-invasive, non-metastatic and slow growing. Uterine adenocarcinoma is locally invasive and metastasis is frequent, often by the time of diagnosis. Metastatic deposits may occur in lymph nodes, other abdominal organs, lung, eye or brain.

Paraneoplastic syndromes

No paraneoplastic syndromes are commonly associated with uterine tumours.

Presentation/signs

Clinical signs associated with uterine tumours are often vague and non-specific but an abdominal mass is sometimes palpable and vaginal discharge or pyometra may occasionally be noted. Increased urinary frequency may be present if the uterine body is very large and applies pressure to the bladder. Advanced cases may present with cachexia or malaise but other cases may be detected incidentally at celiotomy or post mortem examination.

Investigations

Bloods

No specific haematological or biochemical changes are commonly found with uterine tumours.

Imaging techniques

A soft tissue mass in the mid or caudal abdomen may be detected on plain abdominal radiography, or if there is an accompanying pyometra, enlarged coils of uterus may be distinguishable (Fig. 11.4).

Ultrasonography may be useful to distinguish whether an abdominal mass is derived from uterus or cervix.

Table 11.4 Clinical stages (TNM) of tumours of the uterus. Owen (1980).

T	*Primary tumour*
T0	No evidence of tumour
T1	Small non-invasive tumour
T2	Large or invasive tumour
T3	Tumour invading neighbouring structures
N	*Regional lymph nodes (RLN)*
N0	No evidence of RLN involvement
N1	Pelvic RLN involved
N2	Para-aortic RLN involved
M	*Distant metastasis*
M0	No evidence of metastasis
M1	Evidence of metastasis:
M1a	In the peritoneal cavity
M1b	Beyond the peritoneal cavity
M1c	Both peritoneal cavity and beyond

Biopsy/FNA

Ultrasound-guided fine needle aspirate may be possible although many benign mesenchymal tumours do not exfoliate well and cytological examination may be unrewarding. Ultrasound guided biopsy is another option but usually a definitive histological diagnosis is made after ovariohysterectomy and histological examination of the tissues.

Staging

A TNM staging system is available for the uterus (Table 11.4) and requires clinical and surgical examination (celiotomy/laparoscopy) of the primary tumour, regional lymph nodes and distant sites of possible metastasis as well as radiography of the thorax. The regional lymph nodes are the pelvic nodes distal to the bifurcation of the common iliac arteries and the para-aortic nodes proximal to the bifurcation of the common iliac arteries.

Treatment

Surgery

Most uterine and cervical tumours are treated successfully by ovariohysterectomy.

Radiotherapy

Radiotherapy has not been reported for use with uterine tumours.

Chemotherapy

The role of chemotherapy in treating uterine tumours has not been established.

Prognosis

The prognosis for uterine tumours in the dog is good because most are benign. The prognosis for uterine adenocarcinoma in the cat is worse because of its aggressive nature and the tendency for metastases to have occurred by the time of diagnosis.

VAGINA AND VULVA

Epidemiology

The vagina and vulva are the most common sites for reproductive tract tumours in the dog (excluding the mammary gland). Entire, aged dogs (mean age 10–11 years), particularly nulliparous animals, are at risk of benign mesenchymal tumours, whereas lipoma affects a slightly younger age group (mean age six years). Transmissible venereal tumour also affects younger, sexually active or breeding females. In the cat, vaginal and vulval tumours are rare but older, intact animals have been affected.

Aetiology

There is an association between benign smooth muscle tumours and oestrogen production in the dog. Such tumours rarely occur in spayed animals unless they have received oestrogen therapy for some reason.

Pathology

Benign smooth muscle tumours account for 80–90% of vaginal and vulval tumours in the dog

Table 11.5 Tumours of the vagina and vulva.

Benign	Malignant
Leiomyoma	Leiomyosarcoma
Fibroma	Transmissible venereal tumour
Fibroleiomyoma	Adenocarcinoma
Lipoma	Squamous cell carcinoma
	Haemangiosarcoma
	Osteosarcoma
	Mast cell tumour

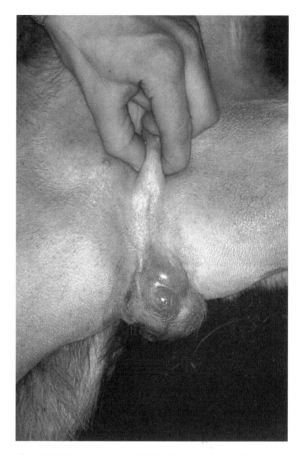

Fig. 11.5 An aggressive SCC of the vulva with metastasis to the inguinal lymph node. (Courtesy of Dr R.A.S. White, Department of Clinical Veterinary Medicine, University of Cambridge.)

and have also been reported in the cat (Table 11.5). Most are situated in the vestibule and may present in one of two ways:

• Extraluminal forms are well encapsulated and poorly vascularised.
• Intraluminal forms are often firm and ovoid, attached to the vestibular or vaginal wall by a thin pedicle. These may be multiple and may ulcerate.

Concurrent mammary gland tumours, ovarian cysts and cystic endometrial hyperplasia may occur with either form. Lipomas arise from the perivascular and perivaginal fat and lie within the pelvis. They are usually slow growing and well circumscribed.

Leiomyosarcoma is the most common malignant tumour of the vagina and vulva although other sarcomas, carcinomas and transmissible venereal tumour have also been reported (Table 11.5). Any type of cutaneous tumours, particularly squamous cell carcinoma and mast cell tumour, may also occur at the vulval labia (Fig. 11.5).

Tumour behaviour

Most mesenchymal tumours of the vagina and vulva are benign, well circumscribed and slow growing. Distant metastases have been reported with leiomyosarcoma.

Paraneoplastic syndromes

No paraneoplastic syndromes are commonly associated with these tumours.

Presentation/signs

Extraluminal tumours present as slow growing perineal masses (Fig. 11.6) whereas intraluminal forms may present as polyps protruding through the vulval lips especially when the animal strains or is in oestrus. These masses may become traumatised and secondarily infected. Other signs may include vulval bleeding or discharge, tenesmus, vulval licking, haematuria, dysuria or even urinary obstruction. In some cases a vulval mass may be noted. In the cat, constipation secondary to compression of the colon has been reported.

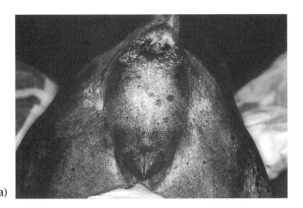

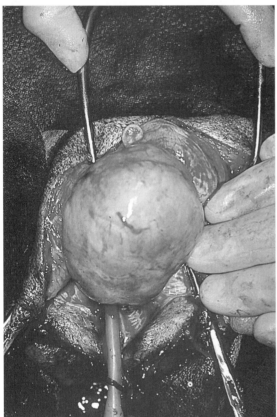

Fig. 11.6 (a) Perineal swelling in a bitch due to a large vaginal fibroma; (b) seen delivered at surgery via an episiotomy. (Courtesy of Dr R. A. S. White, Department of Clinical Veterinary Medicine, University of Cambridge.)

Investigations

Clinical presentation combined with the age of the animal may be sufficient for a preliminary diagnosis. Masses are often palpable per vagina or per rectum.

Bloods

No specific haematological or biochemical changes are commonly associated with these tumours.

Imaging techniques

These are rarely needed but retrograde vaginography or urethrocystography may help to delineate a vaginal mass. Plain caudal abdominal radiography may be useful if the mass extends cranially or to examine sublumbar lymph nodes if malignancy is suspected. Elevation or compression of the rectum, cranioventral displacement of the bladder, and faecal or urinary retention may also be seen on plain films. Thoracic films should be taken for malignant tumours, although these are rare.

Biopsy/FNA

Definitive diagnosis can only be made on histological examination of excised tissue either at biopsy or on complete excision of the tumour.

Chromosome analysis

(See penis/prepuce tumours)

Staging

A TNM staging system is available for vaginal and vulval tumours (Table 11.6) and requires clinical and surgical examination of each category as well as radiography of the thorax. The regional lymph nodes are the superficial inguinal, sacral and internal iliac nodes.

Treatment

Surgery

Surgical resection is the treatment of choice for vaginal and vulval tumours but care should be

Table 11.6 Clinical stages (TNM) of canine tumours of the vagina and vulva. Owen (1980).

T   *Primary tumour*
(add 'm' to the appropriate T category for multiple tumours)
T0   No evidence of tumour
T1   Tumour <1 cm maximum diameter, superficial
T2   Tumour 1–3 cm maximum diameter, with minimal invasion
T3   Tumour >3 cm *or* every tumour with deep invasion
T4   Tumour invading neighbouring structures (skin, perineum, urethra, paravaginal wall, anal canal)

N   *Regional lymph nodes (RLN)*
N0   No evidence of RLN involvement
N1   Movable ipsilateral nodes
N2   Movable bilateral nodes
N3   Fixed nodes

M   *Distant metastasis*
M0   No evidence of metastasis
M1   Distant metastasis detected

taken to identify and preserve the urethral papilla. Most benign mesenchymal tumours are well encapsulated and easily excised but because of the strong association of most tumours with oestrogen production, resection should be combined with ovariohysterectomy to prevent tumour recurrence. A dorsal episiotomy may be needed to access extraluminal tumours. Vaginal carcinomas may be harder to excise surgically because they are rarely as well circumscribed as benign mesenchymal tumours.

Radiotherapy

Post-operative radiotherapy may be appropriate for some vulval carcinomas or mast cell tumours where complete surgical resection has not been possible. Transmissible venereal tumour is also radiosensitive and can be treated successfully with relatively low doses of radiation (15 Gy) if only superficial lesions are present.

Chemotherapy

Chemotherapy is not usually used for the common benign tumours nor for the rarer carcinomas. Transmissible venereal tumour, however, is amenable to weekly therapy with vincristine sulphate (0.5 mg/m^2 q 7 days) with complete responses obtainable in four to six weeks.

Prognosis

Since most vaginal and vulval tumours are benign, surgical resection combined with ovariohysterectomy carries a good prognosis. Malignant tumours such as adenocarcinoma and squamous cell carcinoma carry a poor prognosis because of local recurrence and metastasis.

TESTICLE

Epidemiology

Testicular tumours are the second most common tumours of the male dog and account for 75% of all tumours in the male reproductive tract (Hayes & Pendergrass 1976). Older, intact males (mean 11.5 years) commonly develop interstitial cell tumours in the descended testicle. Cryptorchids have a much greater risk of developing Sertoli cell tumours and seminomas than normal dogs and the average age of affected animals is younger (9 years for Sertoli cell tumours, 10 years seminomas). The right testicle is more often affected than the left (Lipowitz *et al.* 1973). Testicular tumours are rare in the cat and cryptorchidism does not appear to be a risk factor (Mills *et al.* 1992).

Aetiology

Abdominal or inguinal positioning of the testis is important in the development of half of Sertoli cell tumours and two thirds of seminomas in the dog. The higher temperature of the abdomen destroys spermatogenic cells and this may allow Sertoli cells to develop.

Pathology

Testicular tumours can be categorised as gonadostromal (Sertoli and Leydig), or germ cell (seminoma, teratoma). The histological types are listed in Table 11.7.

Table 11.7 Tumours of the testis.

Benign	Malignant
Gonadostromal tissue	
Interstitial cell (Leydig) tumour	Sertoli cell tumour
Germ cell tumours	
Teratoma	Seminoma

Gonadostromal tissue

Interstitial cell tumour/Leydig cell tumour

These arise from the endocrine Leydig cells of the testis. Histologically, tumour cells have foamy cytoplasm, and are sometimes associated with haemorrhage, necrosis or cysts. Grossly, tumours are often encapsulated, remain within the testicle and may be pink to tan in colour. They are usually the smallest, softest tumours to palpate and can be solitary or multiple within the same or the opposite testis. The affected testicle may be enlarged or normal in size.

Sertoli cell tumour

These arise from the Sertoli cells of the testis which supply the nutrients for spermatogenesis. Pallisading rows of elongated Sertoli cells accompanied by fibrous connective tissue are seen histologically. Tumours with the cells arranged in well formed tubules tend to be less malignant than those with more infiltrative cells, arranged in a more diffuse pattern. Grossly they are usually unilateral, often firm and white, with cysts (filled with brown fluid) and fibrous septa enlarging the testis (Fig. 11.7).

Germ cell tumours

Seminoma

Seminomas arise from the primitive gonadal cells of the testis and may appear histologically very similar to dysgerminomas of the ovary. Initially the tumour cells, which are often large and multinucleated, develop within atrophic seminiferous tubules, but later they invade the interstitial stroma and appear more diffuse. Grossly, tumours are usually firm, unencapsulated, lobulated and white to pink-grey in colour.

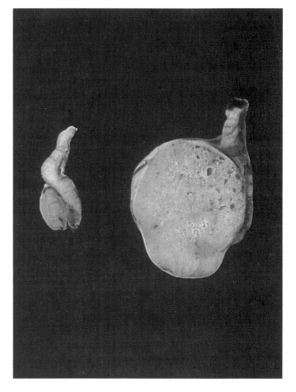

Fig. 11.7 Post mortem picture of a Sertoli cell tumour; the other testicle is atrophied. (Courtesy of Dr P. Nicholls.)

Teratoma

Teratomas are rare in the dog and cat and are almost always benign compared to those in man. They comprise multiple tissues derived from different germ layers and may contain epithelium, bone, cartilage or brain.

Tumour behaviour

Interstitial cell (Leydig) tumours are the most benign testicular neoplasms and do not usually metastasise. Although most Sertoli cell tumours are slow growing and benign, up to 15% of tumours may be malignant and metastasise. Metastasis is usually via the lymphatics to regional lymph nodes, although distant spread to abdominal organs is also reported. A smaller proportion of seminomas are malignant with between 5 and 10% reported to metastasise.

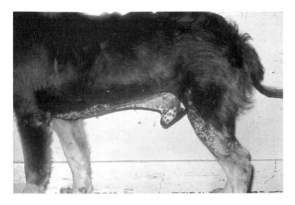

Fig. 11.8 Dog with alopecia and coat changes due to hyperoestrogenism from a Sertoli cell tumour causing feminisation syndrome. (Courtesy of Mr D. Bostock.)

Paraneoplastic syndromes

Sertoli cell tumours may produce oestrogen which causes a feminisation syndrome (Fig. 11.8). Signs may include:

- Bilaterally symmetrical alopecia
- Gynaecomastia
- Pendulous prepuce
- Attractiveness to other male dogs
- Atrophy of the other testis
- Myelosuppression (anaemia, neutropenia and thrombocytopenia).

Any metastases which are present can be secretory and therefore castration to remove the primary tumour may not remove the feminisation signs. Seminomas have also been associated with a feminisation syndrome but much less frequently.

Interstitial (Leydig) cells secrete male hormones in the normal male, but the tumours derived from these cells do not show autonomous secretion. They are often associated with peri-anal adenoma and perineal hernia but these conditions are common in normal male dogs. Hypercalcaemia, however, has been reported as a paraneoplastic syndrome associated with interstitial cell tumours.

Presentation/signs

Affected animals may present with testicles of uneven size or an obvious testicular mass, although many testicular tumours are an incidental finding on clinical examination or at post mortem examination. In cryptorchid dogs, particularly if the descended testicle has been removed, diagnosis may be difficult unless a feminisation syndrome occurs. In this case:

- Bilaterally symmetrical alopecia and possibly pruritus
- Attractiveness to other male dogs
- Lethargy or decreased libido.

may alert the clinician to the possibility of an abdominal testicular tumour. Oestrogen myelotoxicosis may present as a non-regenerative anaemia, thrombocytopenia or neutropenia. Very occasionally, signs of hypercalcaemia such as muscle tremors, weakness, polyuria and polydipsia may be noted with testicular tumours, particularly interstitial cell tumours.

Investigations

Palpation of the testes is usually sufficient to make a presumptive diagnosis of neoplasia, although a definitive diagnosis will require histological analysis of tissue.

Bloods

Unless there are clinical signs of feminisation, blood samples are of limited use. If feminisation is present, plasma concentrations of oestradiol and occasionally progesterone are generally elevated whereas testosterone is low. If increased oestrogen secretion is suspected, haematological assessment is vital to reveal the extent of myelosuppression present. Platelet and neutrophil numbers can fall particularly low, carrying a risk of spontaneous haemorrhage or sepsis.

Imaging techniques

Ultrasonography may help to define the number or extent of testicular lesions but is rarely necessary for a diagnosis. Abdominal radiographs may identify a retained testicle.

Biopsy/FNA

Cytological analysis of a fine needle aspirate may distinguish between the different tumour types but

Table 11.8 Clinical stages (TNM) of canine tumours of the testis. Owen (1980).

T   *Primary tumour*
(add 'm' to the appropriate T category for multiple tumours)
T0   No evidence of tumour
T1   Tumour restricted to the testis
T2   Tumour invading the tunica albuginea
T3   Tumour invading the rete testis and/or the epididymis
T4   Tumour invading the spermatic cord and/or the scrotum

N   *Regional lymph nodes (RLN)*
N0   No evidence of RLN involvement
N1   Ipsilateral RLN involved
N2   Contralateral or bilateral RLN involved

M   *Distant metastasis*
M0   No evidence of metastasis
M1   Distant metastasis detected

this is not usually necessary and a definitive diagnosis is made after castration and histological examination of the tumour tissue. Cytological examination of bone marrow aspirates may be indicated for cases of suspected myelosuppression.

Staging

A TNM staging system is available for testicular tumours (Table 11.8) and requires clinical and surgical examination of primary tumour, regional (sublumbar, inguinal) lymph nodes and sites of distant metastasis, in addition to radiography of the thorax.

Treatment

Surgery

Removal of the primary tumour by castration is usually curative except for the minority of cases which may have metastasised. For scrotal tumours, castration is routine, although cryptorchids will require inguinal or abdominal exploration to locate the retained testicle and tumour. The clinical signs associated with oestrogen production will usually resolve within six weeks after removal of the primary tumour unless metastatic tissue is also present.

Radiotherapy

Radiotherapy is not necessary for testicular tumours since surgical treatment is so effective.

Chemotherapy

Chemotherapy is of limited use for testicular tumours in animals. Although theoretically applicable for tumours which have metastasised, no reports have demonstrated its effectiveness.

Other

For cases with severe myelosuppression due to oestrogen secretion, supportive measures such as broad spectrum antibiotic therapy, platelet infusion or whole blood transfusion may be necessary prior to castration.

Prognosis

The prognosis for most testicular tumours is good since surgical treatment is relatively easy and only a minority of tumours metastasise. If, however, the feminisation signs are not quickly linked to oestrogen secretion from a testicular tumour and myelosuppression is allowed to become severe, fatalities may arise.

PENIS AND PREPUCE

Epidemiology

Penile and preputial tumours are rare except in parts of the world affected by transmissible venereal tumour, namely the Mediterranean countries, south-east USA and the Caribbean. While most tumours are more common in older dogs, transmissible venereal tumour occurs in younger, sexually active dogs, stud dogs or the stray population. Males are often less affected than females.

Aetiology

No aetiology is known for most tumours of the penis and prepuce but transmissible venereal tumour is transmitted by transplantation of cells at coitus. Although a viral aetiology has been proposed, viral particles have only been inconsistently reported on electron microscopy, and the theory has not been unequivocally substantiated.

Pathology

The histological types of tumour occuring on the penis or prepuce are listed in Table 11.9. Squamous cell carcinoma is the most common tumour of the penis of dogs in the UK but papillomas may also occur. Transmissible venereal tumour (TVT) is the predominant tumour type in areas of the world in which it is enzootic. Squamous cell carcinoma occurs as an ulcerated, sessile region of the glans penis or inner lining of the prepuce although it can also more rarely produce a cauliflower-like growth. TVT also produces pedunculated, vegetative, papillary or nodular lesions of the glans or more caudal penis. Histologically ovoid or round cells appear in compact sheets, cords or rows and are scattered with inflammatory cells such as lymphocytes, plasma cells and macrophages.

The prepuce and scrotum may be affected by any skin tumours, but tumours commonly located in this region are mast cell tumours, melanomas and peri-anal gland hepatomas (see Chapter 4).

Table 11.9 Tumours of the penis and prepuce.

Benign	Malignant
Penis	
Papilloma	Squamous cell carcinoma
	Transmissible venereal tumour
Prepuce and scrotum	
Peri-anal gland	
hepatoma	Mast cell tumour

Tumour behaviour

Squamous cell carcinoma of the penis is locally invasive and may spread to the inguinal lymph nodes as well as distant sites if left untreated.

Transmissible venereal tumour does not commonly metastasise but may be transplanted to other areas of the skin, face or nose by trauma and licking. Metastasis to inguinal lymph nodes and abdominal organs does occur infrequently. Since an immune response to the tumour does occur in time, growth usually slows down as this develops and tumour regression may be seen eventually.

Mast cell tumours of the prepuce and scrotum often occur multiply and behave very aggressively, spreading to the inguinal lymph nodes or more distantly even if histologically they do not appear undifferentiated. Local oedema and erythema are common due to mast cell degranulation and may extend down the hind limbs with enlargement of the inguinal lymph nodes due to metastasis.

Paraneoplastic syndromes

Mast cell tumours may be associated with hyper-histaminaemia (see Chapter 2).

Presentation/signs

Tumours of the penis may bleed or become secondarily affected. Clinical signs may include:

- Preputial discharge
- Licking of the region
- Dysuria
- Frank blood in the urine
- Phimosis or paraphimosis (occasionally).

An obvious lesion is not usually apparent unless the penis is fully extruded (Fig. 11.9). Skin tumours of the external prepuce or scrotum are often obvious as discrete masses although mast cell tumours may present with diffuse, inguinal swelling, oedema and erythema and no distinct tumour mass.

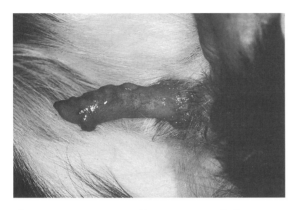

Fig. 11.9 Squamous cell carcinoma of the penis. (Courtesy of Dr R.A.S. White, Department of Clinical Veterinary Medicine, University of Cambridge.)

Table 11.10 Clinical stages (TNM) of canine tumours of the penis (prepuce and glans). Owen (1980).

T   *Primary tumour*
(add 'm' to the appropriate T category for multiple tumours)
T0   No evidence of tumour
T1   Tumour <1 cm maximum diameter, strictly superficial
T2   Tumour 1–3 cm maximum diameter, with minimal invasion
T3   Tumour >3 cm *or* every tumour with deep invasion
T4   Tumour invading neighbouring structures

N   *Regional lymph nodes (RLN)*
N0   No evidence of RLN involvement
N1   Movable ipsilateral nodes
N2   Movable bilateral nodes
N3   Fixed nodes

M   *Distant metastasis*
M0   No evidence of metastasis
M1   Distant metastasis detected

Investigations

Bloods

No specific haematological or biochemical changes are associated with tumours of the prepuce and penis.

Imaging techniques

Imaging techniques are not usually required for these tumours.

Biopsy/FNA

Direct impression smears may be made from ulcerated penile lesions for cytological examination. Alternatively, a small incisional or grab biopsy may be possible. Fine needle aspirates of enlarged inguinal lymph nodes may be helpful in revealing the tumour type if metastasis has occurred and are essential for staging the disease.

Chromosome analysis

Transmissible venereal tumour is characterised by a modal chromosome number of 59 ± 5 instead of the usual 78 seen in normal canine cells (Murray *et al.* 1969). Karyotypic analysis of tumour cells can therefore be used to confirm the diagnosis.

Staging

Tumours of the penis and prepuce can be staged using a TNM staging system (Table 11.10) which involves clinical and surgical examination of all three categories, as well as radiography of the thorax. The regional lymph nodes are the superficial inguinal nodes. A separate staging system is applicable to mast cell tumours of the prepuce or inguinal region (Chapter 4).

Treatment

Surgery

Penile tumours are rarely treated by local surgical excision and penile amputation is usually the recommended option even for early lesions. If the amputation is performed cranial to the bulb, the sheath is left intact but more radical amputation cranial to the scrotum will require a scrotal urethrostomy, castration, scrotal and preputial ablation. Radical surgery is not usually necessary, however, for transmissible venereal tumour.

Treatment of preputial mast cell tumours and melanomas may be attempted but complete surgical excision is rarely possible and metastasis remains a common problem.

Radiotherapy

Radiotherapy is not usually used for squamous cell carcinoma of the penis or preputial tumours. TVT, however, is radiosensitive and will regress in response to relatively low doses (15 Gy).

Chemotherapy

Chemotherapy is not appropriate for squamous cell carcinoma of the penis but TVT will respond well to vincristine therapy. Complete regression will occur with weekly doses of vincristine sulphate at $0.5\,mg/m^2$ q 7 days for a course of four to six weeks.

Poorly differentiated mast cell tumours of the prepuce may be palliated by chemotherapy with prednisolone and/or other cytotoxic drugs (Chapter 4).

Prognosis

The prognosis for squamous cell carcinoma of the penis is favourable if amputation can be performed, although local and distant metastasis may still develop. TVT carries an extremely good prognosis since the response to chemotherapy is usually dramatic. Mast cell tumours of the preputial skin have a very poor prognosis because of their aggressive and malignant nature.

PROSTATE

Epidemiology

Prostatic neoplasia is much less common than hyperplasia in dogs and is extremely rare in cats. Affected dogs are usually old (mean age 10 years) and of medium or large breeds.

Aetiology

Prostatic carcinoma develops independently of hormonal status and occurs in both castrated and entire dogs. This is in contrast to human prostatic carcinoma which is androgen dependent.

Pathology

The most common prostatic tumour is the adenocarcinoma or undifferentiated carcinoma although transitional cell carcinoma and squamous cell carcinoma have also been reported (Table 11.11). Leiomyosarcoma and benign mesenchymal tumours such as leiomyoma and fibroma are rare. Tumours of other pelvic organs may sometimes extend locally to invade the prostate.

Prostatic adenocarcinoma develops from the branching tubuloalveolar glands of the prostate. The prostate is usually enlarged, hard, irregularly nodular and asymmetrical although it may be cystic, haemorrhagic or abscessated and may

adhere to other pelvic structures. Histologically, papillary projections of glandular epithelium are seen within large, irregular alveoli or variably sized acini surrounded by dense, fibrous stroma.

Undifferentiated carcinoma occurs less commonly and consists of scattered carcinoma cells, or cells arranged in solid clusters, strands or syncytia.

Tumour behaviour

Prostatic adenocarcinoma is very invasive locally and may extend to other pelvic organs such as bladder, colon and urethra. It is very malignant and metastasises quickly to sublumbar lymph nodes, abdominal organs and lungs, as well as to the lumbar vertebrae, pelvis and other bones. Approximately 70% of cases will have metastasised by the time of diagnosis.

Table 11.11 Tumours of the prostate.

Benign	Malignant
Leiomyoma	Adenocarcinoma
Fibroma	Undifferentiated carcinoma
	Squamous cell carcinoma
	Transitional cell carcinoma
	Leiomyosarcoma

Paraneoplastic syndromes

No paraneoplastic syndromes are commonly associated with these tumours.

Presentation/signs

Prostatic neoplasia often presents with lower urinary signs such as:

- Haematuria
- Dysuria
- Purulent, penile discharge
- Faecal tenesmus, ribbon-like faeces or constipation (due to constriction of the rectum).

Metastatic lesions to the pelvic bones or spine may be painful and cause hindlimb weakness, lameness or neurological deficits. Although prostatic hyperplasia may also put pressure on the rectum and produce similar faecal signs, it rarely causes urinary signs or pain. An enlarged, painful prostate may be palpable in the caudal abdomen, along with enlarged sublumbar lymph nodes, or alternatively an irregular or enlarged prostate may be palpated per rectum.

Investigations

Rectal examination

A uniform, non-painful enlargement of the prostate is more likely to indicate hyperplasia than neoplasia. Prostatic carcinoma usually produces irregular, asymmetrical, painful enlargement due to secondary abscessation. However, primary prostatic abscesses and paraprostatic cysts may also produce asymmetrical enlargement. Underlying neoplasia may be associated with both these conditions and so the prostate should always be biopsied for a definitive diagnosis. Enlarged sublumbar lymph nodes, common with prostatic neoplasia, may also be palpable per rectum.

Bloods

Haematological and biochemical changes are occasionally associated with prostatic tumours. Renal failure secondary to urinary obstruction may be detected, along with regenerative and non-regenerative anaemia, elevated alkaline phosphatase and ALT, hypoalbuminaemia and hypocalcaemia.

Imaging techniques

The prostate may vary in size on plain abdominal films from normal to grossly enlarged. Although prostatic neoplasia may produce asymmetrical enlargement around the bladder neck, prostatomegaly is not necessarily present. Enlarged sublumbar lymph nodes, lytic or sclerotic bone lesions in the vertebrae or pelvis or pulmonary metastases on thoracic films will help to distinguish prostatic neoplasia from other prostatic conditions (Figs. 11.10 and 11.11). A pneumocystogram or retrograde urethrogram may help to demonstrate cranial displacement of the bladder due to prostatic enlargement, stenosis or irregularity of the urethra in the prostatic region or extravasation of contrast into irregular prostatic crypts.

Ultrasonography will demonstrate changes in the prostatic parenchyma but these are not always distinguishable from other types of prostatic pathology such as prostatitis, abscessation or cystic hyperplasia.

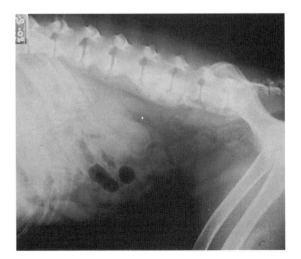

Fig. 11.10 Lateral abdominal radiograph of a dog with a prostatic carcinoma – although the prostate is not grossly enlarged, the tumour has spread locally causing bony changes in the lumbar vertebrae.

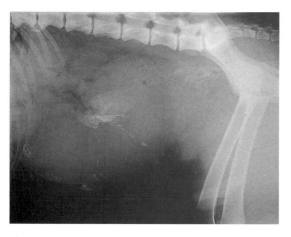

Fig. 11.11 Paraprostatic cysts are a differential diagnosis for caudal abdominal masses in male dogs.

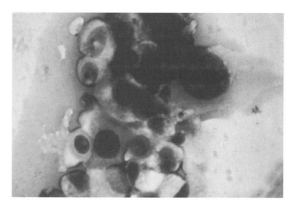

Fig. 11.12 Fine needle aspirate cytology of prostatic adenocarcinoma. (Courtesy of Mrs E. Villiers, Department of Clinical Veterinary Medicine, University of Cambridge.)

Biopsy/FNA

Cytological examination (Fig. 11.2) can be performed on urethral washings obtained by inserting a catheter into the prostatic urethra, inserting a small volume of saline and massaging the prostate per rectum to aid release of cells or by applying negative pressure with a syringe to the catheter to suck in a small tissue sample. Fine needle aspirates or needle biopsies may also be performed through the abdominal wall in the inguinal region if the prostate is palpable and can be fixed, or ultrasound guidance can be used. If the prostate is palpable in the pelvic canal, the needle may have to be inserted through the perineum, although a per rectal technique has also been used. Alternatively, an endoscopic biopsy may be possible with a narrow diameter, flexible endoscope. If none of these methods are successful, an incisional biopsy can be performed at celiotomy (Fig. 11.12).

Staging

There is a TNM staging system specific to the prostate (Table 11.12) which requires clinical and surgical examination, urography, endoscopy and biopsy as well as radiography of the thorax, pelvis and skeleton. The regional lymph nodes are the external and internal iliac nodes.

Table 11.12 Clinical stages (TNM) of canine tumours of the prostate. Owen (1980).

T	*Primary tumour*
T0	No evidence of tumour
T1	Intracapsular tumour, surrounded by normal gland
T2	Diffuse intracapsular tumour
T3	Tumour extending beyond the capsule
T3	Tumour fixed or invading neighbouring structures
N	*Regional lymph nodes (RLN)*
N0	No evidence of RLN involvement
N1	RLN involved
N2	RLN and juxta RLN (lumbar) involved
M	*Distant metastasis*
M0	No evidence of distant metastasis
M1	Distant metastasis detected

Treatment

Surgery

Most prostatic carcinomas are not amenable to successful surgical resection because of their invasive nature and frequent metastasis by the time of diagnosis. Complete resection of the prostate with anastomosis of the urethra has been described but is not compatible with good quality life or urinary continence and is therefore not recommended.

Radiotherapy

Palliative external beam radiotherapy has been used intra-operatively for localised prostatic tumours but with limited sucess (Turrel 1987).

Chemotherapy

Cytotoxic drugs are not usually recommended for the treatment of prostatic neoplasia.

Other

Most prostatic tumours develop independently of hormonal stimulation and appear not to respond to castration or hormonal therapy with anti-androgens.

Prognosis

The prognosis for prostatic tumours is grave because of the lack of surgical options, their highly malignant characteristics and the tendency for early metastasis by the time of diagnosis.

References

Atlee, B.A., DeBoer, D.J., Ihrke, P.J., Stannard, A.A. & Willemse, T. (1991) Nodular dermatofibrosis in German shepherd dogs as a marker for renal cystadenocarcinoma. *Journal of the American Animal Hospital Association*, (27), 481–7.

Hayes, H.M. & Pendergrass, T.W. (1976) Canine testicular tumors: epidemiologic features of 410 dogs. *International Journal of Cancer*, (18), 482–7.

Lipowitz, A.J., Schwartz, A. *et al.* (1973) Testicular neoplasms and concomitant clinical changes in the dog. *Journal of the American Veterinary Medical Association*, 163, 1364–8.

Mills, D.L., Hauptman, J.G. & Johnson, C.A. (1992) Cryptorchidism and monorchism in cats: 25 cases (1980–1989). *Journal of the American Veterinary Medical Association*, (200), 1128–30.

Moe, L. & Lium, B. (1997) Hereditary multifocal cystadenocarcinomas and nodular dermatofibrosis in 51 German shepherd dogs. *Journal of Small Animal Practice*, (38), 498–505.

Murray, M., James, H. & Martin, W.J. (1969) A study of the cytology and karyotype of the canine transmissible venereal tumor. *Research in Veterinary Science*, (10), 565–8.

Owen, L.N. (1980) TNM Classification of Tumours in Domestic Animals. World Health Organisation, Geneva.

Turrel, J.M. (1987) Intraoperative radiotherapy of carcinoma of the prostate gland in ten dogs. *Journal of the American Veterinary Medical Association*, (190), 48–52.

Further reading

Baldwin, C.J., Roszel, J.F. & Clark, T.P. (1992) Uterine adenocarcinoma in dogs. *Compendium of Continuing Education for the Practising Veterinarian*, (14), 731–7.

Bell, F.W., Klausner, J.S., Hayden, D.W. *et al.* (1991) Clinical and pathologic features of prostatic adenocarcinoma in sexually intact and castrated dogs: 31 cases (1970–1987). *Journal of the American Veterinary Medical Association*, (199), 1623–30.

Brodey, R.S. & Roszel, J.F. (1967) Neoplasms of the canine uterus, vagina, vulva. A clinicopathologic survey of 90 cases. *Journal of the American Veterinary Medical Association*, (151), 1294–1307.

Caney, S.M.A., Holt, P.E., Day, M.J., Rudorf, H. & Gruffdd-Jones, T.J. (1998) Prostatic neoplasia in two cats. *Journal of Small Animal Practice*, (39), 140–43.

Gelberg, H.B. & McEntee, K. (1985) Feline ovarian neoplasms. *Veterinary Pathology*, (22), 572–6.

Hargis, A.M. & Miller, L.M. (1983) Prostatic carcinoma in dogs. *Compendium of Continuing Education for the Practising Veterinarian*, (5), 647–53.

Herron, M.A. (1983) Tumors of the canine genital system. *Journal of the American Animal Hospital Association*, (19), 981–94.

Kydd, D.M. & Burnie, A.G. (1986) Vaginal neoplasia in the bitch: a review of 40 clinical cases. *Journal of Small Animal Practice*, (27), 255–63.

Patnaik, A.K. & Greenlee, P.G. (1987) Canine ovarian neoplasms: a clinicopathologic study of 71 cases, including histology of 12 granulosa cell tumours. *Veterinary Pathology*, (24), 509–14.

Richardson, R.C. (1981) Canine transmissible venereal tumors. *Compendium of Continuing Education for the Practising Veterinarian*, (31), 951–6.

Stein, B.S. (1981) Tumors of the female genital tract. *Journal of the American Animal Hospital Association*, (17), 1022–5.

Thatcher, C. & Bradley, R.L. (1983) Vulvar and vaginal tumors in the dog. *Journal of the American Veterinary Medical Association*, (183), 690–92.

Weaver, A.D. (1981) Fifteen cases of prostatic adenocarcinoma in the dog. *Veterinary Record*, (109), 71–5.

12
Mammary Gland

Mammary tumours are very common in both the dog and cat. A wide variety of histological types occur in the dog, although at least half are benign. In the cat, most tumours are malignant and very aggressive.

Epidemiology

Mammary tumours are the second most common tumours in all dogs and the commonest tumours in the bitch. They occur in older animals (mean 10 years), usually those that are entire or have been spayed after numerous seasons. All breeds may be affected.

In the cat, mammary tumours occur less frequently but are still the third most common type of all tumours. Old (mean 10–12 years), entire animals are usually affected and Siamese cats may be more at risk than other breeds.

Aetiology

The production of the female hormones, oestrogen and progesterone, is linked to the development of mammary tumours in both dogs and cats. The relative risk of developing a mammary tumour is related to the number of oestrus cycles a dog has experienced. The risks for spaying prior to first oestrus, after first oestrus or after second oestrus are 0.05%, 8% and 26% respectively (Schneider et al. 1969). In entire cats, there is a seven-fold increased risk of mammary tumours compared to those spayed at puberty (Dorn et al. 1968). Both oestrogen and/or progesterone receptors are present in 40–70% of canine mammary tumours

although at lower concentrations than in human breast tumours (Hamilton et al. 1977; MacEwen et al. 1982; Cappelletti et al. 1988; Sartin et al. 1992). More malignant, undifferentiated tumours tend to be receptor negative. Low concentrations of progesterone receptors are reported in feline mammary tumours and approximately 10% of tumours contain oestrogen receptors (Hamilton et al. 1976; Rutteman et al. 1991).

The administration of some progestagens including medroxyprogesterone acetate, megoestrol acetate and chlormadinone acetate may increase the risk of benign but not malignant mammary tumour development in dogs. Use of progesterone-like drugs in cats may increase development of benign or malignant mammary masses.

Although A-type and C-type retroviruses have been identified in feline mammary carcinomas, their causative role has not been established.

Pathology

The mammary gland consists of epithelial ducts and alveoli situated among stromal connective tissue. Around each alveoli are myoepithelial cells. Tumours arising from epithelial tissues are described as either simple – epithelial elements only – or complex (mixed) – epithelial and myoepithelial elements. Other benign (e.g. lipoma) and malignant mesenchymal tumours (e.g. mast cell tumours) can occur in the mammary gland although they are not strictly mammary tumours.

In dogs, most histopathological studies have shown that approximately 50% of tumours recorded are benign, but this figure may be artificially low because there is a bias towards submit-

Table 12.1 Frequency of histological types of mammary tumours in dogs (Bostock 1986).

Tumour type	Relative frequency/ incidence (%)
Benign	*51.0*
Benign mixed tumours/ fibroadenomas/complex adenomas	45.5
Simple adenomas	5.0
Benign mesenchymal tumours	0.5
Malignant	*49.0*
Solid carcinomas	16.9
Tubular adenocarcinomas	15.4
Papillary adenocarcinomas	8.6
Anaplastic carcinomas	4.0
(Total carcinomas)	(44.9)
Sarcomas	3.1
Carcinosarcoma/malignant mixed tumours	1.0

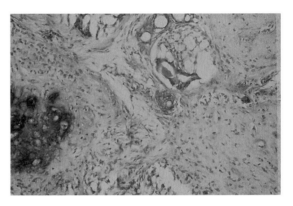

Fig. 12.1 H&E section of a benign mixed mammary tumour. (Courtesy of Mr D. Bostock.)

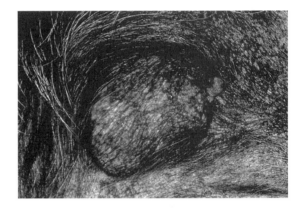

Fig. 12.2 Gross appearance of benign mixed tumour in a bitch. (Courtesy of Mr D. Bostock.)

ting malignant samples for histological analysis. The relative frequency of the various canine tumour types is shown in Table 12.1. Several different tumour types may occur in the same gland or affect different glands in the same animal.

In cats, over 80% of mammary tumours are carcinomas, the rest being mainly fibroadenomas. Lobular hyperplasia (palpable masses in one or more glands) and fibroepithelial hyperplasia (feline mammary hypertrophy) of the mammary gland also occur and are thought to be associated with hormonal stimulation of the glandular tissue.

Benign tumours

Benign tumours are classed as simple adenomas, complex adenomas (benign mixed tumours) or benign mesenchymal tumours. The term fibroadenoma is also used for benign mixed tumours and these are the most common type of benign tumour in dogs and cats. Grossly they may appear firm and nodular and histologically they may contain bone or cartilage (derived from myoepithelial elements) in addition to epithelial elements (Figs 12.1 and 12.2).

Simple adenomas may be classed as lobular if derived from alveolar epithelium or papillary if derived from ductal epithelium. If the ducts appear dilated or cystic they may be classed as cystadenomas.

Malignant tumours

Approximately 90% of malignant tumours are carcinomas although some malignant mixed tumours (sometimes called carcinosarcomas) and some sarcomas do occur.

Carcinomas may be described as:

- Solid (sheets of dense cells)
- Tubular or lobular (derived from alveoli)
- Papillary (derived from ductal epithelium and appearing as branching papillae or cystic)
- Anaplastic (very pleomorphic and lacking any definite pattern).

Occasionally squamous cell carcinoma may develop from squamous metaplasia of ductal epithelium. Grossly, carcinomas may vary from

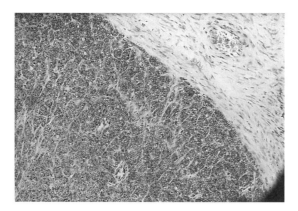

Fig. 12.3 H&E section of a well defined, non-invasive, solid mammary carcinoma; there is a distinct boundary between the tumour and normal tissue. (Courtesy of Mr D. Bostock.)

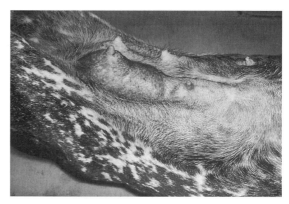

Fig. 12.5 Gross appearance of a mammary carcinoma. (Courtesy of Mr D. Bostock.)

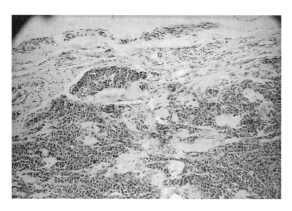

Fig. 12.4 H&E section of a poorly differentiated, invasive mammary carcinoma. Tumour cells are scattered through the adjacent connective tissues with vascular invasion. (Courtesy of Mr D. Bostock.)

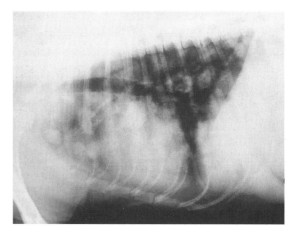

Fig. 12.6 Lateral chest radiograph with multiple 'cannon-ball' type secondary tumours, metastatic from a primary mammary carcinoma.

well circumscribed, small nodules to ulcerated, diffuse and inflamed, infiltrative masses extending into the inguinal region and down the hind legs (inflammatory anaplastic carcinoma) (Figs 12.3, 12.4 and 12.5).

Tumour behaviour

Benign tumours do not invade locally or metastasise but there is a tendency for bitches to develop multiple tumours and for new benign tumours to develop in the same or other glands after excision of an existing nodule.

Malignant tumours may behave relatively benignly or very aggressively. Histologically, the most important feature of carcinomas which will predict their behaviour and likely outcome is whether they appear well differentiated and defined or whether they are infiltrative and invasive (Table 12.2). Those showing local invasion tend to metastasise rapidly to local lymph nodes (superficial inguinal for caudal glands, axillary or cranial sternal for cranial glands) and lungs, although abdominal organs and bone may also be affected (Figs 12.6 and 12.7). Feline mammary carcinomas are especially aggressive and have often metastasised by the time of presentation.

Table 12.2 Tumour behaviour in dogs according to histological type (Bostock 1975).

Histological type	Post surgical death rate (%)		Median survival (weeks)
	1 year	2 year	
Complex adenoma	0	0	125
Benign mixed mammary	6	6	114
Well differentiated, non-invasive carcinoma	21	25	110
Invasive papillary and tubular carcinomas	35	47	40
Invasive solid and anaplastic carcinomas	73	75	20

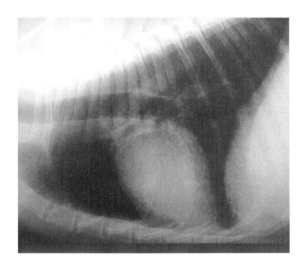

Fig. 12.7 Lateral chest radiograph showing miliary metastases which are sometimes seen with metastatic mammary carcinoma.

Paraneoplastic syndromes

Some dogs with stage IV mammary tumours may have haemorrhagic diatheses or disseminated intravascular coagulation but this is an uncommon clinical problem. A greater proportion of dogs may show subclinical haemostatic abnormalities (Stockhaus *et al.* 1999).

Presentation/signs

The caudal two pairs of mammary glands are most often affected in the dog but the anterior glands are most affected in the cat. Mammary tumours may be single or multiple and are usually easily palpable as discrete nodules or masses within the mammary glands. They may be attached to underlying skin or muscle or may be ulcerated. Small benign masses may be found as incidental findings on clinical examination or at post mortem examination. Occasionally an extremely small primary tumour may be easily missed but an enlarged inguinal lymph node may be palpable. Some aggressive inflammatory carcinomas may present with diffuse mammary swelling, oedema and ulceration. Respiratory distress is rarely noted in dogs with pulmonary metastasis but is common in cats because of pleural carcinomatosis and extensive pulmonary involvement.

Investigations

A presumptive diagnosis of mammary tumour can be made on clinical examination and palpation in most cases. Care should be taken to differentiate mammary hypertrophy and mastitis, however.

Bloods

These are not generally very helpful in the diagnosis of mammary tumours although a recent study has revealed significant haemostatic abnormalities in cases of untreated mammary carcinoma (Stockhaus *et al.* 1999).

Imaging techniques

Radiography of the primary tumour is not necessary, but thoracic films are essential for all malignant tumours to look for pulmonary metastases. These may be discrete nodules or miliary in nature (Figs 12.6 & 12.7). Pulmonary effusion may be present in cats. Abdominal films may show enlarged sublumbar lymph nodes and skeletal surveys may reveal bone metastases. Scintigraphy may also be used to screen for bone metastases.

Biopsy/FNA

Although easy to perform, fine needle aspirates of mammary lesions are not always easy to interpret by cytological examination. They should, however, give an indication of whether the lesion is neoplastic or non-neoplastic. Fine needle aspiration is more helpful to assess regional lymph nodes for metastatic spread. Mammary wedge biopsies may be useful for large lesions but small nodules are often excisionally biopsied as part of the treatment procedure. Biopsy is not usually necessary for mammary tumours since the type of surgical treatment for most cases will not depend on their histological type (see below). It is helpful, however, to distinguish tumours from other non-neoplastic conditions which may not require surgery.

Staging

TNM staging systems are used for mammary carcinomas in both the dog and cat (Tables 12.3 and 12.4). Multiple tumours should be evaluated independently. The primary tumour should be assessed with regard to its size and whether it is fixed to underlying tissues, by clinical and surgical examination. Inguinal and axillary nodes should be examined clinically and surgically to see if they are enlarged or fixed, and thoracic radiographs should be taken to look for pulmonary metastases.

Table 12.3 Clinical stages (TNM) of canine mammary tumours. Owen (1980).

T	*Primary tumour*
(evaluate multiple tumours independently)	
T0	No evidence of tumour
T1	Tumour <3 cm maximum diameter
T1a	Not fixed
T1b	Fixed to skin
T1c	Fixed to muscle
T2	Tumour 3–5 cm maximum diameter
T2a	Not fixed
T2b	Fixed to skin
T2c	Fixed to muscle
T3	Tumour >5 cm maximum diameter
T3a	Not fixed
T3b	Fixed to skin
T3c	Fixed to muscle
T4	Tumour any size, inflammatory carcinoma
N	*Regional lymph nodes (RLN)*
(axillary or inguinal; clinical or histological evaluation)	
N0	No evidence of involvement
N1	Ipsilateral involvement
N1a	Not fixed
N1b	Fixed
N2	Bilateral involvement
N2a	Not fixed
N2b	Fixed
M	*Distant metastasis*
(clinical, radiographic or histological evaluation)	
M0	No evidence of metastasis
M1	Distant metastasis including distant lymph nodes

Group staging can also be performed, as shown in Table 12.5.

Treatment

Surgery

Treatment for most mammary tumours is surgical excision. Options include:

- Nodulectomy/lumpectomy
- Removal of the affected gland (mammectomy)
- Removal of the affected gland along with any glands which drain lymph or blood from it (local mastectomy)
- Mammary strip (total/radical mastectomy).

In dogs, the first three glands drain cranially and glands four and five caudally although there may be lymphatic communication between adjacent glands.

Table 12.4 Clinical stages (TNM) of feline mammary tumours. Owen (1980).

T *Primary tumour*
(evaluate multiple tumours independently)
T0   No evidence of tumour
T1   Tumour <1 cm maximum diameter
  T1a   Not fixed
  T1b   Fixed to skin
  T1c   Fixed to muscle
T2   Tumour 1–3 cm maximum diameter
  T2a   Not fixed
  T2b   Fixed to skin
  T2c   Fixed to muscle
T3   Tumour >3 cm maximum diameter
  T3a   Not fixed
  T3b   Fixed to skin
  T3c   Fixed to muscle
T4   Tumour any size, inflammatory carcinoma

N *Regional lymph nodes (RLN)*
(axillary or inguinal; clinical or histological evaluation)
N0   No evidence of involvement
N1   Ipsilateral involvement
  N1a   Not fixed
  N1b   Fixed
N2   Bilateral involvement
  N2a   Not fixed
  N2b   Fixed

M *Distant metastasis*
(clinical, radiographic or histological evaluation)
M0   No evidence of metastasis
M1   Distant metastasis including distant nodes

Table 12.5 Stage grouping of canine or feline mammary tumours. Owen (1980).

Stage grouping	T	N	M
I	T1a, b or c	N0(−) N1a(−) N2a(−)	M0
II	T0 T1a, b or c T2a, b or c	N1(+) N1(+) N0(+) or N1a(+)	M0
III	Any T3 Any T	Any N Any Nb	M0
IV	Any T	Any N	M1

(−) histologically negative   (+) histologically positive.

Theoretically this necessitates the removal of the adjacent glands for most tumours and a full strip for tumours in gland three. In the dog, no study has shown that the type of surgery performed will influence the outcome dramatically and many surgeons favour simple mastectomy over radical mastectomy, ignoring the drainage patterns. In practice, wherever the tumour is positioned, glands one, two and three are often easily excised as an anatomical unit, and the same for glands four and five. In the cat, communication between glands is less obvious but since size of the primary mass is an important prognostic factor and tumours are usually very aggressive, radical treatment is recommended.

In general, lumpectomy should be regarded as a biopsy procedure or reserved for very small, unfixed lesions less than 0.5 cm diameter. Mammectomy is sufficient for fixed or unfixed tumours centrally positioned within the gland, but most larger and multiple tumours will require local or radical mastectomy depending on their position in the mammary chain. Inguinal lymph nodes are excised as part of gland five but axillary lymph nodes need only be removed if enlarged or shown to contain neoplastic cells cytologically or histologically. It is often easier and quicker to perform a radical mastectomy rather than multiple mammectomies although the influence on survival time may be minimal. Mammary strip has a greater rate of dehiscence and bilateral mammary strip is not recommended. For all radical mammary surgery, an active (preferably) or passive drain should be placed for a few days post-operatively and antibiotic cover used.

There has been much debate on the effect of ovariohysterectomy at the time of excision of a mammary tumour, but it is now generally agreed that it has no effect on development of new benign tumours, the progression of malignant tumours, time to metastasis or overall survival (Fowler *et al.* 1974; Brodey *et al.* 1983; Kitchell 1994; Yamagami *et al.* 1996; Morris *et al.* 1998). In cats, there may be more reason to perform ovariohysterectomy since ovarian and uterine disease occasionally coexist with mammary tumours.

Radiotherapy

Radiotherapy has not been shown to be effective in the treatment of canine or feline mammary tumours.

Chemotherapy

Carcinomas are not particularly chemosensitive tumours and although many chemotherapeutic regimes have been attempted in the treatment of mammary carcinomas, none has shown to be very effective in improving disease free interval or survival beyond that obtained by surgery alone. Doxorubicin appears to have some antitumour effect on mammary tumour cells in vitro but its effect in the clinical situation is variable and needs further evaluation. A combination of cyclophosphamide and 5-fluorouracil with or without doxorubicin may be beneficial but the efficacy still needs to be established in clinical trials. In most cases of invasive carcinoma, the disease is too extensive at the time of diagnosis for chemotherapy to be successful.

In cats, some success has also been claimed with doxorubicin therapy post-surgery (with or without cyclophosphamide) but the drug is nephrotoxic in cats as well as causing anorexia and myelosuppression, and should be administered with caution. The advanced nature of most feline mammary tumours means that in general chemotherapy has a poor response.

Other

Anti-oestrogenic compounds such as tamoxifen are extremely useful for human mammary tumours in delaying recurrence and metastasis. Unfortunately, tamoxifen is metabolised to oestrogenic compounds in the dog, causing pyometra in entire animals and other oestrogenic effects such as vulval swelling, vulval discharge and attractiveness to male dogs in spayed animals (Morris *et al.* 1993). For these reasons, its tumouristatic properties in dogs have not been fully evaluated.

Biologic response modifiers such as Bacillus Calmette-Guerin (BCG), Corynebacterium parvum, neuraminidase or levamisole have been used experimentally to treat mammary tumours, but no clear therapeutic benefit has been demonstrated.

Prognosis

The prognosis for most benign canine mammary tumours which are surgically excised is good, although new tumours may develop and some of these may be malignant.

The prognosis for well differentiated carcinomas is reasonable with survival times over two years for some histological types (Bostock 1975). For invasive carcinomas, however, the prognosis is grave since most will metastasise rapidly despite surgical removal and survival times are short (36 weeks and 11 weeks for solid and anaplastic carcinomas respectively). Sarcomas also have a short survival time (approximately six months).

As well as the histological type and degree of differentiation, other prognostic indicators for canine mammary tumours include:

- Tumour size and volume
- Tumour stage, i.e. nodal metastasis, attachment to underlying structures, ulceration
- Oestrogen receptor positivity (more malignant tumours tend to be oestrogen receptor negative)
- DNA ploidy (aneuploid tumours carry a worse prognosis)
- AgNOR count (high AgNOR count carries a worse prognosis.

In cats, the prognosis for mammary tumours is much more guarded since the majority are highly malignant and local recurrence and metastasis are common. Tumour size, histological grading and the extent of surgery performed are the most important prognostic indicators.

References

Bostock, D.E. (1975) The prognosis following the surgical excision of canine mammary neoplasms. *European Journal of Cancer*, (11), 389–96.

Bostock, D.E. (1986) Canine and feline mammary neoplasms. *British Veterinary Journal*, (142), 506–15.

Brodey, R.S., Goldschmidt, M.H. & Roszel, J.R. (1983) Canine mammary gland neoplasms. *Journal of the American Animal Hospital Association*, (19), 61–90.

Cappelletti, V., Granata, G., Miodini, P., Coradini, D. *et al.* (1988) Modulation of receptor levels in canine breast tumours by administration of tamoxifen and etretinate either alone or in combination. *Anticancer Research*, (8), 1927–1302.

Dorn, C.R., Taylor, D.O.N., Schneider, R. *et al.* (1968) Survey of animal neoplasms in Alameda and Contra Costa Counties, California. II. Cancer morbidity in dogs and cats from Alameda County. *Journal of the National Cancer Institute*, (40), 307–18.

Fowler, E.H., Wilson, G.P., Koestner, A.A. *et al.* (1974) Biologic behaviour of canine mammary neoplasms based on a histogenic classification. *Veterinary Pathology*, (11), 212–29.

Hamilton, M., Else, R.W. & Forshaw, P. (1976) Oestrogen receptors in feline mammary carcinoma. *Veterinary Record*, (99), 477–9.

Hamilton, M., Else, R.W. & Forshaw, P. (1977) Oestrogen receptors in canine mammary tumors. *Veterinary Record*, (101), 258–60.

Kitchell, B.E. (1994) Mammary carcinoma in dogs: update on biology and therapy. *Proceedings of 12th American College of Veterinary Internal Medicine Forum*, 884–6.

MacEwen, E.G., Patnaik, A.K., Harvey, H.J. *et al.* (1982) Estrogen receptors in canine mammary tumours. *Cancer Research*, (42), 2255–9.

Morris, J.S., Dobson, J.M. & Bostock D.E. (1993) Use of tamoxifen in the control of canine mammary neoplasia. *Veterinary Record*, (133), 539–42.

Morris, J.S., Dobson, J.M., Bostock, D.E. & O'Farrell, E. (1998) Effect of ovariohysterectomy in bitches with mammary neoplasia. *Veterinary Record*, (142), 656–8.

Owen, L.N. (1980) TNM Classification of Tumours in Domestic Animals. World Health Organisation, Geneva.

Rutteman, G.R., Blankenstein, M.A., Minke, J. & Misdorp, W. (1991) Steroid receptors in mammary tumours of the cat (Suppl 1). *Acta Endocrinologica*, (125), 32–7.

Sartin, E.A., Barnes, S., Kwapien, R.P. *et al.* (1992) Estrogen and progesterone receptor status of mammary carcinomas and correlation with clinical outcome. *American Journal of Veterinary Research*, (53), 2196–200.

Schneider, R., Dorn, C.R. & Taylor, D.O.N. (1969) Factors influencing canine mammary development and post-surgical survival. *Journal of the National Cancer Institute*, (43), 1249–61.

Stockhaus, C., Kohn, B., Rudolph, R., Brunnberg, L. & Giger, U. (1999) Correlation of haemostatic abnormalities with tumour stage and characteristics in dogs with mammary carcinoma. *Journal of Small Animal Practice*, (40), 326–31.

Yamagami, T., Kobayashi, T., Takahashi, K. & Sugiyama, M. (1996) Influence of ovariectomy at the time of mastectomy on the prognosis for canine malignant mammary tumours. *Journal of Small Animal Practice*, (37), 462–4.

Further reading

Bostock, D.E., Moriarty, J. & Crocker, J. (1992) Correlation between histologic diagnosis, mean nucleolar organiser region count and prognosis in canine mammary tumours. *Veterinary Pathology*, (29), 381–5.

Ferguson, R.H. (1985) Canine mammary gland tumors. *Veterinary Clinics of North America Small Animal Practice*, (15), 501–11.

Giles, R.C., Kwapien, R.P., Geil, R.G. & Casey, H.W. (1978) Mammary nodules in beagle dogs administered investigational oral contraceptive steroids. *Journal of the National Cancer Institute*, (60), 1351–64.

Hahn, K.A., Richardson, R.C. & Knapp, D.W. (1992) Canine malignant mammary neoplasia: biologic behaviour, diagnosis and treatment alternatives. *Journal of the American Animal Hospital Association*, (28), 251–6.

Hahn, K.A. & Adams, W.H. (1997) Feline mammary neoplasia: biological behaviour, diagnosis and treatment alternatives. *Feline Practice*, (25), 5–11.

Hayes, A. & Mooney, S. (1985) Feline mammary tumours. *Veterinary Clinics of North America*, (15), 513–20.

Jeglum, K.A., de Guzman, E. & Young, K.M. (1985) Chemotherapy for advanced mammary adenocarcinoma in 14 cats. *Journal of the American Veterinary Medical Association*, (187), 157–60.

Kurtzman, I.D. & Gilbertson, S.R. (1986) Prognostic factors in canine mammary tumours. *Seminars in Veterinary Medicine and Surgery*, (1), 25–32.

MacEwen, E.G., Hayes, A.A. & Harvey, H.J. (1984) Prognostic factors for feline mammary tumours. *Journal of the American Veterinary Medical Association*, (185), 201–4.

Susaneck, S.J., Allen, T.A., Hoopes, J. *et al.* (1976) Inflammatory mammary carcinoma in the dog. *Journal of the American Animal Hospital Association*, (19), 971–6.

13
Nervous System

The nervous system may be divided into the central nervous system (CNS) comprising the brain (including the optic nerve) and the spinal cord, and the peripheral nervous system (PNS) comprising peripheral nerves and nerve roots, including parts of the autonomic nervous system. By convention tumours of peripheral nerves are included with tumours of the soft tissues, as discussed in Chapter 5. Tumours of the eye will be discussed in Chapter 16. This chapter is devoted to tumours affecting the central nervous system, i.e. the brain and the spinal cord.

BRAIN (INTRACRANIAL) TUMOURS

Epidemiology

Primary tumours of the brain are not common in most epidemiological tumour studies; however with the advent of advanced imaging techniques (CT and MRI), tumours of the brain are assuming more importance in canine and feline medicine. The reported incidence of primary brain tumours is 14.4/100000 dogs and 3.5/100000 cats (Moore *et al.* 1996).

Most primary brain tumours are solitary lesions. They may occur in all breeds of dog but the boxer, golden retriever, dobermann, Scottish terrier and old English sheepdog have been reported to be at increased risk. Primary brain tumours may occur at any age but the incidence increases over five years of age with a median age of nine years reported in dogs (Heidner *et al.* 1991). There does not appear to be any breed predilection for meningioma in the dog but glial cell tumours have a predilection for brachycephalic breeds, particularly the boxer.

Aetiology

The aetiology of brain tumours in cats and dogs is unknown.

Pathology

Intracranial tumours of dogs and cats may be either primary or secondary and are classified on the basis of cytological and histological criteria. Primary tumours arise from tissues of the nervous system: nerve cells, neuroepithelial tissues, neural connective tissues (the glia) and the meninges (as listed in Table 13.1). The most common primary brain tumours in the dog are meningioma, glioma (e.g. astrocytoma) and undifferentiated sarcomas. Tumours of the choroid plexus are also reported. Meningioma is the most common brain tumour in cats and multiple meningiomas may occur in this species.

The brain may be a site for haematogenous

Table 13.1 Classification of intracranial tumours.

Tissue/origin	Tumour	Site/comment
Nerve cells	Ganglioblastoma/gangliocytoma/ ganglioneuroma	Cerebellum & brain stem, mature dogs slow growing, rare
	Neuroblastoma	Cerebellum/olfactory epithelium, rare
	Medulloblastoma	? Origin, young dogs, highly malignant
Neuroepithelial	Ependymoma (neuroepithelioma)	Associated with ependyma of ventricular system in mature brachycephalic dogs. Infiltrating and aggressive
	Chondroid plexus tumours (papilloma)	Usually associated with ventricular system, well defined, slowly growing
Glial	Oligodendroglioma	Rare. Frontal and pyriform lobes of cerebrum, most common site in brachycephalic dogs. Infiltrating growth
	Glioblastoma	Rare but reported in brachycephalic dogs
	Astrocytoma	Common in brachycephalic dogs usually located in cerebellum. Grow by expansion and infiltration
Meningeal	Meningioma	Common in cats and dogs. Sites include base of brain, and convexity of cerebral hemispheres. Growth usually by expansion
	Meningeal sarcoma	Rare, malignant
Nerve sheath	Peripheral nerve sheath tumours (Schwannoma, neurofibroma, neurilemoma, neurofibrosarcoma, malignant schwannoma)	Included because these tumours are associated with nerve tissue but are not usually intracranial in site
		Acoustic neuroma is a notable exception
Neurohypophysis	Pituitary adenoma	
	Posterior pituitary astrocytoma	
Other	Lymphoma	
	Haemangiosarcoma	
	Teratoma/germ cell tumour	
Metastatic tumours	Mammary, prostatic, pulmonary carcinoma	
	Haemangiosarcoma	
	Malignant melanoma	
Tumours which directly invade into the brain from:	Pituitary adenoma/adenocarcinoma Skull Nasal/paranasal sinuses Middle ear	

metastasis of malignant tumours sited elsewhere in the body or may be affected by local extension of tumours of the nasal cavity and paranasal sinuses, from the skull and from the middle ear. Pituitary gland tumours and tumours of the cranial nerves are considered to be secondary tumours as they affect the brain by means of local extension (LeCouteur, 1999).

Tumour behaviour/paraneoplastic syndromes

The distinction between 'benign' and 'malignant' is less relevant for tumours of the brain than for tumours at most other sites. Many intracranial tumours are relatively slow growing but may present with acute or rapidly progressing clinical signs when compensatory mechanisms are overwhelmed. An intracranial tumour may possess cytological features to suggest a benign behaviour, and indeed may not possess the capacity for distant metastasis, but may still be life threatening in biological terms. Some tumours, for example canine meningioma, may be classified as benign but may be locally invasive of normal brain tissue. Feline meningioma are usually well defined with clear demarcation between normal and affected brain tissue. It is rare for primary brain tumours to metastasise outside the cranial cavity.

Primary brain tumours are not usually associated with paraneoplastic syndromes as such although tumours adjacent to or involving the pituitary gland may cause a variety of endocrinopathies as detailed in Chapter 14.

Presentation/signs

Intracranial tumours may manifest in a variety of ways. Behavioural and temperament changes such as:

- Abnormal mental status
- Disorientation
- Loss of trained habits.

are common, but these may be insidious in onset and may be dismissed as ageing in older animals.

More specific neurological signs depend primarily on the site of the tumour within the brain (Table 13.2), its size and rate of growth. Initially such signs may be transient but as the tumour enlarges they may become more severe and permanent. Seizures are common and are often one of the first signs of a tumour of the cerebral cortex. Multiple cranial nerve deficits may be associated with tumours of the ventral brain stem, while dysmetria, intention tremors and ataxia may be seen with tumours of the cerebellum. Visual impairment or blindness may be associated with tumours of the hypothalamus or with meningioma of the optic nerve.

Intracranial tumours may also result in increased intracranial pressure, either due to a mass effect or due to cerebral oedema, ultimately this may lead to herniation of the brain through the foramen magna. Clinical signs of these secondary effects include

Table 13.2 Possible signs of intracranial tumours according to location.

Location of tumour	Associated neurological signs
Cerebral cortex	Abnormal movement, circling (usually towards the side of the tumour) Continual pacing Head pressing Seizures
Hypothalamus	Altered mental status Visual impairment, due to defects in optic (II) nerve at optic chiasm (Diabetes insipidus)
Midbrain	Defects in oculomotor (III): strabismus and abnormal pupil dilation Contralateral spastic hemiparesis
Cerebellum	Dysmetria, ataxia Wide base stance Intention tremor
Vestibular	Head tilt Circling Nystagmus Vestibular strabismus
Ventral brain stem	Cranial nerve deficits (V,VI,VII,IX,X) Hemiparesis to tetraparesis Irregular respiration

altered states of consciousness, lethargy or irritability, compulsive walking, circling, head pressing and locomotor disturbances. Brain herniation will result in respiratory failure and death.

Investigations

A full neurological examination is required in a patient presenting with any of the signs outlined above or in Table 13.2, in order to confirm that the problem is of neurological origin and to attempt to define the location of the lesion.

Bloods

Routine haematological and biochemical analyses are indicated in the investigation of an animal presenting with neurological signs in order to rule out extracranial causes but, with the exception of tumours affecting the pituitary gland, there are no specific changes associated with most intracranial tumours.

Imaging techniques

Plain radiography of the skull is of little value in the detection of most intracranial tumours, although on occasion osteolysis or hyperostosis of the skull may be seen with feline meningioma. Skull radiography may be useful for assessment of tumours of the nasal cavity and paranasal sinuses or tumours of the skull (including the tympanic bullae) that may extend into the cranial vault.

Survey radiographs of the thorax and abdomen and ultrasound evaluation of liver, spleen and other internal organs should be performed as part of the evaluation of the patient to rule out extracranial causes of the neurological problems and the possibility that an intracranial lesion may be a metastatic tumour from elsewhere. Most intracranial tumours do not metastasise so the finding of multiple tumours elsewhere in the body would support a diagnosis of a secondary brain tumour.

Advanced imaging techniques such as CT and MRI have revolutionised the detection of intracranial lesions. Although these techniques are complimentary, MRI is generally superior to CT in providing high quality images of intracranial soft tissues which allow detection of subtle changes such as oedema, changes in vascularity, haemorrhage and necrosis as well as the detection of the primary mass. MRI also permits better definition of the anatomical relationships of a tumour and surrounding normal tissues.

In the absence of a histological diagnosis (see below) the CT or MRI features of a brain lesion are often used to suggest the type of tumour (Table 13.3, Figs 13.1–13.3). However as some non-neoplastic, space-occupying lesions and metastatic

Table 13.3 Presumptive diagnosis of brain tumours based on MRI features (Brearley *et al.* 1999).

MRI features	Likely tumour type
Extra-axial Homogeneously enhancing mass located outside the brain parenchyma (Fig. 13.1)	Meningioma (also Schwannoma and choroid plexus tumour)
Intra-axial Heterogeneously enhancing mass located within the brain parenchyma (Fig. 13.2)	Glial tumour
Pituitary based Homogeneously enhancing mass involving the pituitary gland and extending upwards into the thalamus (Fig. 13.3)	Pituitary macroadenoma

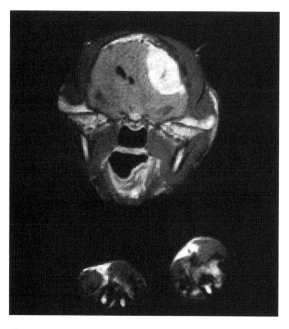

Fig. 13.1 MRI scan showing extra-axial tumour. A large meningioma in a 14 year old domestic short hair cat with seizures. The contrast enhanced transverse T1-weighted scan shows the mass to be extra-axial with dense contrast enhancement. The adjacent cerebrum is compressed and displaced and there is marked overlying hyperostosis. (Courtesy of Ruth Dennis, Centre for Small Animal Studies, Animal Health Trust, Newmarket.)

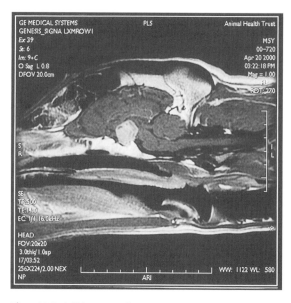

Fig. 13.3 MRI scan showing a pituitary tumour – and MRI scan of a 5 year old Labrador with pituitary dependent hyperadrenocorticism. The image shows a homogeneously enhancing mass involving the pituitary gland and extending upwards into the thalamus. (Courtesy of Animal Health Trust, Newmarket.)

tumours may mimic the CT or MRI appearance of a primary brain tumour, this situation is not ideal.

Biopsy/FNA

Cytological/histological diagnosis of an intracranial tumour requires collection of cells or tissue from the lesion. The brain is not easily accessible for collection of either fine needle aspirates or biopsy specimens. Exploratory surgery carries quite high risks and is generally not undertaken unless there is a reasonable chance of an excisional biopsy of the lesion (see treatment). For this reason many brain

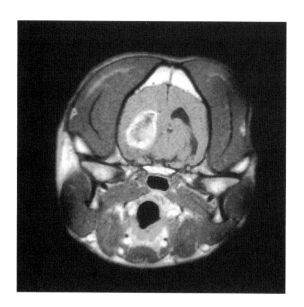

Fig. 13.2 (*Left.*) MRI scan showing intra-axial tumour. MRI scan of an 11 year old collie-cross bitch with seizures. The contrast-enhanced transverse T1-weighted scan shows a large, intra-axial cerebral mass, showing ring enhancement, typical of a glioma. (Courtesy of Ruth Dennis, Centre for Small Animal Studies, Animal Health Trust, Newmarket, previously published by *In Practice* (1998), (20), 117–124, with permission)

'tumours' in cats and dogs are not confirmed histopathologically in life.

Recently a CT-guided stereotactic brain biopsy system has been modified for use in cats and dogs (LeCouter *et al.* 1998) and offers an accurate means of collecting biopsy samples from brain lesions with a low rate of complications.

Other

Several other techniques may be indicated in the evaluation of the patient with neurological signs but none assist specifically in the diagnosis of primary brain tumours.

Cerebrospinal fluid (CSF) analysis

Cerebrospinal fluid (CSF) analysis may be indicated to rule out inflammatory diseases of CNS, for example granulomatous meningioencephalomyelitis (GME), which is an important differential diagnosis for many of the clinical signs listed above. However, it is unusual to find tumour cells in the CSF and so CSF analysis rarely confirms the presence of a tumour. One possible exception is in the case of CNS lymphoma where the CSF may contain significant numbers of abnormal lymphoid cells. Increased CSF protein and normal to increased CSF white cell count are often reported in cases with brain tumours as a result of necrosis or microabcessation associated with the tumour mass. CSF collection should not be performed in animals with suspected brain tumours until after imaging because of the risk that the technique can precipitate herniation of the brain in cases with raised intracranial pressure.

Electrodiagnostic testing

Brainstem auditory evoked potential (BAEP) testing and electroencephalography (EEG) may be used to assess function of the brain stem and the cerebrum, respectively, but neither are widely available. Both techniques can help to locate the site of a lesion but neither provide specific information about the cause of any abnormalities detected (Fischer & Obermaier 1994).

Staging

A clinical staging system has not been devised for primary brain tumours.

Treatment

Surgery

Some primary brain tumours are amenable to surgical resection and this can be an effective treatment for meningiomas, especially those sited over the frontal lobes of the cerebrum in cats. Even partial removal of a brain mass may relieve some of the associated clinical signs, provide tissue for histological diagnosis and allow a better response to subsequent treatment such as radiotherapy.

Neurosurgery is a highly specialised area. Surgical approaches to the brain, anaesthetic considerations and post-operative care are beyond the scope of this book but the following may be useful criteria to aid selection of cases that may be suitable for surgical management:

- Accurate localisation of the mass is essential.
- Nature of tumour – only solitary and non-invasive tumours are suitable
- Site – a tumour that is on or near the surface of the brain is accessible for surgical management. The cerebral hemispheres are the most suitable site for surgical intervention. Significant morbidity may be associated with surgical removal of tumours of the caudal fossa or brain stem.
- Patient status – neurological function must be compatible with life.

Radiotherapy

Radiotherapy is probably the most widely used treatment for brain tumours in cats and dogs and may either be used alone or in conjunction with surgery or chemotherapy. External beam megavoltage radiation provides a deeply penetrating X-ray beam of predictable configuration which allows the tumour volume to be targeted from several treatment ports, while sparing to some degree the adjacent normal tissue (Fig. 13.4). Careful treatment planning is essential, and this is aided by computer planning systems and good quality CT or MRI images of the brain. Brain tissue is quite susceptible to late radiation toxicity resulting in brain necrosis. The optimum fractionation schedule for radiotherapy of brain tumours in animals has not been established. Some authorities favour small daily fractions keeping the normal tissue dose

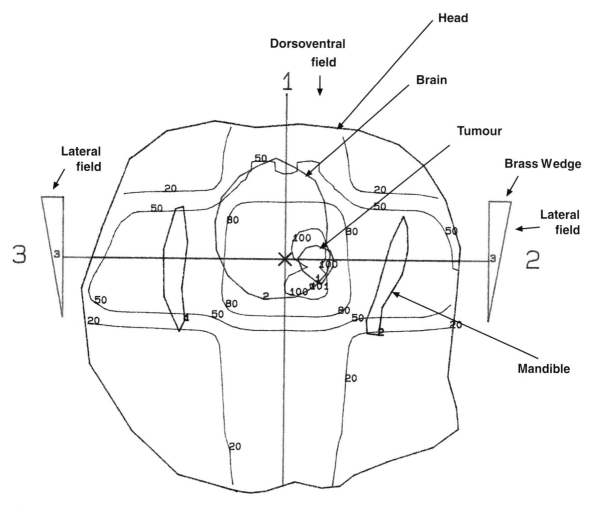

Fig. 13.4 Computer generated treatment plan for a dog with a brain tumour. (See also Colour plate 28, facing p. 162, the key of which follows on here: An MRI scan is digitised into the computer to provide a scaled line drawing of the outline of the dog's head (blue line) and mandibles (blue), the brain (outer red) and the tumour (inner red). The computer predicts the radiation dose deposition, shown as isodose contours (black lines; figures indicate percentage applied radiation dose) based on an isocentric treatment using three portals: dorsoventral and right and left lateral, with brass wedges (green triangles) used to attenuate the lateral beams.)

below 50 Gy (Gavin *et al.* 1995), whilst others have reported similar results with hypofractionated radiotherapy to a total tumour dose of 38 Gy (Brearley *et al.* 1999).

Chemotherapy

The role of chemotherapy in the treatment of brain tumours has not really been established in cats and dogs. Many chemotherapeutic agents do not achieve therapeutic concentrations in the brain because of limited passage of the blood brain barrier. The lipophilic agents BiCNU (carmustine) and CCNU (lomustine) do pass into the CSF in therapeutic concentrations but only rare tumours such as teratoma and dysgerminoma are regarded as potentially curable by chemotherapy in humans. Few chemotherapy studies have been reported in dogs with brain tumours and results have been variable. It is probable that different tumour types differ in their chemosensitivity and there is some evidence that glial cell tumours may show a response to lomustine (Jeffery & Brearley 1993). While lymphoma is chemosensitive, treatment of CNS lymphoma is hampered by drug delivery.

Other

Supportive, symptomatic therapy to control the secondary effects of the tumour can greatly improve the status of patients with brain tumours in the short term.

- Anticonvulsant therapy – may be required to control seizures
- Corticosteroid therapy – reduces tumour associated inflammation and swelling.

These treatments may be required for patients undergoing surgery and/or radiotherapy.

Prognosis

Although many brain tumours are relatively slow growing, most are not diagnosed until they reach an advanced stage and are associated with neurological signs. For those animals that are not treated, or

managed palliatively as above, survival times post diagnosis are short.

Where surgical resection of a brain tumour is possible, e.g. meningioma in cats, long-term survival is possible. In a study of 42 cats with surgically resected cerebral meningiomas, overall survival was 66% at one year and 50% at two years; however, 20% of patients died in the immediate post-operative period (Gordon et al. 1994).

Results of radiotherapy for brain tumours in dogs are variable with median survival times ranging from 20–43 weeks (Heidner et al. 1991; Brearley et al. 1999). It is likely that different tumours may differ in their radiosensitivity and a recent study using hypofractionated radiotherapy has suggested that extra-axial tumours (by inference meningioma) carry a slightly more favourable prognosis than intra-axial tumours (by inference glioma) and that overall, pituitary-based tumours carry a significantly worse prongosis than either (Brearley et al. 1999). However, it should be noted that pituitary-based tumours have a very variable survival rate: those associated with severe neurological problems tend to have a short survival whereas those with mild signs can survive for long periods following radiotherapy (M. Brearley pers. comm.)

SPINAL CORD

Epidemiology

The spinal cord is not a common site for the development of tumours and only a small number of case series have been reported, making unreliable figures for age, breed and sex predisposition. They can be seen in any age of cat and dog; in one study of 29 tumours 27% of animals were three years of age or less (Luttgen et al. 1980). No breed or sex predisposition has been reported in either species although large dogs appear to be at higher risk.

Traditionally tumours affecting the spinal cord are classified according to their location with respect to the cord and dura (Table 13.4). Extradural tumours are the most common, representing up to 50% of all spinal tumours. Intradural-extramedullary tumours comprise up to 30% of tumours at this site.

Aetiology

With the exception of lymphoma in cats (Chapter 15), the aetiology of tumours affecting the spinal cord in cats and dogs is unknown.

Pathology

Extradural

The most common extradural tumours in dogs arise from the vertebrae and include osteosarcoma and other primary bone tumours. The vertebral column may be the site for development of secondary tumours and may also be affected by more generalised neoplastic disease, e.g. multiple myeloma. Extradural liposarcoma and lymphoma have also been reported in dogs. In cats osteosarcoma is the

Table 13.4 Classification of tumours affecting the spinal cord.

Site	Location and origin	Tumour types
Extradural	Located outside the dura mater, arising from mesenchymal elements in the adjacent spinal column	Primary bone tumours (osteosarcoma, chondrosarcoma, fibrosarcoma, haemangiosarcoma) Tumours metastatic to vertebrae (e.g. mammary or prostatic carcinoma) Multiple myeloma Lymphoma (in cats)
Intradural– extramedullary	Located outside the spinal cord but within the dura mater, arising from connective tissues of the dura	Meningioma Peripheral nerve sheath tumours Neuroepithelioma (= ependymoma)
Intramedullary	Sited within the spinal cord, arising from components of the spinal cord	Glial cell tumours Undifferentiated sarcoma Metastatic tumours (haemangiosarcoma, melanoma, mammary carcinoma) Lymphoma

most common extradural tumour; benign tumours such as osteochondroma may affect the vertebral column and extradural lymphoma is of importance. Overall lymphoma is the most common spinal tumour in cats.

Intradural-extramedullary

In dogs meningioma and peripheral nerve sheath tumours are the most common tumours to occur at this site. (The term peripheral nerve sheath tumour encompasses all tumours arising from Schwann cells, also termed neurinoma, neurilemoma, schwannoma, malignant schwannoma, neurofibroma, neurofibrosarcoma – see also Chapter 5.) Neuroepithelioma (also called ependymoma, medulloepithelioma and spinal cord blastoma) has been reported to arise in the T10-L2 segments of the spinal cord in young dogs, especially German shepherds and retrievers (Moissonnier & Abbott 1993). Meningiomas are the most commonly reported intradural-extramedullary tumours in cats but lymphoma may also arise at this site.

Intramedullary

Intramedullary spinal tumours arise from components of the spinal cord and are uncommon in dogs and rare in cats. In dogs glial cell tumours (e.g. astrocytoma) are the most common tumours to

arise at this site. Haemangiosarcoma and other malignant tumours may metastasise to the spinal cord, although this is unusual. The cord may also be affected by lymphoma and occasionally by GME.

Tumour behaviour/paraneoplastic syndromes

Many different patterns of behaviour may be associated with the diverse list of tumours that may affect the spinal cord. All tumours at this site result in spinal cord compression. This may be gradual in the case of a slowly growing extradural tumour but could be acute, due to haemorrhage or ischaemia or where tumour-associated osteolysis of a vertebra results in a pathological fracture or collapse of the bone (Fig. 13.5).

While some of the tumours listed as affecting the spinal cord are malignant, the severity of the local effects on the cord are usually of greater importance than the longer term risk of metastasis.

Primary tumours of the spinal cord are not usually associated with paraneoplastic syndromes.

Presentation/signs

The clinical signs of a spinal tumour are variable and depend to some extent on the location of the lesion and on its rate of growth. The signs may be

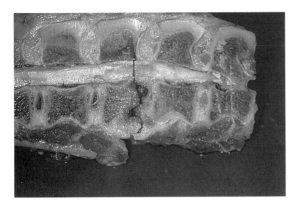

Fig. 13.5 Collapse of an osteolytic myeloma lesion in the lumbar vetebral body, leading to acute onset spinal pain and paresis.

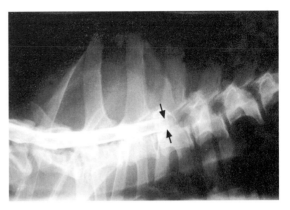

Fig. 13.6 Extradural lesion. On the myelogram, the contrast columns taper and converge slightly at the level of T3 (see arrows). At post mortem examination an epidural mass was located at the level of T3–T4. (Courtesy of Radiology Department, Department of Clinical Veterinary Medicine, Cambridge.)

gradual in onset and progress in severity over a variable period of time, but on occasion (for the reasons outlined above) the onset may be acute.

- Pain is a common feature of extradural and intradural-extramedullary tumours due to involvement of spinal nerves, nerve roots and/or bone.
- Neurological deficits will depend on the site of the lesion. There is usually a progressive loss of neurological function caudal to the lesion, leading to ataxia, paresis or paralysis. This progression can be rapid in the case of intramedullary tumours.

Unilateral spinal cord compression may cause deficits in the opposite limb.

Investigations

A full neurological examination is necessary to locate the site of the spinal lesion but unless there is a large/palpable extradual mass this is unlikely to provide much information on the nature of lesion.

Bloods

Routine haematological and biochemical analyses may be indicated in the initial evaluation of a patient presenting with a potential spinal injury, but there are no specific changes associated with most spinal tumours. Hypercalcaemia and or hypergammaglobulinaemia may be detected in dogs with multiple myeloma.

Imaging techniques

Plain radiographs of the vertebral column may identify an extradural lesion of the axial skeleton but contrast myelography is usually required to locate the lesion in terms of level of cord, site (extradural–intradural) and extent (Figs 13.6 and 13.7). MRI and CT would provide superior detail of the tumour mass and its relationships with surrounding tissues, which would be valuable if planning a surgical approach.

Plain films of the chest and abdomen should be taken to look for primary or secondary tumours.

Biopsy/FNA

Definitive diagnosis of most neoplasms affecting the spinal cord will require a biopsy of the lesion. However, as with tumours of the brain, most spinal tumours are not readily accessible for biopsy or FNA and, by force of necessity, collection of biopsy material becomes part of the therapeutic approach.

Other

CSF may be collected as part of the diagnostic work up, especially if myelography is performed. As with tumours of the brain, neoplastic cells are rarely found in CSF samples from animals with spinal tumours; non-specific changes in protein and cell content may occur in some cases.

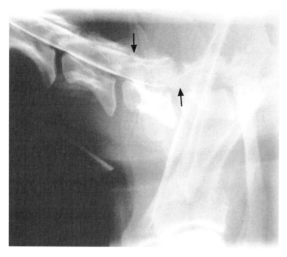

Fig. 13.7 Intradural lesion – myelogram of a dog presented with hemiparesis. The dorsal column stops at C6, the ventral column at C7 (see arrow). The appearance suggests an intramedullary lesion. A nerve root tumour was found at post mortem examination. (Courtesy of Radiology Department, Department of Clinical Veterinary Medicine, Cambridge.)

Staging

A clinical staging system has not been devised for tumours of the spinal cord.

Treatment

Surgery

Where possible surgery is the treatment of choice for most extradural and intradural-exatramedullary tumours. The spinal cord may be approached and the lesion visualised by a dorsal or hemilaminectomy. Complete removal of the tumour mass may be possible at the time of surgery but in cases where this cannot be achieved surgery may still be beneficial for:

- Cytoreduction of the mass
- Provision of biopsy material for histological diagnosis
- Decompression of the cord.

Radiotherapy

There are few reports in the literature concerning the use of radiotherapy in the treatment of tumours of the spinal cord. As with the brain, the spinal cord is reported to be susceptible to late radiation-induced necrosis and is not generally regarded as a good site for radiotherapy, although this may depend on fractionation schedules and total applied dose. One series of nine dogs with assorted tumour types (including six meningioma) suggested that radiotherapy was a useful adjunct to decompressive surgery in these cases and reported a median overall survival time of 17 months (Siegel *et al.* 1996). Radiotherapy has been used in the treatment of spinal cord lymphoma, with or without chemotherapy. The exquisite sensitivity of lymphoma to radiation permits effective treatment at lower radiation doses than would be required for most solid tumours.

Chemotherapy

With the exception of lymphoma, chemotherapy has not been used in treatment of spinal cord tumours.

Other

Glucocorticoids may be used to reduce swelling or compression of the cord in cases with acute onset of problems.

Prognosis

The prognosis for tumours of the spinal cord is very variable depending on the nature and the extent of the lesions. What is clear from the limited literature is that surgical management can be quite successful and even if complete tumour removal is not possible, post-operative radiotherapy can lead to a significant improvement in survival duration.

References

Brearley, M.J., Jeffery, N.D., Phillips, S.M. & Dennis, R. (1999) Hypofractionated radiation therapy of brain masses in dogs: a retrospective anaysis of survival of 83 cases (1991–1996). *Journal of Veterinary Internal Medicine*, (13), 408–12.

Fischer, A. & Obermaier, G. (1994) Brainstem auditory-evoked potentials and neuropathologic correlates in 26 dogs with brain tumours. *Journal of Veterinary Internal Medicine*, (8), 363–9.

Gavin, P.R., Fike, J.R. & Hoopes, P.J. (1995) Central nervous system tumours. *Seminars in Veterinary Medicine & Surgery (Small animal)*, (10), 180–89.

Gordon, L.E., Thatcher, C., Matthiesen, D.T. *et al.* (1994) Results of craniotomy for treatment of cerebral meningioma in 42 cats. *Veterinary Surgery*, (23), 94–100.

Heidner, G.L., Kornegay, J.N., Page, J.N., Dodge, R.K. & Thrall, D.E. (1991) Analysis of survival in a retrospective study of 86 dogs with brain tumours. *Journal of Veterinary Internal Medicine*, (5), 219–26.

Jeffery, N. & Brearley, M.J. (1993) Brain tumours in the dog: treatment of 10 cases and a review of recent literature. *Journal of Small Animal Practice*, (34), 367.

LeCouteur, R.A. (1999) Current concepts in the diagnosis and treatment of brain tumours in dogs and cats. *Journal of Small Animal Practice*, (40), 411–16.

LeCouteur, R.A., Koblik, P.D., Higgins, R.J., Fick, J., Kortz, G.D., Vernau, K.M., Sturges, B.K. & Berry, W.L. (1998) Computed tomography CT-guided stereotactic brain biopsy in 25 dogs and 10 cats using the Pelorus Mark III biopsy system. *Journal of Veterinary Internal Medicine*, (12), 207.

Luttgen, P.J., Braund, K.G., Brauner, W.R. *et al.* (1980) A retrospective study of 29 spinal tumours in the dog and cat. *Journal of Small Animal Practice*, (21), 213–26.

Moissonnier, P. & Abbott, D.P. (1993) Canine neuroepithelioma: case report and literature review. *Journal of the American Animal Hospital Association*, (29), 397–401.

Moore, M.P., Bagley, R.S., Harrington, M.L. & Gavin, P.R. (1996) Intracranial tumours. *Veterinary Clinics of North America: Small Animal Practice*, (26), 759–77.

Siegel, S., Kornegay, J.N. & Thrall, D.E. (1996) Postoperative irradiation of spinal cord tumours in nine dogs. *Veterinary Radiology and Ultrasound*, (37), 150–53.

14
Endocrine System

When tumours develop in endocrine glands, their normal function may be affected in one of two ways:

- Reduced hormone production/secretion may occur if normal tissue is destroyed
- Autonomous hormone secretion may occur if the feedback mechanisms controlling hormone output are altered.

Both scenarios may result in metabolic disorders or 'paraneoplastic syndromes' and the presenting signs characteristic of these disorders should alert the clinician to the possibility of underlying neoplasia. Some endocrine gland tumours, however, do not produce paraneoplastic syndromes and these may remain undetected. Conversely, some endocrinopathies, such as acromegaly in dogs, may be caused by non-neoplastic events, making the diagnosis and management of these conditions quite challenging.

This chapter deals with the tumours which occur in endocrine glands and the endocrinopathies associated with them (Table 14.1). Further information on the medical aspects of these conditions is given in specific medical or endocrinological texts. Other paraneoplastic syndromes which are associated with non-endocrine tumours are discussed in Chapter 2.

THYROID GLAND

Thyroid neoplasms occur in both cats and dogs but the pathological and biological aspects of these tumours differ greatly between the two species. Thyroid tumours in cats are usually benign but functional with significant clinical signs associated with hyperthyroidism. In dogs, thyroid tumours are usually non-functional, and the majority are carcinomas, many of which invade local tissues and metastasise rapidly.

Table 14.1 Paraneoplastic syndromes resulting from tumours of endocrine origin.

Endocrine gland	Syndrome	Tumour(s)	Comment
Thyroid	Hyperthyroidism	Thyroid adenoma (cats) Thyroid adenocarcinoma (dogs and occasionally cats)	Most common endocrine disorder of cats. Much less common in dogs since most tumours are non-functional
Parathyroid	Hyperparathyroidism (hypercalcaemia)	Parathyroid adenoma (dogs and rarely cats)	One of the less common causes of hypercalcaemia
Pituitary	Acromegaly	Pituitary adenoma (cats)	Acromegaly in dogs is caused by high progesterone (endogenous or exogenous) not neoplasia
Pituitary	Hyperadrenocorticism (pituitary dependent)	Pituitary adenoma (dogs and cats)	Most common endocrine disorder of dogs. Pituitary dependent form accounts for approximately 80–85% of cases of hyperadrenocorticism in dogs and cats
Adrenal (cortex)	Hyperadrenocorticism (adrenal dependent)	Adrenal adenoma Adrenal carcinoma (dogs and cats)	Less common cause of hyperadrenocorticism
Adrenal (medulla)	Hypercatecholaminaemia/ hypertension	Phaeochromocytoma (dogs and rarely cats)	Intermittent syndrome due to episodic release of catecholamines
Pancreas (islets)	Hypoglycaemia	Insulinoma (dogs and rarely cats)	Episodic syndrome initially due to fluctuating glucose levels
	Hypergastrinaemia (Zollinger-Ellison syndrome)	Gastrinoma (dogs and cats)	
	Metabolic epidermal necrosis	Glucagonoma (dogs)	Also reported with liver disease and diabetes mellitus

Epidemiology

Thyroid tumours in dogs represent 1–2% of all neoplasms. Old or middle-aged dogs (mean 10 years) are affected, particularly beagles, boxers or golden retrievers, but there is no sex predisposition (Susaneck 1983; Sullivan *et al.* 1987). Thyroid carcinomas in dogs may exist as solitary tumours or as part of a multiple endocrine neoplasia (MEN) syndrome, in conjunction with other primary tumours such as phaeochromocytoma or parathyroid adenoma.

Hyperthyroidism/thyroid adenomas affect middle-aged and old cats (mean age 13 years) but there is no sex or breed predisposition. Thyroid carcinomas, although rare, also occur in old cats (age range 6–18 years), with males over-represented.

Aetiology

The aetiology of canine and feline thyroid tumours is unclear. However, specific chromosome translocations and inversions involving the RET oncogene have been identified in human thyroid carcinomas (Rabbitts 1994).

Pathology

The normal thyroid in the dog and cat consists of two separate lobes which lie lateral to the trachea (approximately from rings three to eight), each lobe being associated with an external parathyroid gland at the cranial pole and an internal parathyroid gland on the medial aspect. Accessory or ectopic thyroid tissue may occur in the pericardial sac, anterior to the heart or at the base of the tongue, and tumours may arise at any of these sites.

Canine thyroid tumours

In dogs, approximately 50–90% of thyroid tumours are carcinomas and the remainder are adenomas. Most carcinomas are large, solid masses, easily noticed by owners. Two thirds are unilateral at initial presentation. Carcinomas are derived from the epithelial cells of the thyroid follicles and microscopically may appear solid, follicular or as a mixture of both patterns. Less commonly, carcinomas may arise from the parafollicular C cells (medullary thyroid carcinoma). Adenomas, on the other hand, are usually small and not readily detected unless they become cystic. Microscopically they are well defined within a capsule and appear distinct from the surrounding compressed parenchyma.

Feline thyroid tumours

The majority of feline thyroid tumours are adenomas (or nodular adenomatous hyperplasia/goitres). Carcinomas are rare in this species, accounting for 1–2% of all thyroid tumours, and usually coexist with adenomatous change. Follicular, papillary or mixed compact patterns of cells are recognised histologically. Pleomorphism, anaplasia and high mitotic rate are not typical of thyroid carcinomas in cats and so degree of invasion, metastasis and biological behaviour have to be used to differentiate them from adenomas (Turrel *et al.* 1988).

Tumour behaviour

Although some thyroid carcinomas are encapsulated and non-invasive, most are large, aggressive tumours which invade local tissues of the neck to a considerable extent, making surgical excision difficult. They metastasise rapidly via lymphatics to the retropharyngeal lymph nodes, lungs, liver and cervical vertebrae and approximately half of all cases will have metastasised by the time of presentation. Thyroid adenomas are small, mobile nodules which do not invade locally or metastasise.

Paraneoplastic syndromes

Hyperthyroidism is the most common endocrine disorder in cats and is reported with both thyroid adenomas and carcinomas. In contrast, hyperthyroidsim in dogs is much less frequently associated with thyroid neoplasia. It is usually associated with carcinomas, not adenomas in this species, and occurs in approximately 6–10% of dogs with thyroid neoplasia. Most dogs with thyroid tumours are euthyroid or if there is significant destruction of normal tissues, hypothyroid.

Medullary thyroid carcinomas may also be functional and secrete calcitonin, somatostatin, serotonin, adrenocorticotrophic hormone (ACTH) or prostaglandins. Calcium concentrations are unaffected, however, and patients are usually eucalcaemic.

Presentation/signs

Dogs and cats with thyroid tumours may present with either:

• The clinical signs of hyperthyroidism (Fig. 14.1)
• A mass in the ventral neck (Figs 14.2 and 14.3).

Most cats present with hyperthyroidism, showing clinical signs such as weight loss, tachycardia, hyperactivity, muscle weakness, diarrhoea, polyuria, polydipsia and poylphagia (Table 14.2). A small, thyroid nodule(s) is often palpable in the ventral neck, sometimes as far as the thoracic inlet, but owners will rarely have noticed it.

Most dogs with thyroid carcinomas present with a firm, painless, mass in the mid-ventral neck which may be attached to underlying structures. Submandibular and retropharyngeal lymph nodes may be enlarged secondary to lymphatic obstruction or metastasis, and coughing, dyspnoea, dysphagia or facial oedema may also be noted if the mass is applying pressure to the trachea or oesophagus. Weight loss, lethargy, anorexia or neck pain may

Table 14.2 Clinical signs associated with hyperthyroidism in cats.

System	Clinical signs	Comment
Metabolic	Weight loss despite polyphagia, heat intolerance	Anorexia in 10% of cases
Urinary	Polyuria and polydipsia	
Neuromuscular	Restlessness, hyperactivity, weakness, muscle wasting, muscle tremors	Depression in 10% of cases
Dermatologic	Unkempt hair coat, alopecia	
Respiratory/cardiovascular	Panting, dyspnoea, tachycardia, gallop rhythm, cardiac murmur, congestive heart failure	Signs due to hypertrophic cardiomyopathy
Gastrointestinal	Bulky faeces and steatorrhoea, vomiting, diarrhoea	

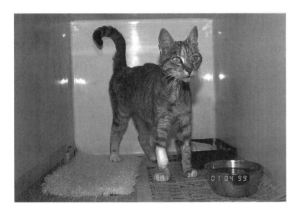

Fig. 14.1 Marked weight loss in this cat was due to hyperthyroidism (picture taken following thyroidectomy).

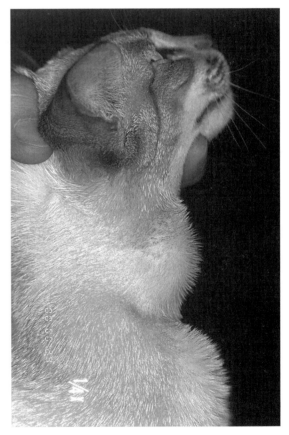

Fig. 14.3 An unusually large thyroid mass in the neck of a cat.

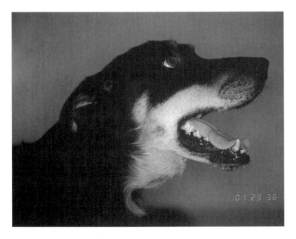

Fig. 14.2 Thyroid carcinoma presenting as a gross mass in the ventral neck of a dog.

also occur. Signs of hyperthyroidism are relatively rare and are less pronounced than in cats. With medullary thyroid carcinomas, diarrhoea is the main presenting sign.

Investigations

Bloods

No specific changes are usually noted on haematological and biochemical analysis, but a stress leucogram may be detected in cats and raised liver enzymes in both species. Hypercalcaemia is uncommon but may be detected in both cats and dogs.

To demonstrate hyperthyroidism, specific tests for thyroid function should be carried out. For cats, measurement of basal plasma thyroxine (T_4) is of most diagnostic use with concentrations increased in 90% of cases with suggestive clinical signs. Normal T_4 concentrations may sometimes be found in early cases and the T_3 suppression test or TRH stimulation test may be needed to confirm the diagnosis in these animals. In dogs, T_4 measurement should be performed if clinical signs are suggestive of hyperthyroidism but in most cases this is not necessary to make a diagnosis of thyroid neoplasia.

Imaging techniques

Thoracic and abdominal radiography should be performed in dogs to look for pulmonary, hepatic or other abdominal metastases. Thoracic radiography in cats (and dogs) may show cardiomegaly due to hypertrophic cardiomyopathy, with or without signs of congestive heart failure such as pulmonary oedema or pleural effusion. Full assessment of cardiac function, however, will require ECG and ultrasonography.

High resolution ultrasonography can be useful in determining whether one or both thyroid lobes are affected in hyperthyroid cats, particularly if no nodule is palpable. For carcinomas in dogs, ultrasonography of the neck will help determine the extent of tumour invasion, will differentiate between solid and cystic masses and will help guide fine needle aspirates.

Thyroid tumours may also be imaged using sodium pertechnetate (^{99m}Tc) scintigraphy since functional thyroid tissue concentrates the isotope and increased uptake is seen with hyperthyroidism.

It is used frequently in hyperthyroid cats prior to thyroidectomy to demonstrate whether one or both thyroid lobes are affected, particularly if no thyroid enlargement can be palpated. It may also be useful if hyperfunctional ectopic thyroid tissue is suspected although this may be confused with metastasis on the basis of the scan alone. Patchy or irregular uptake of ^{99m}Tc is seen with thyroid carcinomas, possibly with extension down the neck. Scintigraphy is not usually necessary to diagnose thyroid tumours in dogs but increased uptake of ^{99m}Tc is seen in hyperthyroid cases.

Radioiodine (^{123}I or ^{131}I) scintigraphy may also be used to image the thyroid with increased uptake seen in hyperthyroid cats (and dogs) compared to normal animals but it is more expensive and is associated with a higher radiation exposure.

Biopsy/FNA

Aspirate or biopsy is not usually performed for feline thyroid neoplasia, but for dogs, fine needle aspirates may be useful to differentiate thyroid carcinomas from non-neoplastic lesions or other tumour types. Haemorrhage is a common problem, however, because thyroid tumours are so vascular, and poor aspirates may be obtained. Histological examination of tumour tissue is the only way to make a definitive diagnosis and to distinguish adenomas from carcinomas. Needle biopsies, like fine needles aspirates, may provoke haemorrhage and so wedge biopsies are recommended.

Staging

A TNM staging system exists for thyroid tumours (Table 14.3) and group staging can also be performed (Table 14.4). Clinical and surgical examination, along with radiography of the thorax and radio-isotope scanning, should be used to assess the primary tumour and look for regional (cervical node) and distant metastasis.

Treatment

The treatment options for feline thyroid tumours include:

• Surgery
• Radioactive iodine (^{131}I) therapy
• Antithyroid drug therapy.

Table 14.3 Clinical stages (TNM) of canine tumours of the thyroid gland. Owen (1980).

T *Primary tumour*
T0   No evidence of tumour
T1   Tumour <2 cm maximum diameter
  T1a   Not fixed
  T1b   Fixed
T2   Tumour 2–5 cm maximum diameter
  T2a   Not fixed
  T2b   Fixed
T3   Tumour >5 cm maximum diameter
  T3a   Not fixed
  T3b   Fixed

N *Regional lymph nodes (RLN)*
N0   No evidence of RLN involvement
N1   Ipsilateral RLN involved
  N1a   Not fixed
  N1b   Fixed
N2   Bilateral RLN involved
  N2a   Not fixed
  N2b   Fixed

M *Distant metastasis*
M0   No evidence of distant metastasis
M1   Distant metastasis detected

Table 14.4 Stage grouping of canine thyroid tumours. Owen (1980).

Stage grouping	T	N	M
I	T1a,b	N0(−) N1a(−) N2a(−)	M0
II	T0 T1a,b T2a,b	N1(+) N1(+) N0(+) or N1a(+)	M0
III	Any T3 Any T	Any N Any Nb	M0
IV	Any T	Any N	M1

(−) histologically negative (+) histologically positive.

The options for canine thyroid carcinoma are slightly more limited with surgery being the main choice, and radiotherapy or chemotherapy used adjunctively.

Surgery

Canine thyroid tumours

Surgical resection is the treatment of choice for canine thyroid tumours, irrespective of whether they are functional or non-functional. Patients with functional tumours (hyperthyroidism) should be stabilised medically prior to the operation to minimise the anaesthetic risk. Benign adenomas are generally well encapsulated and easily resected, as are mobile, non-invasive carcinomas (Klein *et al.* 1995). Most malignant tumours, however, are invasive and in a third of cases they are bilateral, making clean surgical margins difficult to obtain. Surgery is complicated by the vascular nature of most carcinomas and the proximity of important structures such as the recurrent laryngeal nerves, parathyroid glands and major blood vessels. Even if complete excision is unobtainable, surgical debulking is helpful as a palliative measure in many cases, and can be combined with other modalities such as radiotherapy or chemotherapy.

Parathyroid tissue cannot usually be preserved when resecting an invasive thyroid carcinoma but if the tumour is unilateral, hypocalcaemia (and hypothyroidism) are rare complications. With bilateral tumours, both hypoparathyroidism and hypothyroidism must be addressed using calcium and vitamin D (see parathyroid tumours, p. 210) and thyroxine. Other post-operative complications of thyroidectomy may include Horner's syndrome and laryngeal paralysis.

Feline thyroid tumours

Thyroidectomy is also the treatment of choice for benign adenomas in hyperthyroid cats if radioactive iodide therapy is not available (see below). Patients are often stabilised by medical treatment for several weeks prior to the operation to minimise the anaesthetic risk. Scintigraphy may also be performed prior to surgery to see if unilateral or bilateral enlargement of the thyroid gland is present. An intracapsular dissection may be chosen to try and preserve the external parathyroid gland at the cranial end of the thyroid lobe but relapse rates may be worse than with extracapsular surgery. As with thyroid surgery in dogs, unilateral or bilateral thyroidectomy can be performed but careful monitoring of calcium levels is essential post-operatively to detect hypocalcaemia resulting from damaged/excised parathyroid glands. Acute hypocalcaemia will require immediate therapy (see parathyroid tumours, p. 210) but it may be prevented by monitoring plasma calcium concentrations regularly and if they fall below 1.8 mmol/l, supplementing with calcium lactate or carbonate

(50 mg/kg/day) and dihydrotachysterol (0.01 mg/kg/day). Thyroxine supplementation is necessary after bilateral and occasionally unilateral thyroidectomy.

Radiotherapy

External beam hypofractionated radiotherapy should be considered for adjunctive use following surgical resection of an invasive thyroid carcinoma, and may have a palliative role without surgery, as a local treatment for invasive thyroid carcinoma in the dog (Brearley et al. 1999). Side-effects may include oesophagitis, laryngitis, dysphonia and hypothyroidism.

Radioactive iodine (^{131}I) therapy is the treatment of choice for feline thyroid adenomas and hyperthyroidism, since it is a non-invasive procedure which selectively destroys hyperfunctioning thyroid tissue, while preserving the normal thyroid tissue and the parathyroid glands. However facilities are limited to selected referral institutions, and cats must be hospitalised for several weeks while receiving treatment. Dogs with hyperfunctional thyroid tumours may also be treated with radioiodine but treatment is less successful than for cats. Although some canine non-functional tumours may concentrate radioiodine, it is not clear whether they will do so adequately to respond to (^{131}I) therapy.

Chemotherapy

Large, bulky thyroid carcinomas are unlikely to respond to cytotoxic drug therapy, but the metastatic and invasive nature of most tumours means that chemotherapy should be considered following surgical resection. Doxorubicin, cisplatin or a combination of doxorubicin, cyclophosphamide and vincristine (VAC – Table 5.4) have been used adjunctively to surgery to treat thyroid carcinoma in the dog, although controlled trials have not been performed.

Other

Medical management with the antithyroid drugs, methimazole and carbimazole (but not propylthiouracil because of excessive side-effects), may be used to control hyperthyroidism in cats, either as an alternative to surgery or for a period of stabilisation prior to thyroidectomy or (^{131}I) therapy. They are not cytotoxic, however, and will not affect the growth or metastasis of thyroid carcinomas in dogs or cats. Methimazole is associated with more side-effects than carbimazole and these may include anorexia, vomiting, lethargy and haematological abnormalities.

Cardiac drugs such as propranolol or diltiazem may be used in conjunction with antithyroid drugs to control the cardiovascular abnormalities induced by hyperthyroidism.

Prognosis

For thyroid carcinomas in dogs, the histomorphological grade based on the presence of invasion, cellular and nuclear pleomorphism and mitotic rate is the most important prognostic factor. Tumour size also has prognostic significance with the rate of metastasis increasing with larger tumours (Leav et al. 1976). Mean survival times of 36 months have been reported for freely mobile carcinomas without local tissue invasion (Klein et al. 1995), whereas most dogs with fixed, invasive tumours survive for less than 12 months (Carver et al. 1995).

Cats with thyroid adenomas and hyperthyroidism have an excellent prognosis for returning to normal following thyroidectomy or radioiodine treatment, although the complication of hypocalcaemia may arise with bilateral cases treated surgically.

PARATHYROID GLAND

Epidemiology

Parathyroid tumours are uncommon in dogs and rare in cats. They usually occur in older dogs (8–10 years) with a predilection for keeshonds (Berger & Feldman 1987). Older cats are also affected, with a possible predilection for females and Siamese cats (Kallet et al. 1991).

Aetiology

There is no known aetiology for parathyroid tumours in the dog and cat.

Pathology

External and internal parathyroid glands are associated with each thyroid lobe and any one of the four glands may be affected. Tumours derive from the parathormone (PTH) secreting chief cells and adenomas predominate. Multiple nodular hyperplasia of the glands can occur but adenocarcinomas are rare. Ectopic parathyroid tissue may be found in the anterior mediastinum.

Tumour behaviour

Parathyroid adenomas are benign, well encapsulated tumours, whereas adenocarcinomas have the potential for local invasion and metastasis.

Paraneoplastic syndromes

Parathyroid adenomas autonomously secrete PTH to produce hyperparathyroidism and this results in hypercalcaemia (Chapter 2). Hypercalcaemia has also been reported with parathyroid adenocarcinoma.

Presentation/signs

Dogs and cats with functional parathyroid tumours present with the clinical signs associated with hypercalcaemia (see Chapter 2). Parathyroid adenomas are usually small nodules which are rarely palpable in the ventral neck and would go unnoticed if it were not for the signs of hypercalcaemia.

Investigations

Since animals present with hypercalcaemia, the investigation of such cases involves ruling out other more common causes of raised calcium concentrations such as lymphoma, hypoadrenocorticism or adenocarcinoma of the apocrine glands of the anal sac, as detailed in Chapter 2.

Bloods

Raised serum calcium concentrations will be detected on biochemical analysis but values are usually in the region of 3–4mmol/l rather than the very high levels often noted with lymphoma. Phosphate levels are usually low or normal.

Once the more common causes of hypercalcaemia have been eliminated, a PTH assay should be performed to look for increased secretion of PTH. A raised PTH concentration with concurrent hypercalcaemia confirms the diagnosis of hyperparathyroidism and is suggestive of a parathyroid adenoma or hyperplasia. A raised PTH concentration is also present with secondary hyperparathyroidism which may result from renal failure or calcium deficiency during growth. However, in these conditions total calcium is usually normal and ionised calcium may be low; phosphate is usually elevated along with raised urea and creatinine. PTH concentrations are low in cases of hypercalcaemia of malignancy.

Imaging techniques

The parathyroid glands in normal dogs are not routinely visible with ultrasonography, but an enlarged parathyroid gland due to hyperplasia or adenoma can often be detected close to or within thyroid tissue.

Biopsy/FNA

Surgical exploration of the neck to locate an enlarged parathyroid gland/adenoma can be performed as part of the diagnostic investigations of hypercalcaemia, once other more common causes have been excluded, or once a PTH assay has been performed. An excisional biopsy of the enlarged gland is usually performed for a histopathological diagnosis of parathyroid neoplasia.

Staging

There is no specific staging system for parathyroid gland tumours.

Treatment

Surgery

Surgery is the most appropriate treatment for parathyroid adenomas and adenocarcinomas. The affected parathyroid gland can be excised, leaving the other glands to produce PTH. With multiple nodular hyperplasia, more than one gland may be affected and all need to be removed. Calcium concentrations should fall quickly to within the normal range following surgery, although there is a risk of hypocalcaemia initially because the unaffected parathyroid glands will have been suppressed by excess PTH secretion. Calcium concentrations should therefore be monitored carefully post-operatively and prophylactic treatment with vitamin D and calcium supplementation is recommended before hypocalcaemia occurs. If hypocalcaemia causes clinical signs, calcium supplementation should be used as follows:

- Restore normal calcium concentrations with 10% calcium gluconate (0.5–1.5 ml/kg) by i.v. infusion over 10–30 minutes, monitoring heart function by ECG.
- Maintain normocalcaemia with subcutaneous calcium gluconate (diluted 50:50 with 0.9% sodium chloride) every six hours until oral supplementation becomes effective.

- Start oral vitamin D (dihydrotachysterol at 20–30 μg/kg) and calcium carbonate (50–100 mg/kg/day) or calcium lactate (25–50 mg/kg) supplementation.
- Continue treatment for several weeks, maintaining calcium concentration at the lower end of the normal range, then gradually reduce first vitamin D and then calcium supplementation.

There is a danger of inducing hypercalcaemia with dihydrotachysterol therapy and if clinical signs such as polyuria and polydipsia arise, therapy should be discontinued immediately.

Radiotherapy

Radiotherapy has not been used to treat parathyroid tumours in animals.

Chemotherapy

Chemotherapy is not appropriate for treating parathyroid tumours in animals.

Prognosis

The prognosis for parathyroid tumours is excellent since most can be removed surgically. However, complications with post-operative hypocalcaemia may be life-threatening if not recognised and treated immediately.

PITUITARY GLAND

Pituitary gland neoplasms are classified as secondary brain tumours since they affect the brain by local extension. They are discussed here rather than with the nervous system because of the endocrine function of the anterior and posterior lobes.

Epidemiology

Most pituitary adenomas are reported in association with pituitary-dependent hyperadrenocorticism. Dogs with this paraneoplastic syndrome are usually middle-aged or old (median age 10 years), but slightly younger than those with adrenal dependent hyperadrenocorticism. Poodles, dachshunds, beagles, boxers, German shepherd dogs and Boston terriers are frequently affected but both sexes are

affected equally (Peterson 1986; Reusch & Feldman 1991). Cats with pituitary-dependent hyperadrenocorticism also tend to be middle aged or old. Females appear to be predisposed but no particular breeds are affected (Feldman 1995). Cats with acromegaly caused by a pituitary tumour are also middle-aged or old and of mixed breed.

Aetiology

The aetiology of pituitary tumours in animals is not known.

Pathology/tumour behaviour

The pituitary gland consists of two parts:

- The anterior lobe (adenohypophysis) which is a neuroendocrine gland under control of hypothalamic hormones released into the hypothalamic-hypophyseal portal system.
- The posterior lobe (neurohypophysis) which is a neurosecretory system with axons extending directly from cell bodies in the hypothalamus. These release oxytocin and vasopressin.

The cells of the anterior lobe are classified according to their specific secretory products (Table 14.5). Over half are somatotrophs, secreting growth hormone (GH), with the remaining types each representing 5–15% of the gland. Primary tumours may derive from any of these cells but the pituitary is also a possible site for metastatic tumours such as melanoma, or mammary adenocarcinoma.

The most common pituitary tumour in the dog and cat is derived from corticotrophic (chromophobic) cells of the anterior lobe (pars distalis and pars intermedia) which produce adrenocorticotrophic hormone (ACTH). These are benign tumours which may be either microadenomas (less than 1 cm in diameter) or macroadenomas (greater than 1 cm in diameter). They are usually functional, resulting in hyperadrenocorticism, but non-functional tumours also occur. Chromophobe

carcinomas are much less common and are usually non-functional, large and invasive tumours which invade the brain and sphenoid bone, metastasising to lymph nodes, spleen and liver.

In cats, tumours of the somatotrophic cells (which are acidophilic) of the anterior pituitary are often functional and cause acromegaly.

During embryogenesis, the anterior lobe develops from Rathke's pouch, which is derived from the ectoderm of the oropharynx. Tumours which develop from Rathke's pouch are called craniopharyngiomas and they occur in young animals. They are often very large tumours which grow along the ventral aspect of the brain and involve cranial nerves, hypothalamus and thalamus.

Paraneoplastic syndromes

A variety of paraneoplastic syndromes may accompany pituitary tumours, depending on whether hormone production is increased or decreased (see Table 14.5). The most common pituitary related paraneoplastic syndrome in the dog and cat is pituitary-dependent hyperadrenocorticism. The other paraneoplastic syndrome of note, in the cat, is acromegaly.

Table 14.5 Endocrine disorders caused by tumours of the pituitary gland.

Cell type	Hormone	Disorder associated with underproduction	Disorder associated with overproduction
Anterior lobe			
Corticotrophs	ACTH	Secondary hypoadrenocorticism – hypocortisolaemia	Hyperadrenocorticism (Cushing's disease)
Somatotrophs	GH	Possible alopecia due to atrophy of skin and adnexae* (not dwarfism in adults)	Acromegaly (cats not dogs)
Thyrotrophs	TSH	Hypothyroidism	Hyperthyroidism (not reported in dogs and cats)
Gonadotrophs	LH/FSH	Hypogonadism – anoestrus, testicular atrophy	
Lactotrophs	PRL		Galactorrhoea
Posterior lobe			
	Vasopressin	Diabetes insipidus	Syndrome of inappropriate diuresis (SIAD)

* Most 'growth hormone responsive alopecia' of adults is in fact an adrenocortical condition.

Table 14.6 Clinical features of acromegaly in cats.

Type of change	Clinical signs
Physical	Hypertrophy of face and extremities
	Weight gain
	Thickening of skin and development of folds around the head and neck
	Hypertrophy of tongue
	Prognathism and wide interdental spaces
	Hypertrophy of thoracic and abdominal organs
Cardiac	Congestive heart failure
Metabolic	Development of insulin resistance and diabetes mellitus
	Renal failure
Haematological	Increased red blood cell count
Biochemical	Raised concentrations of:
	Glucose
	Liver enzymes
	Phosphate
	Total protein
	Cholesterol
	Elevated basal concentrations of GH or IGF-I or failure to suppress GH concentrations in a glucose suppression test
Diagnostic imaging	Presence of a pituitary mass on CT or MRI

Presentation/signs

Pituitary tumours may present in one of three ways:

- Endocrinologically active tumours may present with specific metabolic disorders due to hormone excess, for example pituitary-dependent hyperadrenocorticism (Fig. 14.4) or acromegaly in cats (Tables 14.5 and 14.6).
- Endocrinologically inactive tumours may present with other metabolic disorders due to insufficiency of one or more hormones. Large, expanding anterior lobe tumours may also reduce hormone production by the posterior lobe if they compress it.
- Other tumours may present as space-occupying lesions with neurological signs due to compression or invasion of the brain. Dogs and cats may present with depression, behavioural changes, disorders of thirst, appetite or temperature regulation, pacing, head pressing and circling.

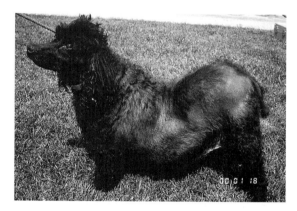

Fig. 14.4 Typical clinical appearance of hyperadrenocorticism in a female poodle (this dog was also diabetic). (Picture courtesy of Mr M. Herrtage, Department of Clinical Veterinary Medicine, University of Cambridge.)

Investigations

Bloods

The presumptive diagnosis of an anterior pituitary tumour may be made on the measurement of peripheral hormone concentrations, for example thyroxine or cortisol, and by stimulation tests with appropriate hypothalamic releasing hormones for assessment of growth hormone (GH), luteinising hormone (LH), adrenocorticotrophic hormone (ACTH) and prolactin (PRL) responses. Inadequate responses may suggest partial or total hypopituitarism. If diabetes insipidus is suspected, plasma vasopressin during osmotic stimulation by hypertonic saline can be measured, or a water deprivation test performed.

Tests for hormone overproduction are numerous (see adrenal cortex tumours later in this chapter for hyperadrenocorticism).

Imaging techniques

Pituitary tumours can only be reliably identified with sophisticated imaging techniques such as contrast-enhanced computed tomography and magnetic resonance imaging (Fig. 14.5).

Biopsy/FNA

Biopsy of pituitary tumours is not possible unless hypophysectomy is attempted.

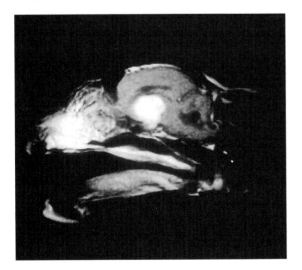

Fig. 14.5 MRI scan showing a pituitary tumour in an 11 year old domestic short hair cat with a long history of polydipsia and lethargy. The contrast enhanced, sagittal T1 weighed scan shows a large, irregularly enhancing mass extending dorsally from the pituitary fossa. (Picture courtesy of Ruth Dennis, Animal Health Trust, Newmarket.)

Staging

No staging system for pituitary tumours has been described.

Treatment

Surgery

Hypophysectomy has been used in the treatment of pituitary-dependent hyperadrenocorticism but the technique does not allow the complete removal of very large pituitary tumours and is not widely practised. With the improvement of diagnostic imaging and surgical techniques, it is possible that in future more dogs may be treated this way and given lifelong supplementation with thyroxine and cortisone.

Radiotherapy

With careful planning of the radiation field based on CT or MRI images, megavoltage irradiation can be used to treat pituitary tumours in both cats and dogs, particularly macroadenomas or tumours causing mild neurological signs (Fig. 14.6; see also Chapter 3) (Dow *et al.* 1990). Radiation will decrease the size of the tumour and resolve neurological signs, but functional tumours may require additional medical treatment, for example mitotane to control hyperadrenocorticism. Radiation side-effects may include hair loss, impaired hearing and

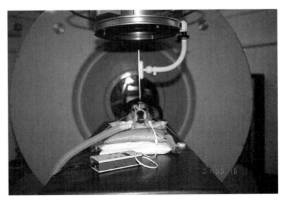

Fig. 14.6 Radiotherapy set up for dog with a brain tumour.

vestibular signs, although brain necrosis has also been reported as a late radiation effect and this causes recurrence of neurological signs.

Chemotherapy

Chemotherapy with mitotane (o,p'-DDD) may be used for pituitary-dependent hyperadrenocorticism to destroy selectively the zona fasiculata and reticularis of the adrenal cortex (see tumours of the adrenal cortex, below).

Other

Anterior pituitary failure can be treated by substituting for the deficient hormone, for example thyroxine or cortisone, but this is usually only a temporary measure until neurological effects develop due to tumour enlargement. Posterior pituitary failure can be treated with the vasopressin analogue, desmopressin (DDAVP), administered topically into the conjunctiva.

Overproduction of hormones may be treated using specific drugs where available, although many are expensive. Cabergoline (galastop), a potent anti-prolactin drug, is licensed for management of pseudopregnancy in bitches. The dopamine agonist, bromocriptine, has been used to counteract the effects of excess prolactin but is only effective in some cases and is not reported to be very effective in counteracting GH excess in acromegalic cats. The somatostatin analogue, octreotide, can be used to lower GH levels, but it is expensive.

Prognosis

The prognosis for pituitary tumours is variable depending on their clinical presentation and whether accompanying endocrine disorders can be controlled. Medical treatment of pituitary-dependent hyperadrenocorticism in dogs can be quite successful with 10% of cases successfully managed for over four years (Peterson 1986). Survival times for cats with acromegaly range from 8 to 30 months.

ADRENAL GLAND

The adrenal gland has two functionally distinct endocrine parts, the medulla and cortex, both of which may become neoplastic.

The adrenal cortex consists of three layers:

- Zona glomerulosa – produces mineralocorticoids
- Zona fasciculata – produces glucocorticoids and androgens
- Zona reticulata – produces androgens but also glucocorticoids.

Adrenocortical tumours of clinical significance are those which over secrete glucocorticoids resulting in hyperadrenocorticism.

The adrenal medulla consists of chromaffin cells of neuroectodermal origin which can be regarded as sympathetic postganglionic neurons without axons. These secrete predominantly epinephrine (adrenaline), but also some norepinephrine, directly into the blood rather than across a synaptic cleft. Tumours derived from the adrenal medulla are phaeochromocytomas.

Tumours of adrenal cortex

Epidemiology/aetiology

Adrenocortical tumours occur in both dogs and cats but there is no known aetiology. They account for 15–20% of cases of hyperadrenocorticism in dogs and 20% in cats. Large breeds of dogs are affected, particularly poodles, German shepherd dogs, dachshunds and Labrador retrievers (Scavelli et al. 1986; Reusch & Feldman 1991). Females are affected more than males.

Cats with hyperadrenocorticism are middle-aged or old (7–15 years). There is no particular breed association but more females than males are affected (Nelson & Feldman 1988).

Pathology/tumour behaviour

Adrenocortical tumours are usually unilateral and solitary, although 10% of cases are bilateral (Ford et al. 1993). With functional unilateral tumours the opposite adrenal gland is atrophied. Both adenomas and carcinomas occur in approximately equal proportions, and some of the latter can be very large, containing areas of haemorrhage and necrosis. They may compress adjacent organs or invade the aorta or vena cava, leading to intra-abdominal haemorrhage. Approximately 50% of cases have liver metastases and invasion of the caudal vena cava and other vessels. Adrenocortical tumours may occur concurrently with phaeochromocytomas in dogs.

Paraneoplastic syndromes

Adrenocortical tumours may be functional and autonomously secrete glucocorticoids. This produces the characteristic signs of hyperadrenocorticism or Cushing's syndrome. Although approximately 80% of Cushing's syndrome cases in the dog and cat are caused by pituitary tumours and are therefore ACTH dependent, the details of Cushing's syndrome are included here, rather than with pituitary tumours.

Presentation/signs

Non-functional tumours may be found incidentally at post mortem examination. Functional tumours, however, present with Cushing's syndrome. The clinical signs of this disease are related to the actions of glucocorticoids and are listed in Table 14.7.

Investigations

Bloods

On haematological analysis high levels of glucocorticoids produce characteristic findings of leucocytosis, neutrophilia, lymphopenia and eosinopenia. Alkaline phosphatase is usually elevated on biochemical analysis in dogs due to the induction of an isoenzyme. ALT may be mildly elevated and raised cholesterol, bile salts and glucose may also be noted. Persistent hyperglycaemia is more common in the cat and, before hyperadrenocorticism is considered, many are diagnosed with diabetes mellitus which is hard to stabilise.

Specific diagnosis of hyperadrenocorticism relies on the following tests for adrenal function:

- ACTH stimulation test – to establish the diagnosis of hyperadrenocorticism (HAC) but false negatives may occur. It will distinguish iatrogenic from spontaneous hyperadrenocorticism and is the most useful test for monitoring treatment with mitotane. ACTH (0.25 mg/dog or 0.125 mg/cat) is administered intramuscularly or intravenously and plasma cortisol is measured one

Table 14.7 Clinical signs of hyperadrenocorticism.

System	Clinical signs	Comment
Metabolic	Polyphagia, hepatomegaly, obesity, pendulous abdomen	Concurrent diabetes mellitus in 5–10% of dogs and 80–100% of cats
Urinary	Polyuria and polydipsia, urinary tract infections, glycosuria	
Neuromuscular	Muscle weakness and atrophy, exercise intolerance, lethargy	
Dermatologic	Bilaterally symmetrical alopecia, pyoderma, seborrhea, skin thinning, hyperpigmentation, calcinosis cutis	Full thickness skin defects in cats
Respiratory/cardiovascular	Hypertension, pulmonary thromboembolism, congestive heart failure	
Reproductive	Anoestrus, testicular atrophy	
Neurologic	Facial nerve paralysis, pseudomyotonia, CNS signs	Less common

hour later (and 1.5 hours for cats). With HAC, cortisol is increased to a much greater extent than in normal animals and exceeds the upper limit of the normal range.

- Low-dose dexamethasone suppression test (dexamethasone screening test) – a more sensitive and less specific way to establish the diagnosis of hyperadrenocorticism. Dexamethasone (0.01 mg/kg) is administered intravenously in the morning and plasma cortisol is measured eight hours later. This is depressed in normal animals due to feedback inhibition of ACTH, but is high in animals with hyperadrenocorticism.
- High dose dexamethasone suppression test – to distinguish between pituitary dependent hyperadrenocorticism and an adrenocortical tumour. Dexamethasone is used (0.1 mg/kg in dogs or 1 mg/kg in cats) and plasma cortisol is usually measured four hours later. With such a high dose of dexamethasone, ACTH secretion can be suppressed in pituitary-dependent hyperadrenocorticism resulting in a decline in baseline cortisol concentration by over 50%. Production of cortisol by adrenocortical tumours, however, is unaffected.
- ACTH assay – if cortisol concentrations are depressed by less than 50%, it is necessary to measure plasma ACTH to differentiate between an adrenocortical tumour and non-suppressible form of pituitary dependent HAC.

Urinalysis

Glycosuria is common in cats and also seen in 5–10% of dogs with HAC. Bacteriuria, or high white cell counts, may be present, indicating urinary infection, and in these cases urine culture and sensitivity should be performed on a cystocentesis sample. Specific gravity is usually low because of polyuria and polydipsia.

Urinary cortisol:creatinine ratio has been used to screen for hyperadrenocorticism but it is not specific and therefore not recommended for routine use.

Imaging techniques

Abdominal radiography may reveal changes due to hyperadrenocorticism such as an enlarged liver, pot-bellied appearance, osteopenia and bladder distension, and in some cases an enlarged or calcified adrenal gland may be detected.

(Adrenal calcification may be noted in normal cats.) Thoracic films may show pulmonary metastases or interstitial lung markings due to poor lung inflation.

Ultrasonography is preferable to survey radiography for visualising the adrenals, and should give information about tumour size and invasion. Unilateral enlargement suggests an adrenal mass, particularly if the contralateral adrenal is atrophied. Bilateral enlargement of the adrenals may be more suggestive of pituitary-dependent hyperadrenocorticism than of bilateral adrenocortical tumours. CT or MRI give the most detailed imaging information about adrenal tumours but they are expensive techniques and not always available.

Biopsy/FNA

A definitive diagnosis of adrenocortical tumour requires histopathological examination. Tissue is usually obtained by excisional biopsy when the tumour is treated surgically.

Staging

A TNM staging system is used for the adrenal gland (Table 14.8). Tumours should be investigated surgically to assess the primary mass, regional (lumbar) lymph nodes and distant sites. Thoracic radiography should be perfomed to look for pulmonary metastases.

Table 14.8 Clinical stages (TNM) of canine tumours of the adrenal gland. Owen (1980).

T	*Primary tumour*
T0	No evidence of tumour
T1	Well-defined tumour
T2	Tumour invading neighbouring structures
T3	Tumour invading blood vessels
N	*Regional lymph nodes (RLN)*
N0	No evidence of RLN involvement
N1	RLN involved
M	*Distant metastasis*
M0	No evidence of distant metastasis
M1	Distant metastasis detected

Treatment

Surgery

Surgical resection is the treatment of choice for unilateral adrenocortical tumours. It may be combined with medical treatment for a few months prior to surgery in order to stabilise debilitated animals which are poor surgical candidates. Removal of adenomas can resolve the hyperadrenocorticism permanently and even with malignant tumours, palliation of the disease or even a surgical cure may be possible. Complications following surgery may be minimal or as high as 50% and may include cardiac arrest, pancreatitis or acute renal failure. There is a danger of post-operative hypoadrenocorticism because of atrophy of the contralateral gland, hence patients must be carefully monitored and supported initially with intravenous fluid therapy and glucocorticoids. Mineralocorticoid supplementation (deoxycorticosterone acetate/pivalate or fludrocortisone acetate) may also be needed, but both glucocorticoids and mineralocorticoids can be tapered over several months. Bilateral tumours may also be resected but long term supplementation with mineralocorticoids is required.

In cats, unilateral adrenalectomy is the treatment of choice for adrenal tumours and since the response to cytotoxic therapy is poor, bilateral adrenalectomy is the best option for hyperadrenocorticism caused by pituitary tumours. Cats with hyperadrenocorticism are often more debilitated than dogs and therefore pose more of a surgical risk. Concurrent diabetes mellitus may also be a problem and so careful management of insulin requirements is essential perioperatively.

Radiotherapy

Radiotherapy has not been used to treat adrenocortical tumours in animals.

Chemotherapy

For inoperable tumours or if owners refuse surgical treatment, it is possible to use medical management in dogs. The condition is poorly responsive in cats. The cytotoxic drug, o,p'-DDD (mitotane) which selectively destroys the zona fasciculata and reticularis of the cortex may be used as for treating pituitary dependent hyperadrenocorticism but higher doses may be necessary. The drug is irritant to the gastrointestinal tract and may produce vomiting and so it is best administered with food. In dogs, the protocol for mitotane is:

- Induction dose of 50–75 mg/kg/day until inappetance, depression, vomiting or diarrhoea or reduced water consumption (below 60 ml/kg/day) occur
- Maintenance dose of 75–100 mg/kg/week, using the ACTH stimulation test to monitor progress and aiming to keep cortisol levels to below the normal pre-treatment range.

Other

Ketoconazole (5 mg/kg BID for seven days then 10 mg/kg BID) may also be used to manage canine hyperadrenocorticism since at high doses it inhibits steroid synthesis. However, it is more expensive than mitotane and requires twice daily dosing, indefinitely. Its use in cats is more disappointing, with only partial responses observed. Side-effects in dogs include anorexia, vomiting and icterus/hepatic necrosis and in cats, depression, anorexia, tremors, low blood cortisol and severe hypoglycaemia.

Metyrapone, a drug which inhibits the conversion of 11b-deoxycortisol to cortisol, has been used successfully to treat hyperadrenocorticism in cats.

Prognosis

The prognosis for adrenocortical adenomas in dogs is very good if surgically removed, but surgical resection of adenocarcinomas is less successful. Dogs treated medically may respond quite well with a mean survival time of 16 months in one study (Kintzer & Peterson 1994).

The prognosis for cats following adrenalectomy is variable, but a median survival time of 12 months was reported in one study (Duesberg et al. 1995). Cats with adrenal tumours have a better long-term survival following adrenalectomy than those with pituitary tumours.

Tumours of adrenal medulla

Epidemiology/aetiology

Phaeochromocytomas are uncommon tumours in dogs and very rare in cats. Older dogs (mean age 10–11 years) and cats are usually affected and boxers may show an increased incidence. They may be solitary tumours or occur with other endocrine and non-endocrine tumours (Barthez *et al*. 1997). There is no known aetiology.

Pathology/tumour behaviour

Phaeochromocytomas derive from adrenomedullary chromaffin cells but they may coexist with tumours of the adrenal cortex. Extra-adrenal phaeochromocytomas (paraganglionas) have also been reported. Phaeochromocytomas are usually unilateral and the affected adrenal appears enlarged with little normal tissue remaining. They are usually slow growing and benign but malignant forms do occur and these may grow quite large. Large tumours may invade local tissues and vessels including the vena cava and produce a tumour cell thrombosis. Distant metastasis to other abdominal organs may occur, particularly the liver, regional lymph nodes, spleen and kidneys.

Paraneoplastic syndromes

Functional phaeochromocytomas over produce catecholamines resulting in overstimulation of adrenergic receptors in different tissues and a syndrome of hypertension and tachycardia (see below).

Presentation/signs

Many phaeochromocytomas go undetected clinically and are found incidentally at exploratory celiotomy or on post mortem examination. Others, however, may present as an acute crisis with cardiovascular collapse or be a cause of sudden death. The most common clinical signs are non-specific and intermittent such as weakness, anorexia, lethargy, depression, panting and polyuria/polydipsia. Tachycardia or other cardiac abnormalities may also occur and an abdominal mass may be palpable in some cases. Occasionally animals may present with haemoperitoneum and abdominal distension due to tumour rupture. Most animals are hypertensive and this may cause retinal haemorrhage or detachment or neurologic abnormalities. The adrenal mass often contains a lot of haemorrhage, possibly due to hypertension.

Investigations

Bloods
At present blood samples are not usually used for diagnosing phaeochromocytomas in dogs and cats since they have not been properly evaluated. Basal catecholamine measurements are of limited use as excessive concentrations are only released intermittently. Measurement of urinary catecholamine concentrations and their metabolites over a 24 hour period may be more useful (Twedt & Wheeler 1984).

Blood pressure
Systemic hypertension is the main clinical feature of phaeochromocytomas but it is often difficult to document because of its episodic nature. Blood pressure should be determined on several occasions if a phaeochromocytoma is suspected.

Imaging techniques
Abdominal radiographs and ultrasonography may be used to detect an enlarged adrenal gland or adrenal mass and to screen for abdominal metastases. Thoracic films should be performed to evaluate cardiac size and signs of congestive heart failure and to look for pulmonary metatases. Caudal vena caval angiography was previously used to detect tumour thrombi but has been surpassed by ultrasonography, which is currently the technique of choice for evaluation of the local extent and anatomic relationships of adrenal tumours. Despite their expense, CT and MRI are being increasingly used and these provide more detailed images of the adrenal glands.

Biopsy/FNA

A definitive diagnosis of phaeochromocytoma requires histological examination of adrenal tissue. Excisional biopsy is usually performed as part of surgical treatment or tissue can be obtained at post mortem examination. Special stains such as chromogranin A and synatophysin may be used to confirm chromaffin cell origin.

Staging

A TNM staging system is available for adrenal tumours (Table 14.8) but no group staging is used. Clinical and surgical examination of primary tumour, regional (lumbar) lymph nodes and other abdominal organs should be performed as well as radiography of the thorax.

Treatment

Surgery

Adrenal phaeochromocytomas have been removed successfully in dogs and cats although dissection is difficult because of their vascular nature and the tendency to invade major blood vessels (Henry *et al.* 1993; Gilson *et al.* 1994). Care is needed to avoid intraoperative hypertension and postoperative hypotension by using a combination of α (phenoxybenzamine) and β blockers (propranolol). Precise monitoring of blood pressure and cardiac function is essential to detect any hypertensive or tachycardic crises.

Radiotherapy

Radiotherapy has not been used to treat phaeochromocytomas in animals.

Chemotherapy

Chemotherapy has not been used to treat phaeochromocytomas in animals.

Other

If surgical resection is not possible, medical management may be used to control blood pressure and cardiac arrhythmias. Cardiac arrhythmias may be treated with a β blocker such as propranolol but only after administration of an α 1 adrenergic blocker to prevent hypertension.

Prognosis

The prognosis for phaeochromocytomas is guarded because of the difficulties associated with surgical treatment and the potential for life-threatening hypertensive and tachycardic events. If surgery is successful, however, long term survival may extend to three years since late metastasis is rare (Barthez *et al.* 1997).

PANCREAS (ENDOCRINE)

Neoplasia of the exocrine pancreas is included with tumours of the gastro-intestinal tract (Chapter 8). Tumours of the endocrine pancreas derive from the Islets of Langerhans. In the dog and cat, these may be classified by immunohistochemical staining as:

- Insulinoma (B cell tumour)
- Gastrinoma (D cell tumour)
- Glucagonoma (A cell tumour)
- Pancreatic polypeptidoma (F or P cell tumour – only one case reported, Zerbe *et al.* 1989).

In reality, pancreatic endocrine tumours often secrete multiple hormones although one cell type usually predominates. Each of the above tumours is associated with a paraneoplastic syndrome (Table 14.1).

Insulinoma

Epidemiology

Insulinoma is the commonest tumour of the pancreatic islet cells. It occurs in medium to large-breed dogs with a mean age of 8–9 years (range 4–13 years) but there is no particular sex or breed predisposition. Insulinoma is rare in cats, with only isolated reports in the literature (Hawks *et al.* 1992).

Aetiology

The aetiology of insulinoma is unknown.

Pathology

Insulinomas may be either benign or malignant, although most tumours in dogs are malignant. Insulinomas are usually solitary and discrete but multiple tumours and diffuse infiltrates are reported. Adenomas are usually spherical nodules on the serosal surface of the pancreas, whereas carcinomas are larger, multilobular masses which invade the parenchyma and contain areas of haemorrhage and necrosis. Both lobes of the pancreas are equally affected in dogs (Caywood et al. 1988).

On immunohistochemical examination, insulinomas stain for not only insulin, but also somatostatin, glucagon and pancreatic polypeptide.

Tumour behaviour

The behaviour of insulinomas is difficult to predict from their histological appearance and some tumours which appear histologically well differentiated may occasionally invade lymphatics. Malignant insulinomas invade surrounding tissues (mesentery and omentum) and metastasise via lymphatics to regional lymph nodes, and liver in approximately 50% of cases.

Paraneoplastic syndromes

Insulinomas autonomously produce insulin despite falling blood glucose concentrations and this results in a paraneoplastic syndrome of episodic hypoglycaemia.

Presentation/signs

The clinical signs associated with insulinomas are caused by intermittent hypoglycaemia. These may be subtle at first and dismissed, but may become more obvious at times of increased glucose consumption such as fasting, exercise, stress or excite-ment, or if insulin release increases after a meal. The central nervous system depends on glucose to function properly and so as glucose concentrations fall, clinical signs such as confusion and bizarre behaviour may become apparent, progressing to epileptiform convulsions if insulinoma is not diagnosed. Other common signs are episodic muscle weakness, tremors, ataxia, hind limb weakness and collapse. Anxiety and restlessness are also reported since counter-regulatory hormones such as glucagon and catecholamines increase in response to hypoglycaemia.

No abnormalities are usually detected on physical examination, apart from weight gain in some animals. Rare cases may show a peripheral neuropathy (Schrauwen 1991; Van Ham et al. 1997).

Investigations

Although persistent hypoglycaemia is suggestive of an insulinoma, other possible causes of hypoglycaemia such as hypoadrenocorticism, liver failure, renal failure or sepsis should be considered as differentials. In these diseases, however, hypoglycaemia is not usually the predominant clinical finding.

Bloods
A diagnosis of insulinoma can be made if hypoglycaemia is detected repeatedly on a fasting blood sample (glucose <3.0 mmol/l) and if accompanying insulin concentrations are high (>10 mU/l). Insulin:glucose, amended insulin:glucose and glucose:insulin ratios may be calculated to confirm the diagnosis but false positives and negatives may occur and use of a single sample to make a diagnosis is often insufficient. A fasting test has been described which measures glucose and insulin in four samples taken from a fasting animal (Siliart & Stambouli 1996). Provocative tests such as glucose and glucagon tolerance tests are unreliable methods of diagnosis and may induce severe hypoglycaemia. Routine haematological and biochemical parameters are often within normal ranges in animals with insulinoma.

Imaging techniques
Abdominal ultrasonography can be used to identify a pancreatic mass and look for metastases, and if

available, more detailed information can be gained by using CT or MRI.

Biopsy/FNA

Histological diagnosis of insulinoma requires biopsy or excision of tumour tissue at exploratory celiotomy but the procedure is not without risks (see surgical treatment below).

Staging

No TNM staging system has been described by the WHO for endocrine tumours of the pancreas, but other authors have used TNM and clinical staging systems (Caywood *et al.* 1988).

Treatment

Surgery

Surgical resection is the preferred method of treatment for insulinomas since it allows a definitive histological diagnosis and better assessment of tumour size and metastatic disease. Partial pancreatectomy is usually performed, however the procedure carries considerable risks of hypoglycaemia and pancreatitis which may be life-threatening. These can be minimised by:

- Intravenous infusion of 5% glucose solution before, during and after surgery
- Hourly monitoring of blood glucose
- Intravenous fluids continued for 48 hours after surgery
- Nil by mouth for 48 hours after surgery
- Minimal manipulation of the pancreas during the surgical procedure.

Some cases may become hyperglycaemic postoperatively and may require insulin therapy for a few days.

The abdomen should be examined carefully for metastases since 40–50% of tumours may have metastasised by the time of surgery and lymph node excision or partial hepatectomy may also be required. If hypoglycaemia persists after surgery, it suggests that resection of the tumour (and metastases) has been incomplete.

Radiotherapy

Radiotherapy has not been used to treat insulinomas in animals.

Chemotherapy

Streptozotocin and alloxan are used to treat pancreatic insulinomas in humans but these drugs are nephrotoxic and are not recommended to treat insulinomas in animals. Medical management with other drugs, however, is appropriate (see below).

Other

Insulinomas may be managed medically prior to surgical resection or as a longer term treatment over several years. Medical management may include:

- Restriction of physical exercise and excitement to reduce the demand for glucose.
- Feeding of four to five small meals a day, of high quality but low carbohydrate content.
- Prednisolone (0.5–1.0 mg/kg/day divided bid) if hypoglycaemia persists or if convulsions occur. Dose may need to be increased gradually.
- Diazoxide (10–60 mg/kg/day divided bid, with food) for longer term management if prednisolone fails to control clinical signs or causes side-effects (hyperadrenocorticism). Diazoxide inhibits insulin secretion and peripheral use of glucose but may cause anorexia, diarrhoea or vomiting, bone marrow suppression or cardiac arrhythmias.
- Octreotide (1 µg/kg tid subcutaneously). This is a somatostatin analogue that inhibits secretion of insulin by normal and neoplastic cells but it is expensive to use and its effectiveness in dogs has not been completely evaluated.

Prognosis

The long term prognosis for dogs with insulinoma is guarded although mean survival times of 12 months can be obtained with medical management. Approximately 40% of canine insulinomas will have metastasised by the time surgical intervention is attempted. Although 10–20% of animals die from surgical complications such as pancreatitis, approximately 40% of cases will survive for at least six months following surgical treatment and mean survival times of 12–18 months may occur (Melhaff et al. 1985; Caywood et al. 1988; Dunn et al. 1993). Metastases frequently develop with recurrence of the signs in most cases treated surgically. Poor prognostic factors for survival time include young age, high preoperative insulin concentrations and presence of regional or distant metastases (Leifer et al. 1986; Caywood et al. 1988).

Gastrinoma

Epidemiology

Gastrinomas are uncommon tumours in dogs and cats. Middle-aged and old animals are affected but there is no sex or breed predisposition.

Pathology/tumour behaviour

Although gastrin is also produced by G cells in the gastric and duodenal mucosa, most gastrin-secreting tumours occur in the pancreatic islets. Gastrinomas may be single or multiple and are often firm to palpate because of fibrous connective tissue in the stroma. They are usually malignant and metastasise to local lymph nodes and the liver.

Paraneoplastic syndromes

Gastrinomas oversecrete gastrin which results in a specific paraneoplastic syndrome, often called Zollinger-Ellison syndrome in humans.

Clinical signs

Gastrinomas are usually small and undetected lesions until the clinical signs of excess gastrin become apparent. Gastric hyperacidity due to excessive gastrin production results in anorexia, weight loss, chronic vomiting and diarrhoea. Reflux oesophagitis and gastroduodenal ulcers may occur, resulting in haematemesis, haematochezia or melaena. Animals are often depressed, emaciated and febrile and abdominal palpation is painful. An abdominal mass is rarely palpable.

Investigations

Bloods

Regenerative anaemia and mild neutrophilic leucocytosis may be detected on haematological analysis. Biochemical evaluation often reveals hyperglycaemia and hypoproteinaemia (hypoalbuminaemia).

Plasma gastrin concentrations are usually significantly elevated but although this is suggestive of a gastrinoma, it is not diagnostic since renal failure, liver disease, chronic gastritis and gastric outlet obstruction may also raise gastrin concentrations. Various provocative diagnostic tests have therefore been described such as the secretin stimulation test, calcium stimulation test, or testing gastrin secretion following a protein rich meal.

Imaging techniques

Contrast radiography with barium may reveal gastric or duodenal ulcers, thickened gastric rugal folds and rapid intestinal transit. Endoscopy will also reveal signs of gastric hyperacidity such as oesophagitis, hypertrophic gastritis and gastroduodenal ulceration. Abdominal ultrasonography can be used to identify a pancreatic mass and look for metastases, but more detailed information is gained by using CT or MRI. Somatostatin receptor scintigraphy with [111]indium pentetreotide has also been described (Altschul et al. 1997).

Biopsy/FNA

Histological confirmation of a gastrinoma requires examination of tissue which is usually obtained at exploratory celiotomy. This is the best method of establishing a definitive diagnosis.

Staging

A specific TNM staging system has not been described for gastrinoma in dogs and cats.

Treatment

Surgery

Surgical resection is the ideal treatment for gastrinomas but it is rarely successful because of unresectable metastases and is therefore a palliative measure.

Radiotherapy/chemotherapy

Radiotherapy and chemotherapy have not been used to treat gastrinoma in dogs and cats.

Other

Unresectable gastrinomas may be managed medically by inhibiting gastric acid secretion. Gastric parietal cells have receptors for histamine and acetylcholine as well as gastrin, and medical management may therefore include:

- Histamine H_2 receptor antagonists (cimetidine, ranitidine)
- Anticholinergics (probantheline bromide)
- Somatostatin analogues (octreotide)
- Proton pump inhibitors (omeprazole).

Gastro-intestinal protectants such as sucralfate may also be used to minimise erosion and ulceration of the mucosa.

Prognosis

The long-term prognosis for gastrinomas is poor because of the high metastatic rate and survival times are short (less than six months).

Glucagonoma

Glucagon-producing tumours of the pancreas are rare, with only isolated cases (all carcinomas) reported in dogs and none reported in cats (Gross *et al.* 1990; Bond *et al.* 1995; Torres *et al.* 1997; Cerundolo *et al.* 1999). All of the dogs with glucagon secreting pancreatic carcinomas presented with the paraneoplastic syndrome of metabolic epidermal necrosis which resembles the condition of necrolytic migratory erythema, associated with glucagonoma in humans. In dogs, metabolic epidermal necrosis has been more frequently reported with other diseases such as chronic liver disease (hepatocutaneous syndrome) and diabetes mellitus, than with glucagonoma (Miller *et al.* 1990) (Fig. 14.7).

Clinical signs

The skin lesions characteristic of metabolic epidermal necrosis are hyperkeratosis and fissuring of the footpads, symmetrical erythema, and ulceration and crusting of the face, feet and external genitalia.

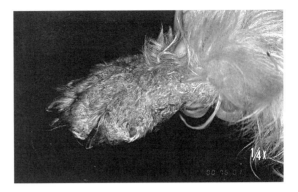

Fig. 14.7 Hepatocutaneous syndrome. Hyperkeratosis and crusting dermatosis of the feet is characteristic of hepatocutaneous syndrome.

These may cause depression and reluctance to walk.

Investigations

A definitive diagnosis of glucagonoma requires histopathological examination of tumour tissue and positive immunohistochemical staining for glucagon, although a tentative diagnosis can be made if a pancreatic neoplasm can be detected using ultrasonography or other diagnostic imaging techniques. Animals may have elevated plasma glucagon levels but this can occur with other diseases such as liver failure as well as with glucagonoma.

Prognosis

The prognosis for dogs with glucagonoma appears to be poor with euthanasia being the likely outcome. Successful excision of the pancreatic tumour was carried out in one dog with subsequent resolution of the skin lesions (Torres *et al.* 1997).

References

Altschul, M., Simpson, K.W., Dykes, N.L., Mauldin, E.A., Reubi, J.C. & Cummings, J.F. (1997) Evaluation of somatostatin analogues for the detection and treatment of gastrinoma in a dog. *Journal of Small Animal Practice*, (38), 286–91.

Barthez, P.Y., Marks, S.L., Woo, J., Feldman, E.C. & Matteucci, M. (1997) Phaeochromocytoma in dogs: 61

cases (1984–1995). *Journal of Veterinary Internal Medicine*, (11), 272–8.

Berger, B. & Feldman, E.C. (1987) Primary hyperparathyroidism in dogs: six cases (1982–1991). *Journal of the American Veterinary Medical Association*, (191), 350–56.

Bond, R., McNeil, P.E., Evans, H. & Screbernik (1995) Metabolic epidermal necrosis in two dogs with different underlying diseases. *Veterinary Record*, (136), 466–71.

Brearley, M.J., Hayes, A.M. & Murphy, S. (1999) Hypofractionated radiation therapy for invasive thyroid carcinoma in dogs: a retrospective analysis of survival. *Journal of Small Animal Practice*, (40), 206–10.

Carver, J.R., Kapatkin, A. & Patnaik, A.K. (1995) A comparison of medullary thyroid carcinoma and thyroid adenocarcinoma in dogs: a retrospective study of 38 cases. *Veterinary Surgery*, (24), 315–19.

Caywood, D.D., Klausner, J.S., O'Leary, T.P., Withrow, S.J. *et al.* (1988) Pancreatic insulin-secreting neoplasms: clinical, diagnostic and prognostic features in 73 dogs. *Journal of the American Animal Hospital Association*, (24), 577–84.

Cerundolo, R., McEvoy, F., McNeil, P.E. & Lloyd, D.H. (1999) Ultrasonographic detection of a pancreatic glucagon-secreting multihormonal islet cell tumour in a dachshund with metabolic epidermal necrosis. *Veterinary Record*, (145), 662–6.

Dow, S.W., LeCouteur, R.A., Rosychuk, R.A.W. *et al.* (1990) Response of dogs with functional pituitary macroadenomas and macrocarcinomas to radiation. *Journal of Small Animal Practice*, (31), 287–94.

Duesberg, C.A., Nelson, R.W., Feldman, E.C. *et al.* (1995) Adrenalectomy for treatment of hyperadrenocorticism in cats: 10 cases (1988–1992). *Journal of the American Veterinary Medical Association*, (207), 1066–70.

Dunn, J.K., Bostock, D.E., Herrtage, M.E., Jackson, K.F. & Walker, M.J. (1993) Insulin-secreting tumours of the canine pancreas: clinical and pathological features of 11 cases. *Journal of Small Animal Practice*, (34), 325–31.

Feldman, E.C. (1995) Hyperadrenocorticism. In: *Textbook of Veterinary Internal Medicine*, (eds S.J. Ettinger & E.C. Feldman), 1538–78. W.B. Saunders, Philadelphia.

Ford, S.L., Feldman, E.C. & Nelson, R.W. (1993) Hyperadrenocorticism caused by bilateral adrenocortical neoplasia in dogs: four cases (1983–1988). *Journal of the American Veterinary Medical Association*, (202), 789–92.

Gilson, S.D., Withrow, S.J. & Orton, E.C. (1994) Surgical treatment of phaeochromocytoma; technique, complications and results in six dogs. *Veterinary Surgery*, (23), 195–200.

Gross, T.L., O'Brien, T.D., Davies, A.P. & Long, R.E. (1990) Glucagon-producing pancreatic endocrine tumors in two dogs with superficial necrolytic dermatitis. *Journal of the American Veterinary Medical Association*, (197), 1619–22.

Hawks, D., Peterson, M.E., Hawkins, K.L. & Rosebury, W.S. (1992) Insulin-secreting pancreatic (islet cell) carcinoma in a cat. *Journal of Veterinary Internal Medicine*, (6), 193–6.

Henry, C.J., Brewer, W.G., Montgomery, R.D., Groth, A.H., Cartee, R.E. & Griffin, K.S. (1993) Adrenal phaeochromocytoma. *Journal of Veterinary Internal Medicine*, (7), 199–201.

Kallet, A.J., Richter, K.P., Feldman, E.C. & Brum, D.E. (1991) Primary hyperparathyroidsim in cats: seven cases (1984–1989). *Journal of the American Veterinary Medical Association*, (199), 1767–71.

Kintzer, P.P. & Peterson, M.E. (1994) Mitotane treatment of 32 dogs with cortisol secreting adrenocortical neoplasms. *Journal of the American Veterinary Medical Association*, (205), 54–9.

Klein, M.K., Powers, B.E., Withrow, S.J. *et al.* (1995) Treatment of thyroid carcinoma in dogs by surgical resection alone: 20 cases. *Journal of the American Veterinary Medical Association*, (206), 1007–9.

Leav, I., Shiller, A.L. & Rijnberk, A. (1976) Adenomas and carcinomas of the canine and feline thyroid. *American Journal of Pathology*, (83), 61–93.

Leifer, C.E., Peterson, M.E. & Matus, R.E. (1986) Insulin-secreting tumor: diagnosis and medical and surgical management in 55 dogs. *Journal of the American Veterinary Medical Association*, (188), 60–64.

Melhaff, C.J., Peterson, M.E., Patnaik, A.K. & Carrillo, J.M. (1985) Insulin-producing islet cell neoplasms: surgical considerations and general management in 35 dogs. *Journal of the American Animal Hospital Association*, (21), 607–12.

Miller, W.A., Scott, D.W., Buerger, R.G. *et al.* (1990) Necrolytic migratory erythema in dogs: a hepatocutaneous syndrome. *Journal of the American Animal Hospital Association*, (26), 573–81.

Nelson, R.W. & Feldman, E.C. (1988) Hyperadrenocorticism in cats: seven cases (1978–1987). *Journal of the American Veterinary Medical Association*, (193), 245–50.

Owen, L.N. (1980) TNM Classification of Tumours in Domestic Animals. World Health Organisation, Geneva.

Peterson, M.E. (1986) Canine hyperadrenocorticism. In: *Current Veterinary Therapy IX Small Animal Practice*, (ed R.W. Kirk) pp. 963–72. W.B. Saunders, Philadelphia.

Rabbitts, T.H. (1994) Chromosomal translocations in human cancer. *Nature*, (372), 143–9.

Reusch, C.E. & Feldman, E.C. (1991) Canine hyperadrenocorticism due to adrenocortical neoplasia. *Journal of Veterinary Internal Medicine*, (5), 3–10.

Scavelli, T.D., Peterson, M.E. & Mattheisen, D.T. (1986) Results of surgical treatment for hyperadrenocorticism caused by adrenocortical neoplasia in the dog: 25 cases (1980–1984). *Journal of the American Veterinary Medical Association*, (189), 1360–64.

Schrauwen, E. (1991) Clinical peripheral neuropathy associated with canine insulinoma. *Veterinary Record*, (128), 211–12.

Siliart, B. & Stambouli, F. (1996) Laboratory diagnosis of insulinoma in the dog: a retrospective study and a diagnostic procedure. *Journal of Small Animal Practice*, (37), 367–70.

Torres, M.F., Caywood, D.D., O'Brien, T.D., O'Leary, T.P. & McKeever, P.J. (1997) Resolution of superficial necrolytic dermatitis following excision of a glucagon-secreting pancreatic neoplasm in a dog. *Journal of the American Animal Hospital Association*, (33), 313–19.

Turrel, J.M., Feldman, E.C., Nelson, R.W. *et al.* (1988) Thyroid carcinoma causing hyperthyroidism in cats: 14 cases (1981–1986). *Journal of the American Veterinary Medical Association*, (193), 359–64.

Twedt, D.C. & Wheeler, S.L. (1984) Phaeochromocytoma in the dog. *Veterinary Clinics of North America, Small Animal Practice*, (14), 767–82.

Van Ham, L., Braund, K.G., Roels, S. & Putcuyps, I. (1997) Treatment of a dog with an insulinoma-related peripheral polyneuropathy with corticosteroids. *Veterinary Record*, (141), 98–100.

Zerbe, C.A., Boosinger, T.R. & Grabau, J.H. (1989) Pancreatic polypeptide and insulin-secreting tumour in a dog with duodenal ulcers and hypertrophic gastritis. *Journal of Veterinary Internal Medicine*, (3), 178–82.

Further reading

Marks, S.L., Koblik, P.D., Hornof, W.J. & Feldman, E.C. (1994) ^{99m}Tc pertechnetate imaging of thyroid tumors in dogs: 29 cases (1980–1992). *Journal of the American Veterinary Medical Association*, (204), 756–60.

Sullivan, M., Cox, F., Pead, M.J. & Mcneil, P. (1987) Thyroid tumours in the dog. *Journal of Small Animal Practice*, (28), 505–12.

Susaneck, S. (1983) Thyroid tumors in the dog. *Compendium of Continuing Education for the Practising Veterinarian*, (5), 35–9.

Wisner, E.R., Nyland, T.G., Feldman, E.C., Nelson, R.W. & Griffey, S.M. (1993) Ultrasonographic evaluation of the parathyroid glands in hypercalcaemic dogs. *Veterinary Radiology and Ultrasound*, (34), 108–11.

15
Haematopoietic System

Haematopoietic tumours are more common in the cat than the dog. Lymphoma is the commonest haematopoietic tumour in both species, with leukaemia, other myeloproliferative disorders and multiple myeloma occurring much less frequently. Haematopoietic neoplasms are the third most common type of tumour diagnosed in the dog, accounting for approximately 8–9% of all canine malignant tumours. In the cat haematopoietic neoplasms are the most common tumour type, accounting for approximately one third of all tumours.

Haematopoietic neoplasms derive from the lymphoid and non-lymphoid cell series. They are described as:
- Lymphoproliferative disease (LPD) – the term used for tumours of solid lymphoid organs (lymphoma) as well as for lymphoid tumours derived from bone marrow (lymphoid leukaemias and multiple myeloma).
- Myeloproliferative disease (MPD) – a spectrum of conditions derived from haematopoietic stem cells located in the bone marrow and including dysplastic or hyperplastic diseases such as myelofibrosis and myelodysplastic syndromes, as well as the non-lymphoid leukaemias.

LYMPHOMA

This disease should strictly be referred to as 'malignant' lymphoma or 'lymphosarcoma', since by convention the ending 'oma' usually refers to a benign tumour. In most of the main oncology texts, however, the term lymphoma is used to mean the malignant lymphoproliferative disease and we have chosen to continue this nomenclature here.

Epidemiology

Lymphoma is the commonest haematopoietic tumour in the dog, accounting for 80–90% of these tumours and 5–7% of all canine neoplasms. Its incidence is reported as 13–24 cases/100 000 dogs/year (Dorn *et al.* 1968). Most cases are middle aged (mean 6–7 years), although young dogs may be affected. 'Histiocytic' lymphoma often affects a younger age group (mean four years). There is no obvious sex predisposition but breeds reported to be at greater risk include Scottish terriers, boxers, basset hounds, bulldogs, Labrador retriever, Airedale terriers and St Bernards (Rosenthal 1982).

In the cat, lymphoma accounts for 50–90% of all haematopoietic neoplasms with an incidence of 200 per 100 000 cats at risk (Essex & Francis 1976). The age distribution is bimodal with the mean age of affected cats ranging from two to three years (FeLV positive) to seven years (FeLV negative). Oriental breeds may be more at risk.

Aetiology

Lymphoma is considered to be a multifactorial disease with no clear aetiology confirmed in the dog. There may be a genetic component, since a familial incidence has been reported in the bullmastiff (Onions 1984).

A C-type retrovirus, feline leukaemia virus (FeLV), is mainly responsible for the disease in the cat with up to 70% of cases testing positive for the viral antigen, p27. The percentage of cats found to be positive for the virus varies with the anatomical site of the disease (Table 15.1). In general, multicentric and mediastinal forms are FeLV positive while cutaneous and alimentary forms are virus negative. Young cats are more frequently virus positive than older cats. More details of FeLV infection are given in Chapter 1 and other texts.

Feline immunodeficiency virus (FIV) may also be responsible for some cases of B cell lymphoma

(often extranodal), either on its own or by coinfection with FeLV (Shelton *et al.* 1990; Hutson *et al.* 1991; Callanan *et al.* 1992; Poli *et al.* 1994). Rather than playing a direct role in tumourigenesis, FIV infection probably induces immune dysfunction and indirect development of lymphoma (Beatty *et al.* 1998).

Pathology

Lymphoma in the dog and cat may be classified by anatomical distribution, morphological cell type and histological appearance, or immunophenotype.

Anatomical classification

Anatomically, tumours may be grouped as:

- Multicentric
- Mediastinal
- Alimentary
- Cutaneous
- Extranodal.

The clinical presentation of each group is discussed in the appropriate section below.

Histopathological classification

In an attempt to link cell type to prognosis, several histological classification schemes have been applied to canine lymphoma. The majority of these are based on those used for human non-Hodgkins lymphoma (Tables 15.2, 15.3 and 15.4). The World

Table 15.1 Variation in FeLV positivity with anatomical site of feline lymphoma. Jarratt (1994) and Vail *et al.* (1998).

Anatomical type	% of cases positive for FeLV	Mean age (years)
Multicentric	30–60	4
Mediastinal	70–80	2.5
Alimentary	5–30	8
Extranodal	20–60	8
All sites	70	

Table 15.2 Rappaport classification of non-Hodgkin's lymphoma.

Nodular
Lymphocytic well differentiated
Lymphocytic poorly differentiated
Mixed lymphocytic and histiocytic
Histiocytic

Diffuse
Lymphocytic well differentiated (± plasmacytoid features)
Lymphocytic poorly differentiated
Lymphoblastic
Mixed lymphocytic and histiocytic
Histiocytic
Undifferentiated

Table 15.3 Kiel Classification of lymphoma.

Low grade malignancy
Lymphocytic (CLL, MF, Sezary)
Lymphoplasmacytic, lymphoplasmacytoid
Centrocytic
Centroblastic/centrocytic (follicular/diffuse)
Unclassified

High grade malignancy
Centroblastic
Lymphoblastic (Burkitt's type, convoluted cell type)
Immunoblastic
Unclassified

Table 15.4 National Cancer Institute Working Formulation for lymphoma.

Low grade malignancy
Small lymphocytic
Follicular predominantly small cleaved
Follicular mixed small cleaved and large cell

Intermediate grade malignancy
Follicular predominantly large cell
Diffuse small cleaved
Diffuse mixed small cleaved and large cell
Diffuse large cell (cleaved/noncleaved)

High grade malignancy
Immunoblastic
Lymphoblastic (convoluted/nonconvoluted)
Small noncleaved (Burkitt's)

Table 15.5 World Health Organisation classification of canine lymphoma (Owen 1980).

Poorly differentiated
Lymphoblastic
Lymphocytic and prolymphocytic
Histiocytic, histioblastic, histiolymphocytic

Health Organization scheme (Table 15.5) which was defined for the dog is rarely used. Using schemes which assess the growth pattern (follicular or diffuse) within the node as well as cell type (lymphocytic, lymphoblastic etc.), approximately 85% of canine lymphomas are classed as diffuse or minimally follicular. The Kiel and National Cancer Institute Working Formulation (WF) schemes are of most prognostic value and, using these schemes, the majority of canine lymphomas are found to

be of high or intermediate grade malignancy and either large cell (WF) or centroblastic (Kiel). The NCI working formulation has been applied to feline lymphoma with just over half of the cases classified as high grade. One third of tumours are immunoblastic cell type (Valli *et al.* 1989).

Immunophenotypic classification

Lymphoma may also be classified by immunophenotype using serum from other species which cross reacts with dog tissue or, more recently, specific canine monoclonal antibodies (Moore *et al.* 1992; Cobbold & Metcalfe 1994). The majority of canine lymphomas are derived from B cells with estimates of T cell lymphomas accounting for between 10 and 38% of cases. There is no correlation between immunophenotype and morphological cell type although T cell lymphomas are often of low or intermediate cytomorphological grade (Teske 1993). Feline lymphomas may also be immunophenotyped. Most feline thymic and multicentric lymphomas are T cell since they are caused by FeLV transformation. Most alimentary lymphomas, however, are B cell derived and test FeLV negative.

Tumour behaviour

Lymphoma arises from the neoplastic transformation and subsequent proliferation of lymphocytes in solid lymphoid organs. The disease may develop in multiple sites simultaneously or originate at one site and progress to others, although this is not metastasis as such. Neoplastic lymphoid cells may circulate in the blood and/or invade bone marrow, resulting in myelosuppression.

Paraneoplastic syndromes

The paraneoplastic diseases commonly seen with canine lymphoma are hypercalcaemia and hypergammaglobulinaemia (see Chapter 2). Both also occur with feline lymphoma but much more rarely than in the dog. Hypercalcaemia is present in 10–40% of canine lymphoma cases and is often associated with mediastinal forms and those thought to be T cell derived. Hypergammaglobulinaemia is less common than hypercalcaemia in the dog.

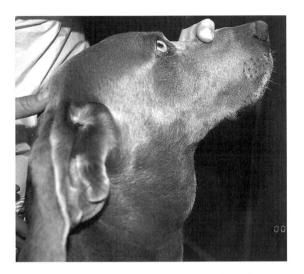

Fig. 15.1 Enlarged submandibular lymph nodes in a weimaraner with multicentric lymphoma.

Presentation/signs

The clinical presentation of lymphoma varies according to the anatomical type. Of the four anatomical groups recognised, the multicentric form is most common in the dog and mediastinal and alimentary forms in the cat.

Multicentric

Animals present with a solitary or generalised lymphadenopathy which may be accompanied by hepatosplenomegaly, involvement of bone marrow or other organs (Fig. 15.1). Lymph nodes are massively enlarged and hard, but usually non-painful to palpate. The majority of cases are clinically well but some cases show non-specific signs such as weight loss, anorexia or lethargy. Approximately 20% of canine cases will show signs of hypercalcaemia such as polydipsia, polyuria, anorexia, vomiting, constipation, depression, muscle weakness or cardiac arrhythmias. Fewer animals will show signs of a monoclonal gammopathy such as bleeding disorders, thromboembolism, ocular lesions (retinal detachment, tortuous blood vessels), neurological signs and infections.

Mediastinal

Cases with mediastinal (thymic) lymphoma have an anterior mediastinal lymphadenopathy, possibly

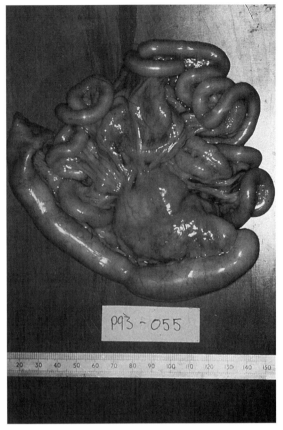

Fig. 15.2 Intestinal lymphoma in a cat (post mortem). (Courtesy of Dr P. Nicholls.)

accompanied by pleural effusion and occasionally bone marrow infiltration. Although occasionally a mass is seen as an incidental finding on thoracic radiography, animals usually present with coughing, dyspnoea, regurgitation or Horner's syndrome and caudal displacement of heart and lung sounds on auscultation. Hypercalcaemia is common with this form of lymphoma in dogs and is often associated with T cell immunophenotype.

Alimentary

Alimentary lymphoma may present as solitary, diffuse or multifocal infiltration of the gastrointestinal tract with or without mesenteric lymphadenopathy (Fig. 15.2). Animals may present with vomiting, diarrhoea, anorexia, weight loss, dyschezia or tenesmus and occasionally peritonitis secondary to complete obstruction and rupture of the gut. An abdominal mass, enlarged mesenteric lymph nodes or thickened bowel loops may be palpable.

Cutaneous

The cutaneous form of lymphoma may be either:

- Primary, that is originating in the skin; *or*
- Secondary, that is associated with lymphoma found predominantly at other body sites.

Primary cutaneous lymphoma includes two forms, both of which are T cell derived and are discussed in detail in Chapter 4. Although these originate in the skin, they may later spread to abdominal viscera, lymph nodes and bone marrow (see Chapter 4). The two forms are:

- *Epitheliotropic form* – 'mycosis fungoides' has T lymphocytes restricted to the epidermis. Cases present with a chronic history of alopecia, depigmentation, desquamation, pruritus and erythema. This progresses over months or years to plaque formation characterised by crusting and ulceration, and finally to tumour formation (nodules or masses). Lesions are often around mucocutaneous junctions or in the oral cavity.
- *Non-epitheliotropic (dermal) form* – a more aggressive disease, spreading rapidly from multiple cutaneous lesions to involve lymph nodes, abdominal viscera and bone marrow.

Secondary cutaneous lymphoma is also characterised by lymphoid cells in the dermis. These often have morphological features similar to those of histiocytes (histiocytic lymphoma) but the immunophenotype may be B or T cell depending on that of the lymphoma at the primary site.

Extranodal

The term extranodal lymphoma is used for lymphoma at sites which are not readily included by the other anatomical classification groups, for example:

- Renal
- Nasopharyngeal
- Ocular
- Neural.

Renal lymphoma is relatively common in cats and clinical signs are related to renal failure since the disease is usually bilateral (Fig. 15.3). Cats present

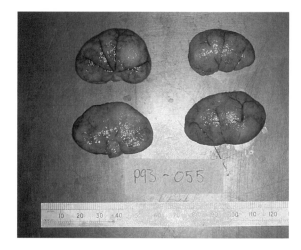

Fig. 15.3 Renal lymphoma in a cat (post mortem). (Courtesy of Dr P. Nicholls.)

with emaciation and pallor (anaemia) and large irregular kidneys may be palpated. Tumour progression to the CNS is commonly found with renal lymphoma.

Animals with nasopharyngeal lymphoma present with upper respiratory signs such as nasal discharge or sneezing and sometimes nasal deformity. Several cases of feline nasopharyngeal lymphoma in our clinic have subsequently developed renal lymphoma.

Ocular and neural lymphoma may be primary or accompany the multicentric form. Ocular lymphoma is more common in cats than dogs and clinical signs associated with it include photophobia, blepharospasm, epiphora, hyphaema, hypopyon, ocular mass, anterior uveitis, chorioretinal involvement or retinal detachment (Fig. 15.4; see also Chapter 16). Neural lymphoma may be solitary or diffuse and involve central or peripheral nervous systems. Presenting signs are variable and include paralysis, paresis, lameness, muscle atrophy or central signs (Chapter 13).

Investigations

FeLV/FIV tests

All cats suspected of having lymphoma should be tested for FeLV and FIV. The most commonly used screening test for FeLV is the enzyme-linked immunosorbent assay (ELISA) which detects free p27 antigen in the blood, but an immunofluorescent

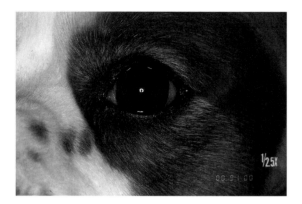

Fig. 15.4 Ocular involvement. This dog presented with sudden onset blindness due to intraocular haemorrhage.

antibody test to detect p27 antigen in blood or bone marrow cells may also be used. The ELISA is available in kit form (CITE test) for use in general practice and is much more sensitive, specific and quick. For a definitive test, virus isolation is necessary, but this is expensive and time-consuming.

An ELISA test is also the most common method used to diagnose FIV infection but the test detects serum antibodies to the virus rather than viral antigen. Western blot and immunofluorescent antibody tests may also be used.

Bloods

All cases of suspected lymphoma require routine haematological analysis:

- To help stage the disease
- To establish a base-line of haematological parameters with which to compare future samples and assess the degree of myelosuppression induced by treatment.

Haematological evaluation may be normal, or if bone marrow involvement is present, may reveal anaemia, thrombocytopenia, neutropenia, lymphocytosis and the presence of immature lymphoid precursors.

Biochemical evaluation should include liver enzymes (ALT and alkaline phosphatase) to detect liver dysfunction, BUN/creatinine to detect renal dysfunction, electrolytes to detect hypercalcaemia, and serum protein electrophoresis to detect a monoclonal gammopathy if the total protein level is raised.

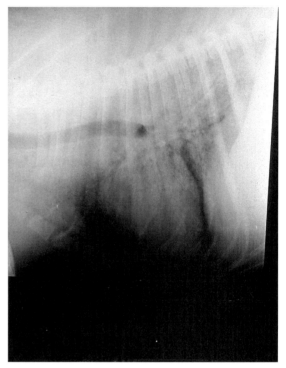

Fig. 15.5 Lateral radiograph of thorax showing diffuse parenchymal involvement in case of multicentric lymphoma (stage V).

Imaging techniques

Radiography is necessary to help with the diagnosis in some anatomical forms of the disease such as mediastinal, renal, spinal or alimentary. Contrast radiography may be required such as a barium series, intravenous urography or myelography. Thoracic and abdominal radiography is also of vital importance to assess lymph node and organ involvement (liver, spleen, lungs etc.) in staging multicentric forms of the disease (Figs 15.5 and 15.6).

Although radiography can show gross enlargement or a change in shape of organs, ultrasonography is of more use for showing a definite infiltration or change of architecture which may be useful for staging the disease. Ultrasonography is also useful for guiding aspirates or biopsies to confirm the diagnosis.

Biopsy/FNA

The quickest and easiest way to confirm the diagnosis of lymphoma is to take a fine needle aspirate

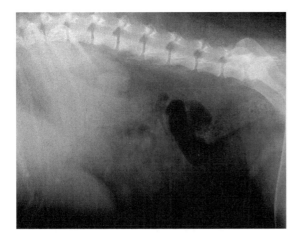

Fig. 15.6 Lateral radiograph of abdomen showing hepatomegaly and sublumbar lymphadenopathy in case of multicentric lymphoma (stage IV).

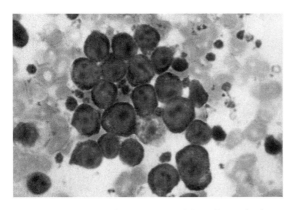

Fig. 15.7 Fine needle aspirate of lymph node from dog with multicentric lymphoma. Cytology reveals a population of large, neoplastic lymphoblasts. (See also Colour plate 29, facing p. 162.)

for cytological evaluation from an enlarged lymph node, mass or affected organ (Fig. 15.7). Alternatively, or additionally if there is any doubt about the cytological diagnosis, biopsy material can be examined histologically. This is also needed for complete histological classification by cell type and growth pattern and also for immunophenotyping. A needle or incisional biopsy may be taken from a mass or affected organ, but for the multicentric form, a whole lymph node (usually the popliteal) is best submitted.

As part of the staging procedure, a bone marrow aspirate or biopsy should also be examined if there

Table 15.6 Clinical stages of lymphoma. Owen (1980).

Stage	Extent of disease
I	Involvement limited to a single node or lymphoid tissue in a single organ (excluding bone marrow)
II	Involvement of many lymph nodes in a regional area (± tonsils)
III	Generalised lymph node involvement
IV	Liver and/or spleen involvement (± stage III)
V	Manifestations in the blood and involvement of bone marrow and/or other organ systems (± stages I–IV)

Subclassify each stage as (a) without systemic signs (b) with systemic signs.

is any evidence of haematological abnormalities. Ideally this should be performed for all cases, since it is possible for bone marrow infiltration to be present without obvious changes to haematological parameters.

Staging

A TNM staging system is not applicable to lymphoma but a group staging system is used instead (Table 15.6). The extent of the disease must be assessed by clinical and radiographic examination, and by haematological and bone marrow evaluation. Most cases of multicentric lymphoma present as stage III, IV or V.

Treatment

Surgery

Surgery is useful in the treatment of certain types of lymphoma. In some cases of anterior mediastinal lymphoma where a diagnosis has not been confirmed by aspirate or biopsy, a thoracotomy may be necessary to obtain tumour material for diagnostic purposes and to remove the mass. Similarly, many cases of alimentary lymphoma will require a celiotomy to obtain biopsy material. For solitary intestinal masses, surgical resection and anastomosis of the gut may be the best treatment option since there is a theoretical risk of gut perforation in cases where the tumour involves the full thickness of the gut wall and which are treated with cytotoxic drugs. Cases of spinal lymphoma or solitary skin masses may also require surgical treatment. If it is likely that not all tumour has been resected or that multicentric disease may develop, surgery should be followed by chemotherapy. A six month course should be sufficient if there is no gross evidence of disease at the start of treatment.

Radiotherapy

Lymphoma is a very radiosensitive tumour and in theory, radiotherapy should be highly successful in treating all forms of the disease. In animals, however, the side-effects associated with whole body or half body radiation are such that multicentric or widespread cutaneous disease is not usually treated in this way. Localised masses, however, can be treated very effectively and radiotherapy can be considered:

• As an alternative for solitary skin masses at sites not amenable to surgery
• For nasal lymphoma
• For some cases of anterior mediastinal lymphoma.

We have also found radiotherapy effective in controlling oral lesions in cases of mycosis fungoides which present with predominantly oral and few skin lesions.

Chemotherapy

The most common method of treatment for lymphoma is combination chemotherapy. If chemotherapy is intended, corticosteroids should not be started before the cytotoxic drugs, since they induce resistance to the cytotoxics and significantly lower the response rate and survival time. Before commencing drug therapy it is essential to establish a baseline of haematological parameters, for future monitoring of treatment associated myelosuppression.

The aims of therapy for most cases of lymphoma are to:

• Induce remission with a chemotherapeutic regime
• Proceed to maintenance treatment once remission is complete
• Intensify the regime if a complete response is not achieved.

The response of the disease to treatment is monitored by lymph node size or a reduction in visible tumour mass (Figs 15.8 and 15.9). Drug side-effects are monitored by haematological parameters and other means specific to the drugs used. Most cases of lymphoma will eventually recur or relapse because treatment is stopped too soon or because of development of resistance to cytotoxic drugs. At this stage 'rescue' treatment is used.

Several combination chemotherapy protocols have been described for treatment of cats and dogs with lymphoma. It is usually recommended to select a protocol and to keep using the same one, in order to familiarise oneself with the drugs and their toxicities. The COAP and COP low dose protocols are often selected for induction because they

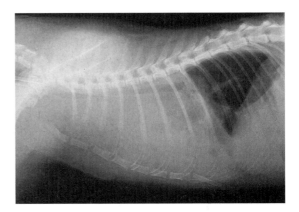

Fig. 15.8 Lateral thoracic radiograph of cat with mediastinal lymphoma.

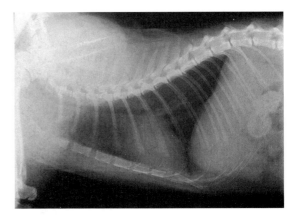

Fig. 15.9 The same cat after four weeks of COP chemotherapy.

Table 15.7 Chemotherapy protocols for the treatment of lymphoma (continuous).

Induction
COAP

Cyclophosphamide	50 mg/m^2 by mouth every 48 hours or for the first 4 days of each week*
Vincristine	0.5 mg/m^2 intravenously every 7 days
Cytosine arabinoside	100 mg/m^2 intravenously daily for first 4 days of protocol (in cats, use subcutaneously for 2 days)
Prednisolone	40 mg/m^2 by mouth daily for 7 days, then 20 mg/m^2 by mouth every 48 hours (with cyclophosphamide)

COP (low dose)

Cyclophosphamide	50 mg/m^2 by mouth every 48 hours or for the first 4 days of each week*
Vincristine	0.5 mg/m^2 intravenously every 7 days
Prednisolone	40 mg/m^2 by mouth daily for 7 days, then 20 mg/m^2 by mouth every 48 hours (with cyclophosphamide)

Maintenance
COP
After 8 weeks of induction with COAP/COP, continue COP as alternate week treatment for 4 months, then 1 week in 3 for 6 months, and reduce to 1 week in 4 after 1 year.

MOP
As for COP, but to reduce the risk of haemorrhagic cystitis, substitute melphalan (2–5 mg/m^2 by mouth) for cyclophosphamide after 6 months.

LMP/LP
After 8–10 weeks of induction with COAP or COP, change to different drugs for maintenance, i.e. chlorambucil and prednisolone ± methotrexate

Chlorambucil	20 mg/m^2 by mouth every 14 days
Methotrexate	2.5 mg/m^2 by mouth 2 to 3 times per week
Prednisolone	20 mg/m^2 by mouth every 48 hours

* In cats, this regime is hard to achieve because cyclophosphamide is only available in the UK as 50 mg tablets which should not be broken. For an average cat of 3–4 kg, a 50 mg tablet is usually equivalent to four or five doses, so pulse dosing may be used – one tablet every 8–10 days. Alternatively, an intravenous dose may be used at 200 mg/m^2 every 2–3 weeks to suit the individual, or the COP (high dose) protocol.

are inexpensive and of low toxicity (Table 15.7), but other protocols based on a 21-day cycle or pulse therapy of a different drug each week are also available (Tables 15.8 and 15.9). For rescue treatment, further protocols may be selected (Table 15.10). For cats, the COP protocol (low or high dose) or pulse therapy (Table 15.9) are most often used. There is some evidence to suggest that protocols including doxorubicin provide longer periods of remission in cats with lymphoma (Moore *et al.* 1996).

Other

Cases of lymphoma presenting with paraneoplastic syndromes may require immediate supportive treatment while the diagnosis is being confirmed. Prolonged hypercalcaemia results in irreversible renal damage and immediate steps should be taken to lower serum calcium levels (Chapter 2). Hypergammaglobulinaemia will also require prompt action if severe.

Some forms of lymphoma, particularly the cutaneous ones, respond poorly to conventional chemotherapy. Other options which have been tried with variable success for mycosis fungoides include retinoids such as isotretinoin or etretinate (White *et al.* 1993) and photodynamic therapy.

A monoclonal antibody called CL/MAb 231 (Synbiotics, California) is available in the USA for use in combination with a non-immunosuppressive chemotherapy regime. The monoclonal acts via complement mediated or antibody dependent cell cytotoxicity (ADCC) pathways which require an intact host immune system. Initial trials showed a significantly increased median survival time compared to controls treated by chemotherapy alone

Table 15.8 Chemotherapy protocols for the treatment of lymphoma (21 day cycles).

Induction

COP (high dose)

Cyclophosphamide	250–300 mg/m^2 by mouth every 21 days
Vincristine	0.75 mg/m^2 intravenously every 7 days for 4 weeks, then every 21 days
Prednisolone	1 mg/kg by mouth daily for 4 weeks, then every 48 hours

COPA

As for COP, except use:

Doxorubicin	30 mg/m^2 intravenously in place of cyclophosphamide every third cycle, i.e. every ninth week

CHOP

Cyclophosphamide	100–150 mg/m^2 intravenously on day 1
Doxorubicin	30 mg/m^2 intravenously on day 1
Vincristine	0.75 mg/m^2 intravenously on days 8 and 15
Prednisolone	40 mg/m^2 daily for 7 days, then 20 mg/m^2 every 48 hours, days 8–21
(Potentiated sulphonamides)	Protocol very myelosuppressive, therefore antibiotic cover advised

PACO

Prednisolone	20 mg/m^2 by mouth every 48 hours	
Actinomycin D	0.75 mg/m^2 intravenously on day 1	repeat every 21 days
Cyclophosphamide	250–300 mg/m^2 by mouth on day 10	
Vincristine	0.75 mg/m^2 intravenously on days 8 and 15	

Maintenance

COP/COPA

After 1 year of induction with COP (high dose) or COPA, use the same cycle every 4 weeks for another 6 months

COP/LMP

After 12 weeks of induction with CHOP, change to low dose COP or LMP for maintenance (see Table 15.7)

PAL

After 12 weeks induction with PACO, change to different drugs, i.e. PAL for maintenance:

Prednisolone	20 mg/m^2 by mouth every 48 hours
Cytosine arabinoside	200 mg/m^2 subcutaneously every 7 days
Chlorambucil	20 mg/m^2 every 14 days

(Jeglum 1991), but further trials have not been published.

Prognosis

Without therapy, the mean survival time for dogs or cats with lymphoma is only six to eight weeks. With corticosteroid therapy alone it may be extended to approximately three months, but with chemotherapy it is usually six to nine months. A variety of protocols are available for treating lymphoma but regardless of which is used, approximately 70–80% of canine cases (65–75% of feline cases) with multicentric lymphoma achieve remission and remain in remission for a mean of six to nine months. Survival times, however, may range from one week to several years. Once relapse occurs, the prognosis worsens since fewer than 50% of cases respond to rescue therapy.

Using large numbers of animals, and multivariate statistical analysis a number of factors have been shown to affect the prognosis for canine multicentric lymphoma:

- Histological grade of malignancy appears to be the most reliable prognostic indicator with high grade tumours giving consistently poorer responses. High grade tumours by the Kiel classification have reduced attainment of complete response (CR) and shorter disease free interval (DFI), whereas high grade tumours by the Working Formulation classification have shorter survival time (Teske *et al*. 1994).
- T cell phenotype is also important and carries a poor prognosis regardless of histological grade (Teske 1993).
- In univariate studies, a higher clinical stage carries a worse prognosis and substage (b) leads to shorter DFI and survival, but the results are

Small Animal Oncology

Table 15.9 Chemotherapy protocols for treatment of lymphoma (weekly pulse therapy/cyclic combination therapy).

Induction

Week 1 (day 1)	Vincristine	0.5–0.75 mg/m^2 intravenously
	L-Asparaginase	400 IU/kg intramuscularly
	± Prednisolone	2.0 mg/kg by mouth daily
Week 2 (day 8)	Cyclophosphamide	200 mg/m^2 intravenously or by mouth
	± Prednisolone	1.5 mg/kg by mouth daily
Week 3 (day 15)	Vincristine	0.5–0.75 mg/m^2 intravenously
	± Prednisolone	1.0 mg/kg by mouth daily
Week 4 (day 22)	Doxorubicin*	30 mg/m^2 intravenously
	± Prednisolone	0.5 mg/kg by mouth daily
Week 5 (day 29)	Vincristine	0.5–0.75 mg/m^2 intravenously
Week 6 (day 36)	Cyclophosphamide**	200 mg/m^2 intravenously or by mouth
Week 7 (day 43)	Vincristine	0.5–0.75 mg/m^2 intravenously
Week 8 (day 50)	Doxorubicin*	30 mg/m^2 intravenously
	or Methotrexate	0.6–0.8 mg/kg (10–15 mg/m^2) intravenously
Week 9 (day 57)	No treatment	

Maintenance
Repeat the 8 week cycle twice with an interval of 2 weeks between each drug administration and then another twice with an interval of 3 weeks between each drug administration. Chlorambucil (1.4 mg/kg by mouth) may be substituted for cyclophosphamide during maintenance cycles

* In cats, methotrexate is often used in weeks 4 and 8. If Doxorubicin is alternated with methotrexate, the dose is 20 mg/m^2 rather than 30 mg/m^2.
** For renal lymphoma in cats, because of the risk of CNS spread, substitute cytosine arabinoside 600 mg/m^2 (30 mg/kg) subcutaneously divided into 4 doses at 12 hour intervals over 48 hours.

Table 15.10 Rescue chemotherapy for relapsed cases of lymphoma.

If response to initial treatment was good, return to original induction protocol until remission achieved and then use maintenance protocol

COAP	Table 15.7
COP (low or high dose)	Tables 15.7 and 15.8
COPA	Table 15.8
CHOP	Table 15.8
PACO	Table 15.8
Cyclic combination	Table 15.9

If response to initial treatment was slow or for a second relapse, change to new drugs for rescue. Return to maintenance once remission complete

Single agents

Doxorubicin	30 mg/m^2 (dogs) or 20 mg/m^2 (cats) intravenously every 21 days
L-Asparaginase	10 000–20 000 IU/m^2 intramuscularly every 14–21 days

ADIC

Doxorubicin	30 mg/m^2 (dogs) or 20 mg/m^2 (cats) intravenously every 21 days
Dacarbazine	1000 mg/m^2 intravenous infusion (over 6–8 hours) every 21 days
CHOP	Table 15.8
PACO	Table 15.8

often inconsistent. Within the T cell lymphomas, however, clinical stage does appear to be important, with higher stages performing worse.
- Of all the proliferation markers available, only AgNOR counts seem to be of prognostic value with a higher count indicating a shorter survival time in some studies.

Age, sex and weight of animals have no prognostic significance and neither does the presence of hyper-calcaemia per se, although many hypercalcaemic cases are of the T cell phenotype and have a worse prognosis because of this.

In cats, stage of disease is considered important for prognosis, along with the severity of haematological and biochemical abnormalities and overall clinical condition. FeLV and FIV status are also important since FeLV related disorders other than neoplasia can influence survival (Mooney *et al.* 1989).

LEUKAEMIA

The term leukaemia is restricted to haematopoietic tumours which are derived from bone marrow and these may be of lymphoid or non-lymphoid origin. They may be classified according to the degree of maturity of the cell type involved as either:

- Acute; *or*
- Chronic.

Acute leukaemias arise from the neoplastic transformation and subsequent proliferation of early haematopoietic precursor cells, leading to the arrest of normal cell lineage differentiation. Chronic leukaemias arise from the neoplastic transformation of late precursor cells leading to proliferation of fairly well differentiated cells. Thus, leukaemia derived from lymphoid series can be classified as either acute lymphoblastic leukaemia (ALL) or chronic lymphocytic leukaemia (CLL). Leukaemia derived from the non-lymphoid series is more variable and difficult to classify, particularly in cats. The disease frequently evolves from one line to another so that one, several or all non-lymphoid cell lines may be affected. Although terms such as acute myeloid leukaemia (AML) and chronic granulocytic leukaemia (CGL) are used, the non-lymphoid leukaemias are often grouped together under the term 'myeloproliferative disease'.

Lymphoid and myeloid leukaemias

The leukaemias included in this section are ALL and CLL, AML and CGL and the monocytic and myelomonocytic leukaemias.

Epidemiology

Acute leukaemias account for less than 10% of all canine haematopoietic neoplasms with acute myeloid cases exceeding acute lymphoid cases in a 3:1 ratio (Couto 1992). Affected dogs are usually young to middle aged (mean 5–6 years for ALL) but the range is wide (1–12 years). More males than females may be affected (3:2 ratio) but there is no breed predisposition. Chronic leukaemias are less common than acute leukaemias in dogs, with cases of chronic lymphocytic leukaemia (CLL) dramatically exceeding those of chronic granulocytic leukaemia (CGL). Most animals are middle-aged to old (mean 9.4 years for CLL) and although a sex ratio of male to females of 2:1 is reported for CLL, there is no breed predisposition.

In cats, leukaemias are more common, accounting for approximately one third of haematopoietic tumours (Theilen & Madewell 1987). Approximately two thirds of cases are myeloid (Couto 1992). Of the lymphoid leukaemias, ALL predominates with CLL occurring more rarely.

Aetiology

The aetiology of canine leukaemias is unknown although a lentivirus has been isolated from one leukaemic dog (Safran *et al.* 1992). Ionising radiation and benzene exposure are proposed for human ALL (Leifer & Matus 1985) and genetic factors for human CLL. There is also an association of human CLL with auto-immune disease suggesting an immunological aberration (Leifer & Matus 1985, 1986).

In cats, FeLV plays an important role in leukaemogenesis since 90% of lymphoid and myeloid leukaemias are FeLV positive. Other factors may be involved, however, since experimental infection with FeLV only causes a low incidence of myeloproliferative disease. Chromosomal aberrations have been reported in feline leukaemia, in both

Table 15.11 Classification of leukaemias.

Acute	Chronic
Lymphoid	
Acute lymphoblastic leukaemia	Chronic lymphocytic leukaemia
Non-lymphoid	
Acute myeloid leukaemia	Chronic granulocytic leukaemia
Acute myelomonocytic leukaemia	
Acute monocytic leukaemia	
Erythremic myelosis (erythroleukaemia)	Primary erythrocytosis (polycythemia vera)
Megakaryocytic leukaemia	Primary (essential) thrombocythemia
	Basophilic leukaemia
	Eosinophilic leukaemia
	Mast cell leukaemia

FeLV positive and FeLV negative cells (Grindem & Bouen 1989; Gulino 1992). It has been proposed that virus infection may cause proliferation of haematopoietic cells, which increases the risk of chromosomal aberrations occurring and it is these which trigger cell transformation. FIV may also be responsible for some cases of myeloproliferative disease, on its own or in conjunction with FeLV (Hutson *et al.* 1991).

Pathology

Acute and chronic leukaemias may arise from lymphoid or non-lymphoid cell lineages (Table 15.11). The distinction between acute and chronic forms is not always precise and some lymphoid leukaemias with predominantly well differentiated cells may also have immature forms, making it difficult to predict how the disease may progress.

For many acute leukaemias, the cells may appear so undifferentiated that it is impossible to decide whether they are lymphoid or myeloid without resorting to special cytochemical or immunocytochemical stains or flow cytometric studies. Use of such stains has shown that many leukaemias previously thought to be lymphoid are, in fact, myeloid and that many myeloid leukaemias show monocytic differentiation. Depending on the cell type involved, acute myeloid leukaemias can be divided into acute myelogenous without differentiation (AML), acute monocytic/monoblastic (AMoL) or acute myelomonocytic (AMML) leukaemias.

In cats, the involvement of multiple haematopoietic cell lines is common and the distinction between myeloid leukaemia and other myeloproliferative diseases is less clear. This is undoubtedly related to the fact that cell lines derive from a common pluripotent myeloid stem cell which may differentiate along various pathways. Erythremic myelosis, for example, may progress to either erythroleukaemia or AML in the cat.

Tumour behaviour

Acute leukaemias are characterised by aggressive biological behaviour and rapid progression. The early blast cells proliferate in the bone marrow at the expense of normal haematopoiesis, spilling over into the blood and infiltrating peripheral organs, e.g. spleen, liver, lymph nodes, bone and nerves. Massive leucocytosis may cause signs of hyperviscosity due to aggregate formation and thrombosis in brain and lungs. Occasionally, neoplastic cells are restricted to the marrow and are not seen in peripheral blood. This is known as an aleukaemic or smouldering leukaemia. Acute leukaemias are usually characterised by severe myelosuppression, i.e. anaemia, thrombocytopenia and lymphopenia or granulocytopenia, and increased susceptibility to infection due to reduced humoral and cellular immunity.

Chronic leukaemias, on the other hand, are characterised by slow progression and relatively mild clinical signs. As for acute leukaemias, the neoplastic cells proliferate in the bone marrow at the expense of normal haematopoiesis, enter the blood and infiltrate peripheral organs, but the degree of myelosuppression is much milder. With CGL, proliferation of blast cells rather than mature cells (a blast cell crisis) may occur as a terminal event, months to years after diagnosis. Secondary infections due to reduced humoral and cellular immunity may also occur.

Paraneoplastic syndromes

A monoclonal gammopathy is associated with 25% of cases of canine CLL although 10% of cases may have reduced immunoglobulin levels. A hyperviscosity syndrome is associated with polycythemia vera.

Presentation/signs

Acute leukaemias present with:

- Non-specific signs including weakness, lethargy, anorexia, vomiting and diarrhoea, pyrexia (more common in AML) or pallor
- Mild lymphadenopathy (much less obvious than with lymphoma), splenomegaly or hepatomegaly may be noted
- Haematological complications may cause bleeding, bruising, joint swelling (haemarthrosis) or DIC (more common in AML).

Other possible signs include:

- Shifting lameness, bone pain (more common in AML)
- Ocular lesions such as retinal and conjunctival haemorrhage, hyphaema, glaucoma, retinal infiltrates (more common in AML)
- Neurological signs, neuropathies, paresis (more common in ALL)
- Secondary infections, e.g. skin lesions.

Half of all cases of CLL may be asymptomatic and only detected on haematological examination. The remaining cases of CLL and all of CGL show mild, progressive disease with vague signs such as lethargy, anorexia, vomiting, pyrexia, polyuria, polydipsia, weight loss, pallor, mild lymphadenopathy (more common in CLL), splenomegaly or hepatomegaly, skin infiltration or hyperviscosity syndrome.

Investigations

A tentative diagnosis of leukaemia may be made, based on clinical signs and haematological assessment (Fig. 15.13), but a definitive diagnosis requires examination of the bone marrow to demonstrate neoplastic changes in one or more of the haematopoietic cell series (Figs 15.10, 15.11 and 15.12).

FeLV/FIV tests
All cats suspected of having leukaemia/myeloproliferative disease should be tested for FeLV antigen and FIV antibodies.

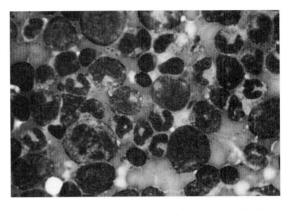

Fig. 15.10 Bone marrow aspirate from dog with AML, showing large undifferentiated myeloblasts. (See also Colour plate 30, facing p. 162.)

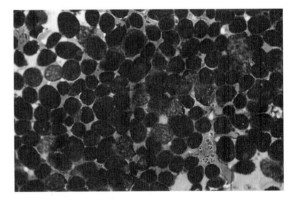

Fig. 15.11 Bone marrow aspirate from dog with ALL. The smear is dominated by medium to large lymphoblasts with very little normal erythroid or myeloid activity. (See also Colour plate 31, facing p. 162.)

Bloods
Haematological evaluation is needed to detect non-regenerative anaemia, thrombocytopenia or neutropenia resulting from myelosuppression (usually more severe cytopenias in acute than chronic leukaemias). Atypical neoplastic cells may be detected in the circulation, i.e. lymphoblasts in ALL, myeloblasts in AML, monoblasts in AMoL, and increased numbers of lymphocytes in CLL or granulocytes in CGL with a left shift to myelocytes or occasionally myeloblasts. With acute leukaemia, a coagulation profile should be carried out to assess clotting function and to look for DIC.

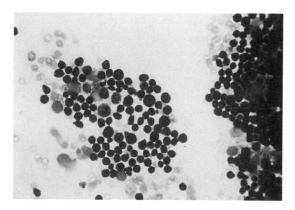

Fig. 15.12 Bone marrow aspirate from dog with CLL. The marrow contains unusually high numbers of small lymphoid cells but normal erythroid and myeloid precursors are also present. (See also Colour plate 32, facing p. 162.)

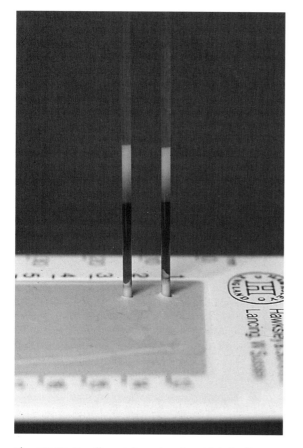

Fig. 15.13 Capillary tubes showing high buffy coat layer; massive leucocytosis may be a feature of some cases of leukaemia.

Biochemical evaluation should include electrolytes to detect hypercalcaemia, liver enzymes to detect liver dysfunction and BUN/creatinine to detect renal dysfunction. Total protein levels and serum electrophoresis are required to detect monoclonal gammopathy in CLL.

Imaging techniques
Abdominal radiography and ultrasonography are useful to confirm hepatosplenomegaly but fine needle aspirates or biopsy are necessary to see if this is due to a neoplastic infiltrate.

Biopsy/FNA
Cytological examination of bone marrow aspirates from leukaemic cases is essential to:

* Confirm the diagnosis of leukaemia
* Assess the degree of normal haematopoiesis
* Determine whether there is a predominance of blast cells (acute leukaemia) or a proliferation of mature lymphoid or myeloid cells (chronic leukaemia).

Special cytochemical and immunocytochemical stains are essential to differentiate blast cell lineage in acute leukaemia since many leukaemias diagnosed as lymphoid are often found to be myeloid on the basis of such stains. The immunophenotype of leukaemias may also be determined by immunocytochemical staining and flow cytometric studies of blood or marrow aspirates (Vernau & Moore 1999).

Staging

No specific staging system is used for leukaemic cases.

Treatment

Surgery
Surgery is not generally indicated for leukaemic cases.

Radiotherapy
Radiotherapy is not generally indicated for leukaemic cases. Irradiation of the bone marrow is associated with side-effects considered unacceptable in animals.

Chemotherapy

Chemotherapy is the treatment of choice for leukaemia although the response to treatment varies considerably with the type of leukaemia. Specific therapy is aimed at destroying the leukaemic cells and allowing normal haematopoiesis to resume and this is more readily achieved with chronic than acute leukaemias. The degree of myelosuppression which is present with most acute leukaemias restricts the use of chemotherapeutic drugs because of the inability to preserve sufficient levels of normal blood cells during treatment. Intensive medical care, bone marrow transplants and extracorporeal treatment of bone marrow are used in human medicine but are not available, nor are they deemed acceptable, for veterinary use. The development of canine and feline recombinant G-CSF and GM-CSF could lead to significant improvements in the treatment of acute leukaemias, but as yet these agents are not available commercially.

Drugs recommended for ALL are similar to those for lymphoma, i.e. vincristine and prednisolone plus an alkylating agent or another drug. Treatment of AML, however, is based on cytosine arabinoside to encourage differentiation of the blast cells, with either prednisolone, mercaptopurine or thioguanine. Induction protocols for acute leukaemia are given in Table 15.12. These are used until the white blood cell count returns to within the normal range and blast cells are no longer seen in peripheral blood. In theory, drug doses and frequencies can then be reduced to maintenance levels, but in practice this is rarely achieved.

Treatment with cytotoxic drugs is usually recommended for chronic leukaemia although frequent

Table 15.12 Chemotherapy protocols for the treatment of acute leukaemia.

Acute lymphoblastic leukaemia (ALL)

Basic induction protocol

Vincristine	$0.5 \, \text{mg/m}^2$ intravenously every 7 days
Prednisolone	$40 \, \text{mg/m}^2$ by mouth daily for 7 days, then $20 \, \text{mg/m}^2$ every 48 hours

Additional agents

Cyclophosphamide	$50 \, \text{mg/m}^2$ by mouth every 48 hours* (see Table 15.7)
Cyclophosphamide and cytosine arabinoside	$50 \, \text{mg/m}^2$ by mouth every 48 hours* (see Table 15.7) $100 \, \text{mg/m}^2$ subcutaneously or intravenously daily for 2 days (cats) or 4 days (dogs) (use divided doses if given intravenously)
L-Asparaginase	$10\,000–20\,000 \, \text{IU/m}^2$ intramuscularly every 2–3 weeks

Acute myeloid leukaemia (AML)

Basic protocol

Cytosine arabinoside	$100 \, \text{mg/m}^2$ subcutaneously or intravenously daily for 2–6 days

Additional agents

Prednisolone	$40 \, \text{mg/m}^2$ by mouth daily for 7 days, then $20 \, \text{mg/m}^2$ every 48 hours
6-Thioguanine	$50 \, \text{mg/m}^2$ by mouth daily or every 48 hours
6-Thioguanine and doxorubicin	$50 \, \text{mg/m}^2$ by mouth daily or every 48 hours $10 \, \text{mg/m}^2$ intravenously every 7 days
Mercaptopurine	$50 \, \text{mg/m}^2$ by mouth daily or every 48 hours

Alternative protocols

Cytosine arabinoside	$5–10 \, \text{mg/m}^2$ subcutaneously twice daily for 2–3 weeks, then on alternate weeks
Doxorubicin	$30 \, \text{mg/m}^2$ (dogs) or $20 \, \text{mg/m}^2$ (cats) intravenously every 3 weeks or $10 \, \text{mg/m}^2$ every 7 days

Maintenance

Any of the above combinations of drugs used for induction reduced to a dose and frequency which maintain white blood cell counts within the normal range monitoring and haematological screens without actual therapy may be sufficient for asymptomatic cases of CLL. The alkylating agent chlorambucil combined with prednisolone is the usual therapy for CLL, whereas the drug of choice for CGL is either hydroxyurea or busulphan (Table 15.13). The aim is to restore the peripheral blood counts to within the normal range and response to treatment is monitored by haematological findings. Once remission is achieved, maintenance therapy is continued at reduced doses and frequencies of the appropriate drugs, in order to keep the white blood cell counts within the normal range.

Other
Paraneoplastic complications such as hypercalcaemia and hypergammaglobulinaemia may need to be addressed before specific chemotherapy commences (see Chapter 2). In addition, various supportive measures may be needed for acute leukamias such as fluid therapy for dehydration or anorexia, blood transfusion for severe loss of red cells or platelets, and antibiotic therapy for secondary infections.

Prognosis

The prognosis for all acute leukaemias is poor due to:

- Failure to induce and maintain remission
- Organ failure which enhances the cytotoxic effects of the drugs
- Septicaemia secondary to the disease or treatment
- DIC.

The prognosis for dogs with ALL is slightly better than for AML; 20–40% of cases of ALL go into remission, usually with short survival times between one and three months (Couto 1992) but occasionally for longer (MacEwen *et al.* 1977; Matus *et al.* 1983; Gorman & White 1987). Survival times for AML rarely exceed three months (Couto 1985; Grindem *et al.* 1985). The prognosis for

Table 15.13 Chemotherapy protocols for chronic leukaemia.

Chronic lymphocytic leukaemia (CLL)

Basic induction protocol

Chlorambucil	2–5 mg/m^2 by mouth daily for 7–14 days, then 2 mg/m^2 every 48 hours or 20 mg/m^2 by mouth as a single dose every 14 days
± Prednisolone	40 mg/m^2 by mouth daily for 7 days, then 20 mg/m^2 every 48 hours

Additional agent

Vincristine	0.5 mg/m^2 intravenously every 7 days

Alternative protocols

Vincristine	0.5 mg/m^2 intravenously every 7 days
Cyclophosphamide	50 mg/m^2 by mouth every 48 hours*
Prednisolone	40 mg/m^2 by mouth daily for 7 days, then 20 mg/m^2 every 48 hours
Vincristine	0.5 mg/m^2 intravenously every 14 days (weeks 2 and 4)
Cyclophosphamide	200–300 mg/m^2 by mouth or intravenously every 14 days (weeks 1 and 3)
Prednisolone	40 mg/m^2 by mouth daily for 7 days, then 20 mg/m^2 every 48 hours

Chronic myeloid leukaemia (CML)

Hydroxyurea	50 mg/kg by mouth daily for 1–2 weeks, then every 48 hours, or 80 mg/kg by mouth every 3 days until remission achieved, or 1 g/m^2 by mouth daily until remission achieved
Busulphan	2–6 mg/m^2 by mouth daily until remission achieved

Maintenance
Any of the above combinations of drugs used for induction reduced to a dose and frequency which maintain white blood cell counts within the normal range

* see Table 15.7.

chronic leukaemias in dogs is much more favourable than for acute leukaemias. Mean and median survival times for CLL may exceed one year (Leifer & Matus 1985, 1986) but are usually shorter for CGL, which has a greater risk of blast cell crisis.

In cats, fewer cases of leukaemia (27%) than lymphoma (64%) respond to chemotherapy when given a COP protocol (Cotter 1983). In general, survival times are better for ALL (one to seven months) than AML (two to ten weeks) (Couto 1992). Responses to treatment for CLL are good but reports of CGL are scarce.

Other myeloproliferative diseases

Eosinophilic and basophilic leukaemia

Eosinophilic and basophilic leukaemias are rarely reported in the dog and cat but are characterised by high white blood cell counts with a high proportion of either basophils or eosinophils. Eosinophilic leukaemias are difficult to distinguish from other hypereosinophilic syndromes and basophilic leukaemias are often confused with mast cell leukaemias. Treatment of both leukaemias is with corticosteroids or hydroxyurea.

Megakaryoblastic leukaemia/primary thrombocytosis

Megakaryoblastic or megakaryocytic leukaemia is rare in dogs and cats and may be associated with platelet dysfunction. Abnormal megakaryocytic hyperplasia is seen in the bone marrow and thrombocytosis or thrombocytopenia may be present. Primary thrombocytosis or essential thrombocythemia has also been infrequently reported, and is characterised by excessively high platelet counts, bizarre giant platelets with abnormal granulation and increased numbers of megakaryocytes in the bone marrow. It must be distinguished from secondary or reactive thrombocytosis.

Erythroid leukaemias

These include erythremic myelosis and erythroleukaemia which are relatively common in cats,

and polycythaemia vera which is rare in both dogs and cats. Erythremic myelosis is characterised by excessive proliferation of early erythroid precursors and nucleated red blood cells in bone marrow with severe anaemia, increased numbers of circulating nucleated red blood cells, moderate to marked anisocytosis, and increased mean corpuscular volume. Transformation of erythremic myelosis to erythroleukaemia may occur. Essentially, this is very similar to erythremic myelosis but myeloblasts are present in low numbers along with the erythroid precursors.

Polycythemia vera or primary erythrocytosis is rare in both cats and dogs and must be distinguished from relative and secondary absolute polycythemia and is characterised by persistently elevated PCV (65–85%) with low or normal erythropoietin activity. There is proliferation of the erythroid series with differentiation to mature red blood cells. Repeated phlebotomy and replacement of blood with colloids and electrolyte solutions may be necessary (see Chapter 2) but a more gradual reduction in the PCV can be obtained using hydroxyurea.

Myelodysplastic syndromes (preleukaemia)

Myelodysplastic syndromes are vague clinical conditions presenting as lethargy, anorexia, depression and pyrexia and are associated with bone marrow which is normocellular or hypercellular but not overtly neoplastic. They are relatively common in cats (80% FeLV positive) but less common in dogs. Maturation arrest of granulocytes and increased numbers of immature precursors are seen. The bone marrow changes may be reflected by haematological abnormalities such as cytopenias or presence of bizarre cells in the blood and physical findings may include pallor, hepatosplenomegaly, lymphadenopathy, recurrent infections or weight loss. These changes may wax and wane, without ever progressing, but a proportion of cases will develop into aleukaemic leukaemia or overt myeloid leukaemia eventually. In cats, this is less likely since many are euthanased because of their FeLV status.

Treatment of such preleukaemic conditions with

chemotherapy is contraversial since not all will progress to full leukaemia, but regular monitoring and supportive therapy with fluids and antibiotics

is recommended. Differentiating agents (cytosine arabinoside), haematopoietic growth factors or anabolic steroids may also be tried.

MULTIPLE MYELOMA

Epidemiology

Multiple myeloma accounts for 8% of haematopoietic tumours and 4% of all bone tumours but less than 1% of all canine malignant tumours. It occurs in older dogs (mean 8.3 years, range 2–15 years) but there is no sex or breed predisposition.

Plasma cell myeloma is very rare in the cat and represent less than 1% of all haematopoietic tumours. Affected cats are generally old (range 6–13 years) but there is no sex predisposition.

Aetiology

No aetiology has been proposed for multiple myeloma in the dog or cat although chronic antigen stimulation associated with desensitisation of allergies has been implicated in man. C type retroviruses have been implicated in mice but not cats, and feline cases are generally FeLV negative (MacEwen & Hurvitz 1977; Matus & Leifer 1985).

Pathology and tumour behaviour

Multiple myeloma arises from the neoplastic proliferation of plasma cells (B lymphocytes) predominantly in bone marrow (Fig. 15.14), although spill over into blood and infiltration of peripheral lymphoid organs may occur. In classical cases the plasma cells retain their secretory function and produce monoclonal immunoglobulin (sometimes called the M protein). IgA and IgG have equal prevalence in canine multiple myeloma (Hammer & Couto 1994) whereas production of IgM is often called primary macroglobulinaemia.

Abnormal immunoglobulin coats red blood cells causing a Coombs' positive anaemia and occasionally haemolysis. Antibody coating of platelets leads to poor platelet aggregation, release of platelet factor 3 and inhibition of coagulation protein function resulting in bleeding disorders and hyperviscosity syndrome. Hyperviscosity is usually

associated with IgM which is the largest immunoglobulin molecule, or with IgA dimers which can polymerise. As well as inhibiting haemostasis, increased blood viscosity reduces oxygen perfusion due to sludging of blood vessels in the vasculature, and interferes with cardiac function due to increased peripheral resistance. Normal immunoglobulin levels are depressed in multiple myeloma and this results in impaired phagocytosis, granulocytopenia and depressed cell mediated immunity, which cause an increased susceptibility to infection.

Immunoglobulin light chains, known as Bence-Jones proteins, are excreted in urine, and later in the disease albumin is also lost as glomerular damage proceeds. Renal tubular damage may be caused by several mechanisms such as direct plasma cell infiltration or hypercalcaemia, but most damage results from reabsorption and catabolism of immunoglobulin molecules by the tubular cells. As tubules are damaged and more light chains excreted, they precipitate to form casts which impair renal function even more. Pyelonephritis is common due to an increased susceptibility to infec-

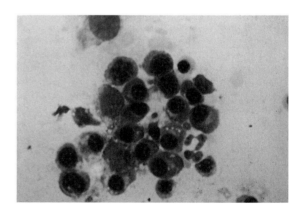

Fig. 15.14 Bone marrow aspirate from dog with multiple myeloma, showing a cluster of plasma cells, some with secretory vacuoles in their cytoplasm. (See also Colour plate 33, facing p. 162.)

tion but glomerular amyloidosis, although present in humans, is rare in dogs.

Proliferation of neoplastic plasma cells in the marrow may cause myelosuppression resulting in anaemia, thrombocytopenia and leucopenia. It may also produce skeletal lesions, usually in long bones or vertebrae, due to increased osteoclast activity. Occasionally a solid plasma cell mass may occur, for example in the extra-dural space, leading to spinal compression.

Paraneoplastic syndromes

Numerous paraneoplastic syndromes may accompany multiple myeloma. Hypergammaglobulinaemia causes bleeding disorders in a third of canine cases and hyperviscosity syndrome in 20% of cases. Hypercalcaemia may occur in 15–20% of cases and polyneuropathy has also been reported (Villiers & Dobson 1998).

Presentation/signs

Affected animals usually present with non-specific signs including pyrexia, pallor, lethargy or depression. They may have a mild lymphadenopathy or hepatosplenomegaly. Cases with bleeding disorders may have epistaxis, gingival bleeding, bruising, petechiae, echymoses or gastro-intestinal bleeding (Figs 15.15 and 15.16) while those with hyperviscosity may also show:

- Cerebral dysfunction (ataxia, dementia, coma)
- Ocular changes or sudden blindness (retinal detachment, venous dilation and tortuosity)
- Congestive heart failure (exercise intolerance, syncope, cyanosis).

Some animals may present with signs of hypercalcaemia (Chapter 2) or renal failure, while others with skeletal lesions (over 50% of cases) may show lameness, pain, paresis or pathological fracture.

Investigations

Bloods

Haematological evaluation is essential for cases of suspected multiple myeloma. Abnormalities likely to be detected include a mild to moderate non-

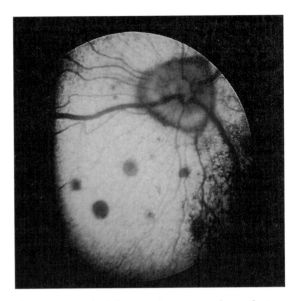

Fig. 15.15 Retinal haemorrhages may be a feature of myeloma as a result of hyperviscosity or thrombocytopenia. (Courtesy of Mr M. Herrtage, Department of Clinical Veterinary Medicine, Cambridge) (See also Colour plate 34, facing p. 162.)

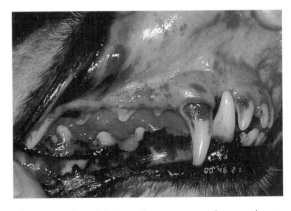

Fig. 15.16 Petechiation of mucous membranes due to thrombocytopenia associated with multiple myeloma. (See also Colour plate 35, facing p. 162.)

regenerative anaemia (70% canine cases) or a Coombs' positive anaemia, leucopenia (25% canine cases), thrombocytopenia (16–30% canine cases) or peripheral plasmacytosis (10% canine cases). Coagulation parameters should also be assessed to detect bleeding diatheses.

Hyperproteinaemia will invariably be detected on biochemical evaluation and an assessment of the albumin : globulin ratio will give an indication of the degree of immunoglobulin secretion and albumin loss. Serum protein electrophoresis should be done to differentiate a monoclonal from a polyclonal gammopathy. BUN and creatinine are needed to assess renal function which is impaired in a third of cases, and electrolyte analysis should be performed to look for hypercalcaemia.

Urinalysis

Urinalysis is necessary to look for proteinuria caused by renal damage and Bence Jones proteins. Although albumin is detected using a dipstick, Bence Jones light chains must be detected by a heat precipitation test. The chains precipitate at 40–60°C, dissolve on boiling and reform a precipitate on cooling. Urine electrophoresis should reflect the monoclonal gammopathy seen on serum electrophoresis.

Imaging techniques

Radiography is useful in multiple myeloma cases to screen vertebrae, pelvis and long bones for skeletal lesions. These may appear as localised multiple punctate lesions or generalised osteoporosis (Fig. 15.17).

Biopsy/FNA

Cytological examination of bone marrow aspirates is necessary to look for sheets of neoplastic plasma cells and to assess the degree of myelosuppression. In cases of multiple myeloma, plasma cells usually account for 5–10% of bone marrow cells.

None of the above investigations are satisfactory

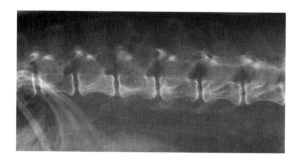

Fig. 15.17 Lateral radiograph of the lumbar spine of a dog with multiple myeloma, showing punched out osteoltic lesions.

on their own to make a diagnosis of multiple myeloma. A definitive diagnosis requires three of the following four parameters:

- Plasma cells in the bone marrow
- Osteolytic bone lesions
- Monoclonal immunoglobulin in serum or urine
- Bence-Jones proteinuria.

Staging

There is no TNM or clinical staging system for multiple myeloma.

Treatment

Surgery

Surgical treatment is not usually needed for multiple myeloma except to repair pathological fractures.

Radiotherapy

Radiotherapy may be used to treat localised bone lesions and give pain relief but there is a danger of inducing a pathological fracture if the bone is very lytic.

Chemotherapy

Specific treatment for multiple myeloma uses combination chemotherapy based on alkylating agents (melphalan or cyclophosphamide) and corticosteroids to target the neoplastic plasma cells (Table 15.14). The response to treatment is assessed by monitoring total protein levels and the presence of a monoclonal spike on serum protein electrophoresis. Examination of bone marrow aspirates may also be used. Once the immunoglobulin concentration is within normal limits, drug doses and frequency are reduced to a maintenance level which keeps the immunoglobulin within these limits.

Other

For cases presenting with hypercalcaemia, immediate supportive therapy may be needed to maintain

Table 15.14 Chemotherapy protocols for the treatment of multiple myeloma.

Induction

Basic protocol

Melphalan	$2.0\,\text{mg/m}^2$ by mouth daily for 7–14 days, then every 48 hours**
Prednisolone	$40\,\text{mg/m}^2$ by mouth daily for 7–14 days, then $20\,\text{mg/m}^2$ every 48 hours

*Additional agent
(if response is inadequate)*

Vincristine	$0.5\,\text{mg/m}^2$ intravenously every 7 days

*Alternative protocols
(if response is inadequate)*

Cyclophosphamide	$50\,\text{mg/m}^2$ by mouth every 48 hours*
Prednisolone	$40\,\text{mg/m}^2$ by mouth daily for 7–14 days, then $20\,\text{mg/m}^2$ every 48 hours
± Vincristine	$0.5\,\text{mg/m}^2$ intravenously every 7 days
or	
Chlorambucil	$2–5\,\text{mg/m}^2$ by mouth every 48 hours
Prednisolone	$40\,\text{mg/m}^2$ by mouth daily for 7–14 days, then $20\,\text{mg/m}^2$ every 48 hours
± Vincristine	$0.5\,\text{mg/m}^2$ intravenously every 7 days

Maintenance
Use prednisolone in combination with either melphalan, cyclophosphamide or chlorambucil at a dose rate and frequency sufficient to maintain plasma immunoglobulin concentration within normal limits

* see Table 15.7.
** Alternative dose for cats is 0.1 mg/kg orally for 10 days, then 0.05 mg/kg daily.

renal function (Chapter 2). If hyperviscosity-induced neurological signs and cardiac changes are very severe, plasmapheresis may be necessary. Antibiotic therapy should be used if the animal is febrile or there is evidence of secondary infection.

Bisphosphonate or mithramycin therapy has been used to prevent further bone lesions by reducing osteoclast activity and to reduce hypercalcaemia, although it is not an essential part of treatment.

Prognosis

The prognosis for multiple myeloma is reasonably good with over 75% of canine cases responding to treatment and median survival times between 12 and 18 months (MacEwen & Hurvitz 1977; Matus & Leifer 1985; Matus *et al.* 1986). A good initial response to treatment is considered a favourable prognostic indicator whereas hypercalcaemia, the presence of Bence-Jones proteinuria, azotemia or extensive bone lesions reduce survival times. The immunoglobulin type is not related to prognosis.

The prognosis for cats is less favourable since some appear not to respond to therapy (MacEwen & Hurvitz 1977).

References

Beatty, J.A., Lawrence, C.E., Callanan, J.J. *et al.* (1998) Feline immunodeficiency virus (FIV)-associated lymphoma: a potential role for immune dysfunction in tumourigenesis. *Veterinary Immunology and Immunopathology*, (65), 309–22.

Callanan, J.J., McCandlish, I.A.P., O'Neil, B. *et al.* (1992) Lymphosarcoma in experimentally induced feline immunodeficiency virus infection. *Veterinary Record*, (130), 293–5.

Cobbold, S. & Metcalfe, S. (1994) Monoclonal antibodies that define canine homologues of human CD antigens: summary of the first international canine leukocyte antigen workshop (CLAW). *Tissue Antigens*, (43), 137–54.

Cotter, S.M. (1983) Treatment of lymphoma and leukemia with cyclophosphamide, vincristine, and prednisolone: II. Treatment of cats. *Journal of the American Animal Hospital Association*, (19), 166–72.

Couto, C.G. (1985) Clinicopathologic aspects of acute leukemias in the dog. *Journal of the American Veterinary Medical Association*, (186), 681–5.

Couto, C.G. (1992) Leukemias. In: *Essentials of Small Animal Internal Medicine*, (eds R.W. Nelson & C.G. Couto), pp. 871–8. Mosby Year Book, St. Louis.

Dorn, C.R., Taylor, D.O.N., Schneider, R. *et al.* (1968) Survey of animal neoplasms in Alameda and Contra Costa Counties, California. II. Cancer morbidity in dogs and cats from Alameda County. *Journal of the National Cancer Institute*, (40), 307–18.

Essex, M. & Francis, D.P. (1976) The risk to humans from malignant diseases of their pets: an unsettled issue. *Journal of the American Animal Hospital Association*, (12), 386–90.

Gorman, N.T. & White, R.A.S. (1987) Clinical management of canine lymphoproliferative diseases. *Veterinary Annual*, (27), 227–42.

Gulino, S.E. (1992) Chromosomal abnormalities and oncogenesis in cat leukemias. *Cancer Genetics and Cytogenetics*, (64), 149–57.

Grindem, C.B. & Bouen, L.C. (1989) Cytogenetic analysis in nine leukaemic cats. *Journal of Comparative Pathology*, (101), 21–30.

Grindem, C.B., Stevens, J.B. & Perman, V. (1985) Morphological classification and clinical and pathological characteristics of spontaneous leukemia in 17 dogs. *Journal of the American Animal Hospital Association*, (21), 219–26.

Hammer, A.S. & Couto, C.G. (1994) Complications of multiple myeloma. *Journal of the American Animal Hospital Association*, (30), 9–14.

Hutson, C.A., Rideout, B.A. & Pederson, N.C. (1991) Neoplasia associated with feline immunodeficiency virus infection in cats in Southern California. *Journal of the American Veterinary Medical Association*, (199), 1357–62.

Jarratt, O. (1994) Feline Leukaemia virus. In: *Feline Medicine and Therapeutics*, (eds E.A. Chandler, C.J. Gaskell & R.M. Gaskell), 2nd edn, pp. 473–87.

Jeglum, K.A. (1991) Monoclonal antibody treatment of canine lymphoma. *Proceedings of the Eastern States Veterinary Conference*, (5), 222–3.

Leifer, C.E. & Matus, R.E. (1985) Lymphoid leukaemia in the dog. *Veterinary Clinics of North America: Small Animal Practice*, **15** (4), 723–39.

Leifer, C.E. & Matus, R.E. (1986) Chronic lymphocytic leukaemia in the dog: 22 cases (1974–1984). *Journal of the American Veterinary Medical Association*, (189), 214–17.

MacEwen, E.G. & Hurvitz, A.I. (1977) Diagnosis and management of monoclonal gammopathies. *Veterinary Clinics of North America*, **7** (1), 119–32.

MacEwen, E.G., Patnaik, A.K. & Wilkins, R.J. (1977) Diagnosis and treatment of canine haematopoietic neoplasms. *Veterinary Clinics of North America*, **7** (1), 105–18.

Matus, R.E. & Leifer, C.E. (1985) Immunoglobulin-producing tumors. *Veterinary Clinics of North America: Small Animal Practice*, **15** (4), 741–53.

Matus, R.E., Leifer, C.E. & MacEwen, E.G. (1983) Acute lymphoblastic leukaemia in the dog: a review of 30 cases. *Journal of the American Veterinary Medical Association*, (183), 859–62.

Matus, R.E., Leifer, C.E., MacEwen, E.G. & Hurvitz, A.I. (1986) Prognostic factors for multiple myeloma in the dog. *Journal of the American Veterinary Medical Association*, (188), 1288–92.

Mooney, S.C., Hayes, A.A., MacEwen, E.G. *et al.* (1989) Treatment and prognostic factors in lymphoma in cats:

103 cases (1977–1981). *Journal of the American Veterinary Medical Association*, (194), 696–9.

Moore, P.F., Rossitto, P.V., Danilenko, D.M. *et al.* (1992) Monoclonal antibodies specific for canine CD4 and CD8 define functional T-lymphocyte subsets and high-density expression of CD4 by canine neutrophils. *Tissue Antigens*, (40), 75–85.

Moore, A.S., Cotter, S.M., Frimberger, A.E., Wood, C.A., Rand, W.M. & L'Heureux, D.A. (1996) A comparison of doxorubicin and COP for maintenance of remission in cats with lymphoma. *Journal of Veterinary Internal Medicine*, (10), 372–5.

Onions, D.E. (1984) A prospective study of familial canine lymphosarcoma. *Journal of the National Cancer Institute*, (72), 909–12.

Owen, L.N. (1980) *TNM classification of tumours in domestic animals.* World Health Organization, Geneva.

Poli, A., Abramo, F., Baldinotti, M. *et al.* (1994) Malignant lymphoma associated with experimentally induced feline immunodeficiency virus infection. *Journal of Comparative Pathology*, (110), 319–28.

Rosenthal, R.C. (1982) Epidemiology of canine lymphosarcoma. *Compendium of Continuing Education for the Practising Veterinarian*, (10), 855–61.

Safran, N., Perk, K. & Eyal, O. (1992) Isolation and preliminary characterisation of a novel retrovirus from a leukaemic dog. *Research in Veterinary Science*, (52), 250–55.

Shelton, G.H., Grant, C.K., Cotter, S.M. *et al.* (1990) Feline immunodeficiency virus (FIV) and feline leukemia virus (FeLV) infections and their relationships to lymphoid malignancies in cats: a retrospective study (1968–1988). *Journal of Acquired Immune Deficiency Syndrome*, (3), 623–30.

Teske, E. (1993) *Non-Hodgkin's lymphoma in the dog: characterisation and experimental therapy.* PhD Thesis, University of Utrecht, printed by OMI Offset, Utrecht.

Teske, E., van Heerde, P., Rutteman, G.R., Kurzman, I.D., Moore, P.F. & MacEwen, E.G. (1994) Prognostic factors for treatment of malignant lymphoma in dogs. *Journal of the American Veterinary Medical Association*, (205), 1722–8.

Theilen, G.H. & Madewell, B.R. (1987) Haemolymphatic neoplasms, sarcomas and related conditions. Part II Feline. In: *Veterinary Cancer Medicine*, 2nd edn, pp. 354–81. Lea & Febiger, Philadelphia.

Vail, D.M., Moore, A.S., Ogilvie, G.K. & Volk, L.M. (1998) Feline lymphoma (145 cases): Proliferation indices, cluster of differentiation 3 immunoreactivity, and their association with prognosis in 90 cats. *J. Veterinary Internal Medicine*, (12), 349–54.

Valli, V.E.O., Norris, A., Withrow, S.J. *et al.* (1989) Anatomical and histological classification of feline lymphoma using the National Cancer Institute Working Formulation. *9th Annual Conference of the Veterinary Cancer Society*.

Vernau, W. & Moore, P.F. (1999) An immunophenotypic study of canine leukaemias and preliminary assessment of clonality by polymerase chain reaction. *Veterinary Immunology and Immunopathology*, (69), 145–64.

Villiers, E. & Dobson, J.M. (1998) Multiple myeloma with associated polyneuropathy in a German shepherd dog. *Journal of Small Animal Practice*, (39), 249–51.

White, S.D., Rosychuk, R.A.W., Scott, K.V., Trettien, A.L., Jonas, L. & Denerolle, P. (1993) Use of isotretinoin and etretinate for the treatment of benign cutaneous neoplasia and cutaneous lymphoma in dogs. *Journal of the American Veterinary Medical Association*, (202), 387–91.

Further reading

Carter, R.F., Harris, C.K., Withrow, S.J., Valli, V.E.O. & Susaneck, S.J. (1987) Chemotherapy of canine lymphoma with histopathological correlation: doxorubicin alone compared to COP as first treatment regimen. *Journal of the American Animal Hospital Association*, (23), 587–96.

Cotter, S.M. (1983) Treatment of lymphoma and leukemia with cyclophosphamide, vincristine, and prednisolone: I. Treatment of dogs. *Journal of the American Animal Hospital Association*, (19), 159–65.

Cotter, S.M. (1986) Clinical management of lymphoproliferative, myeloproliferative, and plasma cell neoplasia. In: *Contemporary Issues in Small Animal Practice 6, Oncology*, (ed. N.T. Gorman), pp. 169–94. Churchill Livingstone, London.

Couto, C.G. (1985) Canine lymphomas: something old, something new. *The Compendium of Continuing Education for the Practising Veterinarian*, (7), 291–302.

Couto, C.G., Rutgers, H.C., Sherding, R.G. & Rojko, J. (1989) Gastrointestinal lymphoma in 20 dogs. *Journal of Veterinary Internal Medicine*, (3), 73–8.

Crow, S.E. (1982) Lymphosarcoma (malignant lymphoma) in the dog: diagnosis and treatment. *The Compendium of Continuing Education for the Practising Veterinarian*, (4), 283–92.

Dobson, J.M. & Gorman, N.T. (1993) Canine multicentric lymphoma 1: Clinicopathological presentation of the disease. *Journal of Small Animal Practice*, (34), 594–8.

Facklam, N.R. & Kociba, G.J. (1986) Cytochemical characterisation of feline leukemic cells. *Veterinary Pathology*, (23), 155–61.

Grindem, C.B., Perman, V. & Stevens, J.B. (1985) Mor-

phological classification and clinical and pathological characteristics of spontaneous leukemia in 10 cats. *Journal of the American Animal Hospital Association*, (21), 227–36.

Hahn, K.A., Richardson, R.C., Teclaw, R.F., Cline, J.M., Carlton, W.W., DeNicola, D.B. & Bonney, P.L. (1992) Is maintenance chemotherapy appropriate for the management of canine malignant lymphoma? *Journal of Veterinary Internal Medicine*, (6), 3–10.

Hardy, W.D. (1981) Haematopoietic tumors of cats. *Journal of the American Animal Hospital Association*, (17), 921–40.

Jeglum, A.K., Whereat, A. & Young, K. (1987) Chemotherapy of lymphoma in 75 cats. *Journal of the American Veterinary Medical Association*, (190), 174–8.

Leifer, C.E. & Matus, R.E. (1986) Canine lymphoma: clinical considerations. *Seminars in Veterinary Medicine and Surgery (Small Animal)*, (1), 43–50.

Loar, A.S. (984) The management of feline lymphosarcoma. *Veterinary Clinics of North America: Small Animal Practice*, (14), 1299–330.

MacEwen, E.G., Brown, N.O., Patnaik, A.K., Hayes, A.A. & Passe, S. (1981) Cyclic combination chemotherapy of canine lymphosarcoma. *Journal of the American Veterinary Medical Association*, (178), 1178–81.

Madewell, B.R. (1975) Chemotherapy for canine lymphosarcoma. *American Journal of Veterinary Research*, (36), 1525–8.

Mooney, S.C., Hayes, A.A., Matus, R.E. & MacEwen, E.G. (1987) Renal lymphoma in cats: 28 cases (1977–1984). *Journal of the American Veterinary Medical Association*, (191), 1473–7.

Ogilvie, G.K. (1993) Recent advances in cancer, chemotherapy and medical management of the geriatric cat. *Veterinary International*, (5), 3–12.

Price, G.S., Page, R.L., Fischer, B.M., Levine, J.F. & Gerig, T.M. (1991) Efficacy and toxicity of doxorubicin/cyclophosphamide maintenance therapy in dogs with multicentric lymphosarcoma. *Journal of Veterinary Internal Medicine*, (5), 259–62.

Rosenthal, R.C. & MacEwen, E.G. (1990) Treatment of lymphoma in dogs. *Journal of the American Veterinary Medical Association*, (196), 774–81.

Weller, R.E. & Stann, S.E. (1983) Renal lymphosarcoma in the cat. *Journal of the American Animal Hospital Association*, (19), 363–7.

16
The Eye and Orbit

Epidemiology

The eye is not a common site for development of tumours in cats and dogs, neither are tumours a common cause of ocular disease in these species. Nevertheless, tumours of the eye and surrounding structures are important because of the threat they may pose to the patient's vision, quality of life and survival. The eyelids are the most common site for ocular tumours in the dog and the majority of these tumours are benign. Tumours of the eyelids and conjunctiva are less common in cats but there is a higher incidence of malignant tumours, especially SCC. Tumours of the third eyelid are rare in both cats and dogs. Primary intraocular tumours are not common in either species, although a variety of tumours have been described affecting the cornea, sclera, iris and ciliary body (Table 16.1). The eye may also be a site for secondary tumours or may be involved in systemic neoplastic disease, e.g. multi-centric lymphoma.

Aetiology

The aetiology of most ocular tumours is not known. Prolonged exposure to sunlight is important in the development of SCC of the eyelids in white cats and possibly in some dogs, as previously described (Chapter 1). Previous trauma and/or chronic inflammation have been reported to incite invasive ocular sarcomas in cats (Dubielzig *et al.* 1990). Genetic factors are known to be important in the development of retinoblastoma in children where the role of the hereditary retinoblastoma gene (Rb) is well documented. However retinoblastoma is very rare in domestic species.

TUMOURS OF THE EYELID AND CONJUNCTIVA

Pathology

Meibomian (sebaceous) gland adenomas are the most common tumour affecting the eyelids in the dog, accounting for 60% of eyelid tumours in one study (Roberts *et al.* 1986). They tend to affect older animals; no sex predisposition has been reported. These tumours arise from the meibomian glands sited at the eyelid margin. Most are benign,

Table 16.1 Summary of tumours affecting the eye and orbit.

Site		
Extraocular	Eyelids	SCC and BCC – cats and dogs
		Meibomian/sebaceous gland adenoma (adenocarcinoma) – dogs
		Melanoma
		MCT and other skin tumours
	Third eyelid	Primary tumours
		Melanoma
		Haemangioma
		BCC and SCC
		Adenoma/adenocarcinoma
		Viral papilloma
		Secondary
		Lymphoma
	Conjunctiva	SCC
		Melanoma
		Systemic histiocytosis
	Orbit	Primary connective tissue tumours, e.g. rhabdomyosarcoma, fibrosarcoma
		Primary tumours of skull, e.g. multilobular osteochondrosarcoma
		Local invasion by tumours of nasal cavity, frontal sinus and caudal maxilla
	Optic nerve	Optic nerve meningioma
Ocular	Cornea and sclera	Melanoma (limbal or epibulbar)
		SCC
	Iris and ciliary body	Ciliary body adenoma/adenocarcinoma
		Multicentric lymphoma
		Melanoma
		Medulloepithelioma
		Metastatic tumours (mammary carcinoma, haemangiosarcoma, malignant melanoma)
	Retina and choroid	(Retinoblastoma)
		(Melanoma)

although occasionally meibomian gland adenocarcinoma is reported. Viral papillomas may occur in younger dogs and SCC in older animals. SCC is the most common tumour of the eyelid in cats. Other tumours of the skin, for example mast cell tumours, basal cell tumours and melanoma, may affect the skin of the eyelids and epitheliotrophic lymphoma may affect the mucocutaneous junction of the lid margin (Chapters 4 and 15).

Tumours of the third eyelid and conjunctivae are rare but melanoma, haemangioma, histiocytoma, adenoma, adenocarcinoma and basal and squamous cell tumours may arise at this site, as may, rarely, mast cell tumours. Secondary involvement from multicentric lymphosarcoma may be seen as a bilateral nodular form affecting the third eyelid (Fig. 16.1) or a more diffuse inflamed and swollen

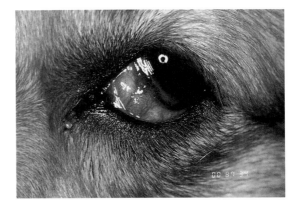

Fig. 16.1 Lymphoma presenting as raised nodules on the third eyelid in a dog.

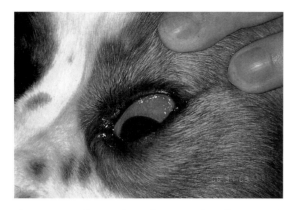

Fig. 16.2 A dog with multicentric lymphoma with ocular involvement causing inflammation of the conjuctiva and sclera.

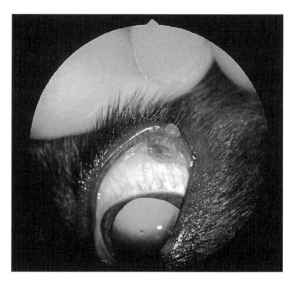

Fig. 16.3 Meibomian gland adenoma in an English springer spaniel. (Courtesy of Dr S. Petersen-Jones, Department of Small Animal Clinical Sciences, Veterinary Medical Centre, Michigan State University.)

conjunctiva (Fig. 16.2). Ocular signs are also seen in systemic histiocytosis, a rare familial condition in the Bernese mountain dog. In addition to skin lesions (Chapter 4) affected animals often show signs of scleritis, episcleritis and conjunctivitis. Conjunctival biopsies show a diffuse infiltrate of histiocytic cells.

Presentation/tumour behaviour/ paraneoplastic syndromes

Meibomian gland tumours usually arise on the margin of the eyelid but often extend into the eyelid where they present as a bulging of the conjunctiva (Fig. 16.3). These are slowly growing tumours that range in size from 1–10 mm. They may cause ocular irritation or discomfort leading to ocular discharge and blepharospasm and may ultimately lead to corneal damage and ulceration. Meibomian gland tumours are mostly adenomas which are non-invasive and follow a benign course.

SCC of the eyelids is an invasive tumour often presenting as an ulcerated mass causing distortion and destruction of adjacent soft tissues (Figs 16.4 and 16.5). Although locally aggressive, the rate of metastasis is low.

Melanoma of the eyelid may follow a benign course, especially if the tumour is cutaneous, heavily pigmented and well differentiated histologically. Tumours sited at the mucocutaneous junction

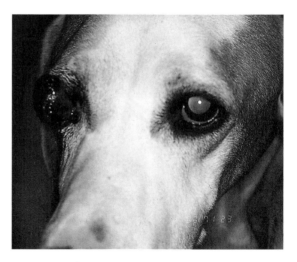

Fig. 16.4 A large squamous cell carcinoma affecting the upper eyelid in a dog.

of the lid and tumours affecting the conjunctivae tend to be more anaplastic morphologically and malignant in their behaviour with a high rate of distant (haematogenous) metastasis.

Paraneoplastic syndromes are not commonly associated with primary tumours of the eyelids.

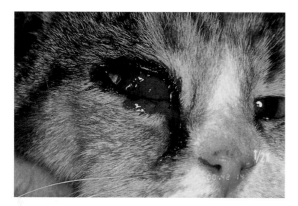

Fig. 16.5 An ulcerated squamous cell carcinoma of the third eyelid in a cat.

Investigations

In the case of meibomian gland tumours and other primary tumours of the eyelids a presumptive diagnosis of a neoplasia may be made on clinical examination. Lymphoma of the third eyelid or conjunctiva may be confused with inflammatory conditions of these tissues.

Bloods

These are not generally indicated in the diagnosis of primary tumours of the eyelids, although they would be included in the work-up of cases with lymphoma.

Imaging techniques

Radiography/ultrasonography of the primary tumour is not necessary. Thoracic films are important to look for metastases in cases of malignant tumours, but most tumours at this site have low metastatic potential.

Biopsy/FNA

FNAs may be difficult to perform safely at this site unless the patient is anaesthetised, in which case it is probably preferable to collect a total excisional biopsy of the lesion for histological diagnosis. Cytological preparations from impression smears and tissue scrapings are of limited diagnostic value. Many meibomian gland tumours are small at initial presentation and as they are non-invasive an excisional biopsy would be justified in such cases. Incisional or punch biopsies are indicated for ulcerative lesions, suspicious of SCC or other malignant tumours, and for multiple or diffuse lesions prior to treatment.

Staging

There is no staging system specific to the eyelids but the clinical staging system for tumours of the skin (Table 4.2) is applicable to this site.

Treatment

Surgery

Most solitary tumours of the eyelids are amenable to surgical resection. Cryosurgery may be preferred for treatment of small, benign lesions as this may provide better preservation of the eyelid margin. Cryosurgery may also be used for early, superficial, non-invasive SCC in the cat. In any tumour of the eyelid it is preferable to treat early, upon initial detection of the problem. Smaller tumours can be resected with minimal damage to the lids; removal of larger tumours may require substantial reconstructive eyelid surgery. In the case of meibomian gland adenoma the surgical resection needs to include any extension of the tumour into the conjuctiva. Larger benign tumours that involve less than 25% of the margin, may be excised by a partial or full thickness wedge resection. Radical surgical resection is required for carcinomas and other malignant tumours of the eyelid and this will require complex reconstructive techniques (Bedford 1999). Removal of the eye may be considered as a salvage procedure for treatment of advanced tumours or those with extensive conjunctival involvement.

Radiotherapy

External beam radiation is rarely used in the treatment of periocular tumours because of the damaging effects of radiation on the tissues of the eye (Chapter 3). Brachytherapy offers a more localised form of radiotherapy that may have a role in the management of periocular carcinomas. Implantation techniques are not widely used in small animals due to lack of specialist containment facilities, although irridium brachytherapy is used in treatment of periocular SCC in horses (Fig. 3.7). Strontium 90 provides a superficial source of radiotherapy which could be applied to perioribital tumours, but this technique has not been widely used in small animals.

Chemotherapy

The main indication for chemotherapy in the treatment of eyelid tumours is in the management of lymphoma as described in Chapter 15. A cream containing a 5% solution of the antimetabolite 5-Fluorouracil is available for topical treatment of superficial squamous and basal cell tumours and has been used for SCC of the third eyelid in horses. This agent must not be used (even topically) in cats.

Other

Manual expression of meibomian gland adenomas may release trapped secretions and provide short term alleviation of ocular discomfort prior to surgical management. Photodynamic therapy may offer an alternative to surgical excision or cryosurgery for treatment of early, superficial SCC (Chapter 3).

Prognosis

The prognosis for tumours of the eyelids depends on the histological type. Most meibomian gland tumours are benign and the prognosis following surgical resection or cyrosurgery is very good. The prognosis for early SCC (in both cats and dogs) following surgery is also favourable due to the low rate of metastasis from this site. More advanced and invasive SCC carry a guarded prognosis as local recurrence may result from inability to achieve adequate margins of excision. The prognosis for melanoma of the eyelid is guarded because while most are benign, a proportion of such tumours follow a malignant course with haematogenous metastasis.

TUMOURS OF THE ORBIT

Tumours of the orbit are not common but neoplasia is the most common cause of orbital disease. Tumours affecting the orbit may be:

- Primary, usually soft tissue tumours, e.g. fibrosarcoma, mast cell tumour, arising within the retrobulbar space
- Tumours of the adjacent skull, e.g. osteosarcoma, multilobular osteochondrosarcoma, which extend into the orbit
- Local extension of tumours arising in the nasal cavity and paranasal sinuses (e.g. nasal carcinoma – dog) and local extension of tumours of the oral cavity (e.g. squamous cell carcinoma – cat).

Most tumours of the orbit are thus malignant.

Tumour behaviour/paraneoplastic syndromes

The behaviour of tumours which may affect the orbit has been discussed in previous chapters: Chapter 4, Skin; Chapter 5, Soft tissues; Chapter 6, Skeletal system; Chapter 7, Head and neck. Para-

neoplastic syndromes are not commonly associated with most of these tumours.

Presentation/signs

Most orbital or retrobulbar tumours are relatively slow growing and usually present as gradual onset exophthalmos with or without conjunctival swelling or chemosis. This may first be noticed as a widening of the palpebral fissure and is clinically detectable as a reduced ability to retropulse the affected eye. As the globe is gradually displaced by the increasing retrobulbar mass, deviation of the eye from its normal axis will result in strabismus. In cases where the tumour is anterior to the midpoint of the globe its growth may cause enophthalmos, but this would be unusual. Conjunctival swelling and oedema may be marked and in some cases may obscure the globe. Unless there are secondary complications (e.g. corneal ulceration or glaucoma) the eye is not usually painful and this lack of pain is a useful sign to distinguish retrobulbar neoplasia from a retrobulbar abscess. However, some retrobulbar tumours, e.g. carcinomas that erode into the orbit from adjacent sites, may be more acute in onset than outlined above and these may be associated with considerable pain. Retrobulbar mast cell tumours can also have a more acute presentation due to inflammation mediated through local release of histamine with sporadic massive chemosis.

Investigations

A complete ophthalmic examination with pupil dilation is important in the investigation of cases presenting with exophthalmos, as is a full examination of the head and mouth. The main differential diagnoses for exophthalmos are:

- Retrobulbar abscess
- Foreign body
- Cellulitis
- Zygomatic salivary gland inflammation or mucocele.

Bloods

These are not generally indicated in the diagnosis of tumours of the orbit. A neutrophilia with a left shift might support a differential diagnosis of infection or abscessation, but a similar picture may occur in tumours containing areas of necrosis.

Imaging techniques

Radiography of the skull including the nasal and paranasal sinuses, the orbit and the maxilla may be useful in the evaluation of tumours involving these sites. Ultrasound is a more useful technique for evaluation of the soft tissues of the orbit and retrobulbar space (Fig. 16.6). CT or MRI images can provide excellent detail of the eye and adjacent structures (Fig. 16.7).

Biopsy/FNA

FNA is a useful technique in investigation of an orbital lesion. Cytological examination of FNA samples may at least differentiate between inflammatory and neoplastic conditions and in some cases provide a cytological diagnosis (Boydell 1991). Ultrasound guidance for aspirate collection is useful both to direct the needle to the abnormal

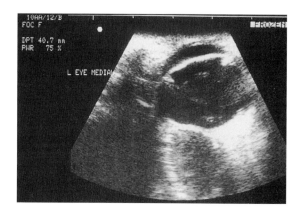

Fig. 16.6 Ultrasonogram of the eye and retrobulbar mass, showing a discrete hyopechoic mass in the medial aspect of the orbit. (Courtesy of Ruth Dennis, Animal Health Trust, Newmarket, previously published in *Journal of Small Animal Practice* (2000), (41), 145–55, with permission.)

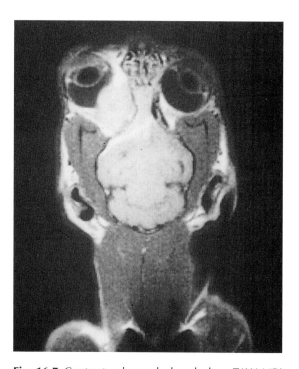

Fig. 16.7 Contrast enhanced, dorsal plane T1W MRI scan of a cat with an orbital mass. Enhancement of frontal lobe tissue indicates intracranial extension of the tumour. The final diagnosis was lymphoma. (Courtesy of Ruth Dennis, Animal Health Trust, Newmarket, previously published in *Journal of Small Animal Practice* (2000), (41), 145–55, with permission.)

tissue and to aid avoidance of the globe, optic nerve and major blood vessels. A needle biopsy (e.g. tru-cut) may be considered if there is a large mass to provide tissue for histological diagnosis but an exploratory orbitotomy may be preferable for providing representative biopsy material (Slatter & Abdelbaki 1979).

Staging

There is no clinical staging system described for tumours of the orbit in cats or dogs.

Treatment

Surgery

Surgical resection is the theoretical treatment of choice for most primary tumours of the orbit, e.g. fibrosarcoma (Gilger *et al*. 1994). The surgical approach will often necessitate removal of the eye and supporting structures but because of the relatively advanced stage of many tumours by the time of diagnosis, it may not be possible to achieve the margins required for complete eradication of the tumour. Surgical resection of tumours which have invaded into the orbit from the nasal or oral cavity is rarely feasible.

Radiotherapy

The use of radiotherapy in the orbit is limited by the sensitivity of the eye to radiation (Chapter 3).

Radiotherapy may have a role as an adjunct to cytoreductive surgery (including removal of the eye) in the management of locally invasive retrobulbar tumours, especially soft tissue sarcomas. Radiotherapy has been used alone for treatment of carcinomas of the nasal and paranasal sinuses with retrobulbar involvement, but such treatment is only palliative and carries a high risk of radiation-induced keratitis, keratoconjunctivitis sicca and corneal ulceration.

Chemotherapy

With the exception of lymphoma, most tumours involving the orbit are not amenable to chemotherapy.

Prognosis

Irrespective of tumour type, most tumours affecting the orbit carry a guarded to poor prognosis because:

- Most tumours at this site are malignant and although distant metastasis is not usually a major problem, the locally invasive nature of their growth precludes adequate surgical resection.
- Diagnosis is often delayed until the tumour has reached a relatively advanced stage.
- Treatment is complicated by the proximity of critical structures such as the eye and brain.

OCULAR TUMOURS

Melanoma and lymphoma are the two most important tumours of the globe in cats and in dogs. Melanoma is the most common primary tumour in both species and usually affects the iris and ciliary body (i.e. intra-ocular melanoma). In dogs melanoma may also be limbal (epibulbar) and in rare cases, arise in the choroid. Ocular lymphoma is usually a manifestation of systemic or multicentric disease which may involve the conjunctiva, the iris, the choroid and the retina. Primary epithelial tumours of the iris and ciliary body are not common in either species although adenoma and adenocarcinoma have been reported and rarely, in young dogs, medulloepithelioma (Dubielzig 1990;

Dubielzig *et al*. 1998). In cats an invasive soft tissue sarcoma may arise secondary to lens rupture several years following ocular trauma. Primary tumours of the choroid and retina are rare in the cat and the dog.

Presentation/signs

Primary ocular tumours are usually unilateral.

In dogs ocular melanoma usually presents as a nodular pigmented lesion. Epibulbar or limbal tumours may be detected by the owner as a non-painful, pigmented mass bulging from the sclera,

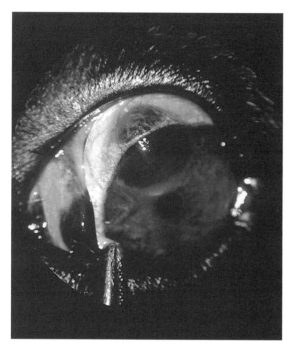

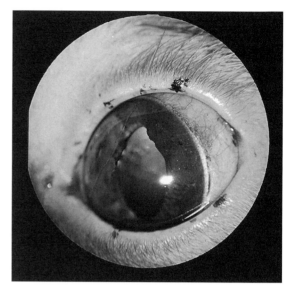

Fig. 16.9 Diffuse iris melanoma in a cat. (Courtesy of Dr S. Petersen-Jones, Department of Small Animal Clinical Sciences, Veterinary Medical Centre, Michigan State University.)

Fig. 16.8 Epibulbar or limbal melanoma in a three year old German shepherd dog. (Courtesy of Dr S. Petersen-Jones, Department of Small Animal Clinical Sciences, Veterinary Medical Centre, Michigan State University.)

adjacent to the cornea (Fig. 16.8). An increased incidence of epibulbar melanoma has been reported in German shepherd dogs and other breeds, e.g. cocker spaniel, standard schnauzer and poodle, may also be predisposed (Diters *et al.* 1983). Intra-ocular melanomas affect the iris and ciliary body. Most but not all tumours at these sites are heavily pigmented lesions causing thickening of the iris and irregularity of the pupil. Blindness, ocular pain and glaucoma may result from the expanding tumour mass restricting aqueous drainage, or from tumour infiltration.

Feline ocular melanoma usually presents in a more diffuse form, with tumour infiltration causing a diffuse darkening, thickening and distortion of the iris (Fig. 16.9). Secondary glaucoma, due to infiltration of the filtration apparatus, is common. Feline melanoma can present as a solitary mass which may be difficult to differentiate from a benign naevus.

Other primary iridociliary epithelial tumours may present as a white, pink, red or pigmented mass visible in the pupil, as a result of distortion of the iris or as a result of secondary ocular changes. In cats, spindle cell sarcoma and osteosarcoma have been reported in animals with a history of ocular trauma, 1–10 years prior to the onset of tumour. Post-traumatic sarcomas present as a firm, swollen, opaque, usually non-painful globe (Dubielzig *et al.* 1990).

In cats and dogs with lymphoma, ocular involvement is more likely to be bilateral and diffuse in nature. Infiltration of the iris may lead to a detectable change in the eye, the iris becoming paler and assuming a swollen appearance. More often, though, such cases present with signs of anterior uveitis, hyphema or hypopyon (Fig. 16.10). Other tumours which metastasise to the eye, e.g. haemangiosarcoma, are also more likely to show a bilateral presentation and intraocular haemorrhage as a common feature.

Tumour behaviour/paraneoplastic syndromes

While the biological behaviour of an ocular tumour in terms of malignancy is important for overall

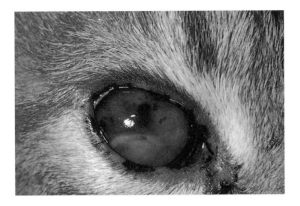

Fig. 16.10 Ocular lymphoma with cellular infiltrate and haemorrhage in the anterior chamber. (Courtesy of Mr D. E. Bostock.)

prognosis it is important to appreciate that even benign intra-ocular tumours can cause severe intra-ocular damage and blindness due to space occupying and pressure effects.

Canine ocular melanomas may be described as benign or malignant according to histological criteria (e.g. cellular anaplasia, presence of mitoses); however, local infiltration and progressive destruction of the eye are features common to both benign and malignant variants. Although there was a popular perception of canine ocular melanoma as a malignant tumour with a high risk of systemic metastasis, clinical studies have shown that limbal and benign uveal melanomas do not metastasise. Even in those tumours with histological features of malignancy, the actual incidence of metastasis is low (Wilcock & Peiffer 1986). In contrast, feline ocular melanomas are truly malignant tumours; they are locally destructive of adjacent ocular structures and the development of systemic metastases, especially to the liver, has been documented (Acland *et al.* 1980).

Benign and malignant variants of iridociliary epithelial tumours have been described. Invasive behaviour is one criterion used to make this distinction, with tumours demonstrating scleral invasion being designated as malignant (i.e. adenocarcinoma) although the actual rate of metastasis in such cases appeared to be very low in one study, if it occurred at all (Dubielzig *et al.* 1998).

Feline ocular sarcomas are aggressive, infiltrating tumours that invade the retina and optic nerve early in the course of the disease. Tumour extension along the course of the optic nerve may lead to involvement of the optic chiasm, thus affecting vision in the other eye. Orbital extension of the tumour is also possible.

Investigations

A complete ophthalmic examination with pupil dilation is important in the investigation of cases presenting with an ocular mass, or with less specific signs of ocular disease.

Bloods

These are not generally indicated in the diagnosis of ocular tumours, although would be indicated in the investigation of animals with lymphoma and are important in pre-surgical assessment of the patient.

Imaging techniques

Radiography is of little value in the evaluation of ocular tumours, but thoracic and abdominal films would be required in the evaluation of animals with malignant or systemic tumours. Ultrasound is a more useful technique for evaluation of the eye and can provide detail on the size and position of a mass and its relationship with adjacent structures. CT or MRI images can be useful where orbital extension is possible.

Biopsy/FNA

While FNA or biopsy via iridectomy might assist in the diagnosis of some ocular tumours, most ocular tumours are diagnosed following either an excisional biopsy or, in more advanced cases, following enucleation of the eye.

Staging

There is no clinical staging system described for ocular tumours in cats or dogs. In animals with lymphoma, ocular involvement would signify stage V disease according to the WHO stage grouping (Owen 1980).

Treatment

Surgery

Surgical resection is the treatment of choice for most primary ocular tumours. In some cases, small, localised lesions of the iris can be excised successfully without loss of the eye. Limbal melanomas in dogs and cats may also be treated by local surgical excision. Most cases, however, will require at least enucleation of the eye and in cases where the tumour has invaded the sclera and extraocular tissues, exenteration of the orbit is recommended.

Radiotherapy

Most ocular tumours are not amenable to radiotherapy although radiotherapy may have a role as an adjunct to cytoreductive surgery (including removal of the eye) in the management of locally invasive tumours, such as ocular sarcomas.

Chemotherapy

With the exception of lymphoma, ocular tumours are not amenable to chemotherapy. In dogs and cats with multicentric lymphoma, ocular lesions may improve following systemic chemotherapy with any of the protocols described in Chapter 15, although the prognosis for animals with ocular involvement (i.e. stage V lymphoma) is very guarded. Survival times tend to be shorter than those for stage III or IV lymphoma and recurrence of ocular signs often heralds systemic relapse.

Other

Non-invasive diode laser photocoagulation has been used for treatment of solitary lesions of the iris in dogs, presumed to be melanoma, and this would appear to be a safe and effective alternative for isolated lesions (Cook & Wilkie 1999).

Prognosis

The prognosis for ocular tumours depends on histological type and species. Irrespective of whether the tumour is described as benign and malignant it would seem that most canine ocular melanomas carry a favourable prognosis following enucleation. In contrast most feline ocular melanomas are malignant and the prognosis for such cases is poor due to a high risk of systemic metastasis.

The prognosis for iridociliary epithelial tumours is favourable in both species but feline ocular sarcomas are aggressive tumours and are unlikely to be cured by surgical resection.

The prognosis for ocular lymphoma is poor for the reasons outlined above.

References

Acland, G.M., McLean, I.W., Aguirre, G.D. *et al.* (1980) Diffuse iris melanoma in cats. *Journal of the American Veterinary Medical Association*, (176), 52–6.

Bedford, P.G.G. (1999) Diseases and surgery of the canine eyelids. In: *Veterinary Ophthalmology*, 3rd edn, (ed. K.N. Gelatt), pp. 535–68. Williams & Wilkins, Lipincott. Chapter 14.

Boydell, P. (1991) Fine needle aspiration biopsy in the diagnosis of exophthalmos. *Journal of Small Animal Practice*, (32), 542–6.

Cook, C.S. & Wilkie, D.A. (1999) Treatment of presumed iris melanoma in dogs by diode laser photocoagulation: 23 cases. *Veterinary Ophthalmology*, (2), 217–25.

Diters, R.W., Dubielzig, R.R., Aguirre, G.D. *et al.* (1983) Primary ocular melanoms in dogs. *Veterinary Pathology*, (20), 379–95.

Dubielzig, R.R. (1990) Ocular neoplasma in small animals. In: *Small Animal Ophthalmology, Veterinary Clinics of North America, Small Animal Practice*, (eds N.J. Millichamp & J. Dziezyc), 20 (3), 837–48. W.B. Saunders, Philadelphia.

Dubielzig, R.R., Everitt, J., Shadduck, J.A. *et al.* (1990) Clinical and morphological features of post-traumatic ocular sarcomas in cats. *Veterinary Pathology*, (27), 62–5.

Dubielzig, R.R., Steinbery, H., Garvin, H., Deehr, A.J. & Fischer, B. (1998) Iridociliary epithelial tumours in 100 dogs and 17 cats: a morphological study. *Veterinary Ophthalmology*, 1 (4), 223–31.

Gilger, B.C., Whitley, R.D. & Mc Laughlin, S.A. (1994) Modified lateral orbitotomy for removal of orbital neoplasms in two dogs. *Veterinary Surgery*, (23), 53–8.

Owen, L.N. (1980) *TNM Classification of Tumors in Domestic Animals*. World Health Organization, Geneva.

Roberts, S.M., Severin, G.A. & Lavach, J.D. (1986) Prevalence and treatment of palpebral neoplasms in the dog: 200 cases (1975–1983) *Journal of the American Veterinary Medical Association*, (189), 1355–9.

Slatter, D.H. & Abdelbakl, Y. (1979) Lateral orbitotomy by zygomatic arch resection in the dog. *Journal of Veterinary Medical Association*, (175), 1179–82.

Wilcock, B.P. & Peiffer, R.L. (1986) Morphology and behaviour of primary ocular melanomas in 91 dogs. *Veterinary Pathology*, (23), 418–24.

17
Miscellaneous Tumours

Most neoplasms of cats and dogs have been included within the body systems presented in the preceding chapters. However, a small number of tumours arising at specific sites have not been considered. This chapter draws these together.

THYMOMA

Epidemiology

Thymoma is an uncommon tumour in dogs and cats and there are few population-based reports on the incidence of this tumour. In one study of cats and dogs with 'thymic disease', thymoma was diagnosed in 5 of 30 cats and 18 of 36 dogs (Day 1997). Thymoma is usually a disease of the older animal, affecting medium to large breeds of dog, with a female predisposition. However in Day's study the 18 dogs were aged from 10 months to 12 years with a mean of 7.5 years. Labradors, Labrador-crosses and German shepherd dogs were over represented, as were females. The five cats in the same study were aged from 5 to 14 years (mean 9.10 years), four were male, three were domestic short hair, one domestic long hair and one Siamese.

Aetiology

The aetiology of thymoma in cats and dogs is unknown.

Pathology

The thymus is sited in the cranial mediastinum and this is the site of development of the tumour mass. The normal thymus consists of two cell types:

• Epithelial cells derived from the embryonic pharyngeal pouches
• T-lymphocytes.

In thymoma the epithelial cells are the neoplastic element but are accompanied by a benign proliferation of small, well differentiated, mature lymphoid cells. Thymoma may be predominantly epithelial or predominantly lymphoid according to the relative proportions of the two cell types. Subclassification of thymoma according to the organization of the epithelial elements (spindle cell, epithelial, pseudorosette) has not been shown to be of prognostic value in animal tumours.

Tumour behaviour/paraneoplastic syndromes

Thymoma is typically a slowly growing tumour of relatively benign behaviour. Most tumours are quite well encapsulated but some may be locally invasive of adjacent structures. Metastasis is rare.

Thymoma may be associated with autoimmune paraneoplastic syndromes, in particular myasthenia gravis and occasionally polymyositis, and with an increased incidence of non-thymic neoplasms (lymphoma, pulmonary adenocarcinoma and haemangiosarcoma) (Aronsohn 1985a). The association between thymoma and myasthenia gravis is well recognised in dogs, especially German shepherd dogs and thymoma associated myasthenia has also been reported in the cat (Scott-Moncrieff *et al.* 1990; Rusbridge *et al.* 1996). On occasion, myasthenia gravis has been observed to develop after surgical resection of thymoma in humans, dogs and cats (Gores *et al.* 1994). Paraneoplastic hypercalcaemia is rare in dogs with thymoma.

Presentation/signs

As a result of the slow growth rate of most thymomas, clinical signs may not be apparent until the tumour has reached massive proportions (Fig. 17.1). The most common clinical signs result from the presence of a large mass in the cranial mediastinum causing pressure on adjacent organs and structures. These include:

- Respiratory – cough, dyspnoea
- Cardiovascular – obstruction of the cranial vena cava, impairing venous return to the heart leading to 'precaval syndrome' with facial and/or forelimb oedema (Fig. 17.2) and enlarged, prominent jugular veins
- Salivation, regurgitation or vomiting could result from direct pressure on the oseophagus,

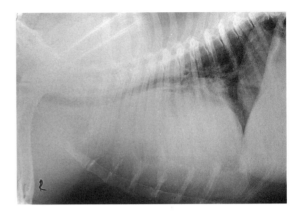

Fig. 17.1 Lateral thoracic radiograph of dog with a large cranial medistinal mass, causing elevation of the trachea and caudal displacement of the heart. The mass was diagnosed as a lymphocytic thymoma following surgical excision.

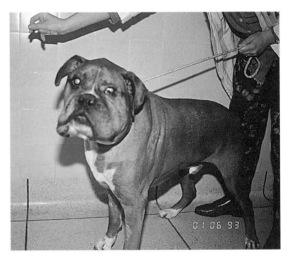

Fig. 17.2 Oedematous swelling of the head and neck, anterior caval syndrome.

but such signs may also be a manifestation of myasthenia.

Those animals with paraneoplastic myasthenia gravis may present with signs of:

- Muscle weakness
- Regurgitation and possibly aspiration pneumonia due to megaoesophagus (dogs).

On auscultation the chest is dull cranially and ventrally, and heart sounds are muffled and often displaced caudally. In cats there may be reduced compressibility of the cranial chest.

Investigations

Further investigations are indicated in order to:

- Confirm the presence of a mediastinal mass
- Determine the histological type.

The main differential diagnoses for a mediastinal mass are listed in Table 17.1. Lymphoma is the most common tumour at this site in dogs and cats and can be difficult to distinguish from lymphocytic thymoma.

Bloods

Routine haematological/biochemical analyses are not generally very helpful in establishing a definitive diagnosis of thymoma. Lymphocytosis has been reported but this is neither a consistent nor a specific finding (Atwater *et al.* 1994). However, such investigations would be indicated to rule out concurrent problems and in the pretreatment evaluation of older animals. Leucocytosis with a left shift may occur in the presence of aspiration pneumonia.

Imaging techniques

On plain lateral thoracic radiographs animals with thymoma usually have an obvious soft tissue mass in the cranial mediastinum (Fig. 17.1). The tumour is usually of sufficient size to cause dorsal dis-

Table 17.1 Differential diagnoses of a cranial mediastinal mass.

Neoplastic
Lymphoma
Chemodectoma (aortic/carotid body tumours)
Ectopic thyroid tumour
Ectopic parathyroid tumour
Thymoma
(Soft tissue sarcoma)
(Tumour metastasis in mediastinal/presternal lymph
　node)

Non-neoplastic
Abscess
Granuloma

---

placement of the trachea and caudo-dorsal displacement of the heart. A pleural effusion may be present but this is not a consistent finding. Megaoesophagus and aspiration pneumonia may also be apparent on plain radiographs in dogs with myasthenia gravis.

Tracheo-bronchial lymph nodes are not usually enlarged in cases with thymoma, an observation that may assist in differentiation between thymoma and mediastinal lymphoma.

Ultrasound may be useful to distinguish between fluid and soft tissue in cases with pleural effusion, but although some thymomas may contain cystic clefts and cavities as opposed to the more homogeneous appearance of lymphoma, the texture of these tumours varies considerably and ultrasound does not provide a definitive guide to the likely histology of the mass. Ultrasound is useful to assess the capsule of the tumour for local invasion, to assess relationships with adjacent structures and to aid collection of biopsy or aspirate material.

Biopsy/FNA

Fine needle aspiration is the least invasive method of obtaining cytological material from a mediastinal mass and with the aid of ultrasound guidance this is a relatively safe technique. However, although cytology can be useful in the diagnosis of mediastinal lymphoma (on the basis of finding large numbers of lymphoblasts) it is not a reliable method for diagnosis of thymoma. Thymomas do not exfoliate very well and samples collected by FNA may yield non-diagnostic material or tend to contain predominantly lymphocytes (and often mast cells) rather than the epithelial component of the tumour.

Definitive diagnosis of thymoma depends on examination of biopsy material. Tumour material may be collected under ultrasound guidance by a transthoracic needle biopsy technique, or at thoracotomy.

Other

Diagnosis of generalised myasthenia gravis may be confirmed by observing a rapid reversal of clinical signs following administration of a test dose of an anticholinesterase drug e.g. edrophonium. Alternatively acetylcholine receptor autoantibodies may be detected in the patient's serum (Hopkins 1993).

Table 17.2 Clinical staging of canine thymoma.

Stage	Description
I	Growth completely within intact thymic capsule
II	Pericapsular growth into mediastinal fat tissue, adjacent pleura and/or pericardium
III	Invasion into surrounding organs and/or intrathoracic metastases
IV	Extrathoracic metastases

The presence and extent of the paraneoplastic syndrome can be indicated by:
P_0 – no evidence of paraneoplastic syndrome
P_1 – myasthenia gravis
P_2 – non-thymic malignant tumour

Staging

Clinical staging of thymoma requires assessment of the tumour capsule, tumour invasion into adjacent tissues/structures and the presence of metastasis. Ultrasound is the most useful technique for clinical staging of a thymic tumour prior to thoracotomy and gross inspection. A clinically relevant staging system for canine thymoma based on human and veterinary literature was proposed by Aronsohn (1985a) as shown in Table 17.2.

Treatment

Surgery

Surgical resection, thymectomy, is the definitive treatment for thymoma and is the treatment of choice for stage I and II tumours. Median sternotomy is the favoured approach to give best exposure, especially for larger tumours and those with pericapsular invasion. The feasibility of complete tumour resection can often only be assessed at the time of surgery when tumour adhesion to major veins, the pericardium and oesophagus become apparent. Surgical debulking of unresectable tumours is often not very successful and may lead to considerable post-operative morbidity. Thus it is advisable to discuss the possibility of inability to remove the tumour with the client prior to surgery and to formulate a plan for such an eventuality. If the tumour is not resectable and further treatments (see below) are to be attempted a reasonable sized biopsy should be collected from the tumour mass prior to closure.

Radiotherapy

There is little information on the use of radiotherapy in the treatment of canine or feline thymoma, although in theory radiation might be expected to reduce the lymphoid component of the tumour mass. In human patients with invasive or metastatic tumours radical surgery followed by radiation has been shown to produce longer survival times than surgery alone and it is possible that this would be the case in animals.

Chemotherapy

Chemotherapy has not been used successfully in treatment of canine or feline thymoma. Indeed because of the difficulty encountered in some cases in distinguishing between thymic lymphoma and lymphocytic thymoma without resorting to incisional biopsy, on occasion response to chemotherapy may be used to assist the diagnosis. The majority of thymic lymphomas will respond rapidly to chemotherapy, and thymoma should therefore be suspected in cases where the thymic mass remains relatively unchanged after two to three weeks of combination chemotherapy.

Other

If myasthenia gravis is present this should be treated with immunosuppressive doses of prednisolone and anticholinesterase therapy (pyridostigmine).

Prognosis

The prognosis for thymoma depends on the feasibility of surgical resection and the presence of paraneoplastic myasthenia gravis. The prognosis for stage I uncomplicated thymoma is good with long term remissions or even cure likely to be achieved following thymectomy. In one study a one year survival rate of 83% was reported for dogs with a resectable tumour and without megaoe-sophagus (Atwater *et al.* 1994). Surgical resection of thymoma in cats also appears to lead to a favourable prognosis with median survival approaching two years in one study (Gores *et al.* 1994). Stage III and IV tumours carry a guarded to poor prognosis due to lack of effective treatment but because of the slow growth rate some animals may survive many months untreated. The presence of myasthenia gravis, megaoesophagus and aspiration pneumonia all lead to an increasingly guarded prognosis.

CARDIAC TUMOURS

Neoplasia is not a common cause of heart disease in cats or dogs but cardiac muscle, vessels and connective tissues may be the site for development of both primary and secondary tumours. Such lesions may be intracavitary, intramural or pericardial in location.

Epidemiology

Primary cardiac tumours are uncommon in dogs and rare in cats. The most common cardiac tumour in the dog is haemangiosarcoma, to which the German shepherd dog appears predisposed. Aortic body tumours (chemodectoma) are the second most common canine cardiac tumour; these tend to occur in older (10–15 years) brachycephalic dogs, with males at greater risk. Primary cardiac tumours are so rarely reported in cats that no age, sex or breed associations have been observed.

Aetiology

The aetiology of primary cardiac tumours is unknown, although the breed/type predispositions noted above might suggest a genetic influence in certain breeds or types of dog.

Pathology

Primary tumours of the heart may be benign or malignant. As already stated, haemangiosarcoma is the most common primary cardiac tumour in the dog. In most cases the tumour is sited in the right atrium or the right auricle, or both (Aronsohn 1985b). Chemodectoma of the aortic body arises at the base of the heart ('heart-base tumour') and is usually located either at the base of the aorta or between the aorta and pulmonary artery. (Carotid body tumours, also chemodectoma, arise near the bifurcation of the carotid artery in the neck and present as a cranial cervical mass.) Isolated case reports have documented the occurrence of a number of other primary cardiac tumours in the dog, as listed in Table 17.3.

Primary cardiac tumours are extremely rare in cats, two cases of chemodectoma have been reported (Tilley *et al.* 1981). Mesothelioma may affect the pericardium in both cats and dogs, as discussed in a later section.

Cardiac muscle and the pericardium may also be the site for development of secondary, metastatic tumours including lymphoma, as listed in Table 17.4. Lymphoma is the most common tumour affecting the heart in cats.

Table 17.3 Cardiac tumours – primary tumours reported in the dog.

Haemangiosarcoma
Chemodectoma
Fibroma
Fibrosarcoma
Haemangioma
Rhabdomyosarcoma
Chondroma
Chondrosarcoma
Myxoma
Teratoma
Granular cell tumour

Table 17.4 Canine and feline cardiac tumours – tumours reported to have metastasised to the heart.

Haemangiosarcoma
Lymphoma
Mammary carcinoma
Pulmonary carcinoma
Salivary adenocarcinoma
Malignant melanoma
Mast cell tumour

Tumour behaviour/paraneoplastic syndromes

The behaviour of cardiac tumours varies according to tumour type, but irrespective of the degree of malignancy, all tumours at this site have potentially life-threatening consequences through interference with cardiac function.

Haemangiosarcoma is a highly malignant tumour and widespread haematological dissemination occurs early in the course of the disease. The primary tumour or the presence of metastases may act as a trigger for disseminated intravascular coagulation (Chapter 2).

Chemodectoma is less aggressive than haemangiosarcoma and some tumours follow a benign course. However 40–50% of tumours display local invasion and infiltration, and metastasis (to the lungs, mediastinal lymph nodes, left atrium, pericardium, kidney, liver, spleen and other distant sites) may occur in up to 22% of cases (Patnaik *et al.* 1975). The histological appearance of the tumour does not appear to correlate with clinical behaviour. Chemoreceptors are part of the parasympathetic nervous system but tumours in cats and dogs do not appear to be functional. However, concurrent endocrine tumours (including testicular, thyroid and pancreatic tumours) appear to be quite common in dogs with chemodectoma (Owen *et al.* 1996).

Presentation/signs

Most animals with cardiac tumours present as a result of the effects of the tumour on the function of the heart. Clinical signs can be variable and depend on the size and location of the primary tumour.

Haemangiosarcoma is usually sited in the right atrium/auricle. Presenting signs may include:

- Sudden death from rupture of the tumour or cardiac dysrhythmia
- Pericardial haemorrhage, cardiac tamponade and signs of right-sided heart failure:
  - Dyspnoea, cough
  - Exercise intolerance
  - Syncope
  - Ascites, possibly pleural effusion
  - Muffled heart sounds
  - Dysrhythmias and pulse deficits
  - Weight loss
- Haemorrhagic diathesis due to disseminated intravascular coagulation.

Chemodectoma usually causes signs of right-sided congestive heart failure due to pressure on the aorta and/or vena cava, although it may also be associated with pericardial effusion.

Myocardial infiltration by lymphoma or metastatic tumours is likely to cause rhythm disturbances.

Investigations

The diagnosis of a cardiac tumour may be difficult, as the clinical signs are non-specific and usually only indicate the presence of heart disease. In many cases a definitive diagnosis may not be possible before exploratory thoracotomy or necropsy.

Bloods

Routine haematological/biochemical analyses are not generally very helpful in establishing a definitive diagnosis of cardiac tumours, although such investigations may be helpful in ruling out differential diagnoses. Clotting studies would be indicated if there were a suspicion of DIC.

Imaging techniques

Plain thoracic radiography may be normal or may indicate non-specific changes associated with heart disease:

- Cardiomegaly
- Globular cardiac silhouette with pericardial effusion
- Pulmonary oedema.

Heart-base tumours may be visualised on plain radiographs as a soft tissue mass extending from the base of the heart into the cranial mediastinum, causing dorsal displacement of the trachea (Fig. 17.3). Contrast techniques, e.g. angiography, may assist better definition of a tumour mass. In cases with pericardial effusion, pneumopericardiography may be performed following drainage of the effusion to outline a right atrial mass. However, such techniques have been superseded by ultrasonography. Plain thoracic radiographs are indicated for evaluation of metastases.

Ultrasound, echocardiography, is the most useful, non-invasive technique to define the presence, location and size of cardiac masses and to confirm the presence of pericardial effusion or myocardial infiltration. Echocardiography can also provide information on the effect of the tumour on the haemodynamics and function of the heart. Although echocardiography cannot provide a definitive diagnosis of tumour type, the site of a cardiac mass is an important indicator of its likely histogenesis. Ultrasound may also be used to assess feasibility of surgical excision of a solitary mass and to examine local lymph nodes as potential sites of metastasis.

Biopsy/FNA

Histological diagnosis of cardiac tumours is usually made on tissue collected at exploratory thoracotomy or at post mortem examination. Fine needle aspiration and non-surgical biopsy of suspected vascular tumours carry high risks and are not advised. In cases with pericardial effusions, cytological examination of pericardial fluid is of limited diagnostic value (Sisson *et al.* 1984).

Other

Electrocardiography may show a number of abnormalities:

- Low voltage QRS complexes and electrical alternans associated with pericardial effusion
- Dysrhythmias associated with myocardial disease, which may correlate with the specific location of the tumour or be secondary to myocardial ischaemia and hypoxia.

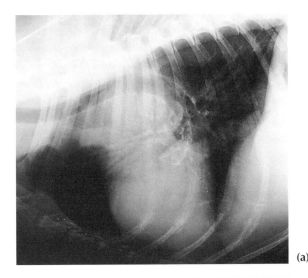

(a)

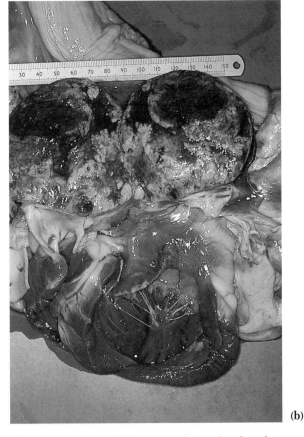

(b)

Fig. 17.3 (a) Lateral thoracic radiograph of a dog, demonstrating a large soft tissue mass sited at the base of the heart which is extending into the cranial mediastinum and elevating the trachea. **(b)** Gross appearance of this same heart base tumour at post mortem examination.

Table 17.5 Clinical staging for canine haemangiosarcoma.

T   *Primary tumour*
T0 = no evidence of tumour
T1 = tumour confined to primary site
T2 = tumour confined to primary site but ruptured
T3 = tumour invading adjacent structures

N   *Lymph nodes**
N0 = no evidence of lymph node involvement
N1 = regional lymph node involvement
N2 = distant lymph node involvement

M   *Metastasis*
M0 = no evidence of metastatic disease
M1 = metastasis in same body cavity as primary tumour
M2 = distant metastasis

Stage
I = T0 or T1, N0, M0
II = T1 or T2, N0 or N1, M1
III = T2 or T3, N1 or N2, M2

* Haemangiosarcoma usually metastasises via the haematogenous route. Local or regional lymph node involvement is uncommon.

Staging

Clinical staging of cardiac tumours requires assessment of the primary tumour and evaluation of possible sites of lymphatic and haematogenous metastasis. Ultrasonography and radiography may both contribute to this process. A clinical staging system for canine haemangiosarcoma which is applicable to cardiac tumours has been described (Brown *et al.* 1985; Table 17.5).

Treatment

Surgery

Surgical resection of cardiac tumours is only successful in a small number of cases with non-invasive primary tumours. Considerable skill and expertise is required in the surgical procedure and in the perioperative care of the patient (Aronsohn 1985b).

Radiotherapy

There are few reports on the use of radiotherapy in the treatment of cardiac tumours in animals, although in humans radiation may be used as a palliative measure in patients with inoperable or recurrent chemodectoma. Four dogs with aortic body tumours were reported to respond well to radiotherapy (Turrell 1987) but further studies are necessary to evaluate the efficacy of radiotherapy in such tumours.

Chemotherapy

Chemotherapy with doxorubicin alone or combined with cyclophosphamide and vincristine (VAC protocol, Table 5.4) is used to treat haemangiosarcoma at other sites, often in an adjuvant setting following surgical resection of the primary tumour. Reports on the use of chemotherapy for cardiac haemangiosarcoma are few but combination chemotherapy with vincristine, doxorubicin and cyclophosphamide produced a partial remission of a right atrial haemangiosarcoma in one dog and resulted in resolution of an associated pericardial effusion. However, the dog succumbed to pulmonary metastasis and died after 20 weeks (de Madron *et al.* 1987). There is no evidence that chemodectoma is sensitive to chemotherapy.

Other

In most cases treatment is limited to symptomatic medical management of cardiac failure and dysrhythmias.

Prognosis

The prognosis for many animals with cardiac tumours is poor. Surgical resection of the tumour is not possible in most cases and these do not usually respond well to medical management.

Haemangiosarcoma is a highly malignant tumour and even if the primary tumour can be treated surgically, the prognosis remains poor due to early onset metastatic disease. In one study of 38 dogs with right atrial haemangiosarcoma it was possible to resect the tumour by removing part of the right atrium in nine cases but the surgery was not without complications that required prolonged hospitalisation and the mean survival time for this group was only four months (Aronsohn 1985b). None of these animals were treated with adjuvant chemotherapy.

Local invasion often prevents surgical management of aortic body tumours and studies on postoperative survival times are not available.

MESOTHELIOMA

Epidemiology

Mesothelioma is a rare tumour in cats and dogs. Although this tumour usually arises in older animals, a juvenile form is recognised in ruminants. No breed or sex predispositions have been established in cats and dogs.

Aetiology

In humans, mesothelioma is associated with occupational exposure to airborne asbestos fibres and asbestos may be implicated in the aetiology of some tumours in dogs. Dogs with pleural mesothelioma were shown to have higher levels of asbestos in their lungs than normal controls and their owners often had a history of contact with asbestos (Glickman *et al.* 1983). The aetiology of mesothelioma at other sites is not known.

Pathology

Mesothelioma arises from the serosal lining of body cavities. Pleural, pericardial and peritoneal sites are those most frequently affected in cats and dogs but the tumour can also occur in the scrotum and tunica vaginalis in dogs.

Grossly the tumour forms a diffuse, often nodular proliferation covering the surface of the body cavity; this is usually associated with a significant effusion into the affected cavity. The effusion is usually haemorrhagic in nature, but may become chylous if the tumour causes lymphatic obstruction.

Normal mesothelial cells are of mesodermal origin although their morphological appearance is epithelial. Histologically epithelial, mesenchymal, sclerosing and mixed types of mesothelioma are described.

Tumour behaviour/paraneoplastic syndromes

Mesothelioma is considered to be malignant because of its ability to seed throughout the affected body cavity. Tumours may spread by local extension and invasion. Pleural mesothelioma has been reported to metastasise beyond the pleural cavity (Morrison & Trigo 1984). No paraneoplastic syndromes are commonly associated with mesothelioma.

Presentation/signs

Mesothelioma is a highly effusive tumour and it is the effusion that is the most common presenting sign:

• Pleural effusion – dyspnoea
• Pericardial effusion – cardiac tamponade and signs of right-sided heart failure
• Peritoneal effusion – abdominal distension.

Investigations

The diagnosis of mesothelioma can be challenging. In most cases investigations will be directed towards establishing the cause of the presenting effusion and because mesothelioma is one of the less common causes of this (Table 17.6), the suspicion of mesothelioma may only be reached follow-

Table 17.6 Major differential diagnosis for mesothelioma.

Pleural effusion
Haemangiosarcoma
Metastatic carcinoma
Feline infectious peritonitis
Infections (pyothorax)

Pericardial effusion
Pericardial cyst
Traumatic pericardial haemorrhage
Coagulopathy
Haemangiosarcoma
Idiopathic pericardial haemorrhage

Peritoneal effusion
Peritonitis
Feline infectious peritonitis

ing exclusion of more common causes or persistent recurrence of the effusion.

Bloods

Routine haematological/biochemical analyses are not generally very helpful in establishing a diagnosis of mesothelioma although such investigations may be helpful in ruling out other causes of effusions.

Imaging techniques

Survey radiographs of the thorax and abdomen will indicate the presence of fluid in the affected cavity, or a pericardial effusion, but are unlikely to show evidence of the tumour.

Pleural, pericardial or peritoneal masses may be visualised on ultrasound but can be difficult to detect in early cases or where the tumour is very diffuse.

Biopsy/FNA

Analysis of the fluid collected by pleural, pericardial or peritoneal drainage can be useful to establish:

- The nature of the fluid – in dogs the effusion associated with mesothelioma is most commonly haemorrhagic, sterile and non-clotting. In cats the nature of the fluid is more variable, ranging from haemorrhagic to chylous.
- Cell content – cytological examination of the effusion can be very useful to diagnose or rule out other effusive conditions, e.g. lymphoma, infection. However, the cytology of the effusion is of limited value in the diagnosis of mesothelioma because, although neoplastic mesothelial cells readily exfoliate into the fluid, it is very difficult to distinguish between neoplastic and reactive mesothelial cells on the basis of cell morphology. Reactive mesothelial cells are commonly found in effusions and are often of bizarre appearance.

Where a mass is visible on ultrasonography, fine needle aspirates of the lesion may provide adequate samples for cytological diagnosis within the limitations set out above. In most cases, definitive diagnosis of mesothelioma depends on histopathological examination of biopsy samples. Collection of representative tissue usually requires exploratory thoracotomy or celiotomy to allow direct visualisation of the lesion. The techniques of thoracoscopy and laparasocopy may provide a less invasive alternative in the future.

Staging

By virtue of the diffuse and effusive nature of mesothelioma, it is usually assumed that the affected body cavity is contaminated with tumour and no clinical staging systems have been described.

Treatment

An effective method for treatment of mesothelioma has not been established.

Surgery

Treatment of pericardial mesothelioma by pericardiectomy has been described (Closa *et al.* 1999) but surgical resection is not possible in most cases due to the widespread nature of mesothelioma.

Radiotherapy

Radiotherapy is not a realistic option in most cases as irradiation of the entire thorax or abdomen would cause unacceptable toxicity.

Chemotherapy

Chemotherapy with cisplatin or other agents may have a role in the management of mesothelioma. Intracavitary administration of cisplatin was useful in palliation of mesothelioma in a small number of cases by controlling the malignant effusion and retarding tumour progression without undue toxicity (Moore *et al.* 1991).

Prognosis

In the absence of a successful method of treatment, the prognosis for mesothelioma is poor. Survival figures are sparse as many animals are euthanased upon diagnosis. On the basis of small numbers of animals, intracavitary chemotherapy does appear to be of palliative value with survival times from 129 days to 27 months (Moore *et al.* 1991; Closa *et al.* 1999).

SPLENIC TUMOURS

As one of the major reticuloendothelial organs of the body, the spleen is an important site for the development of primary tumours and is also a common site for development of metastatic tumours and tumours of the haematopoietic system. Although most of these tumours have been covered elsewhere, splenic haemangiosarcoma and splenic sarcoma warrant individual consideration. Tumours affecting the spleen are summarised in Table 17.7 (canine) and 17.8 (feline).

Epidemiology

Splenic abnormality, most commonly spleno-megaly, is frequently recognised in dogs, and pathological reviews of splenic biopsies/splenectomies suggest that neoplasia is the cause of the abnormality in between 43–75% of such cases (Frey & Betts 1977; Day *et al.* 1995). Haemangiosarcoma is the most common tumour of the canine spleen. It affects older dogs and the German shepherd is at greater risk than other breeds. Non-angiomatous mesenchymal tumours (splenic sarcoma – see below) are also recognised with some frequency in the spleen of older dogs, especially retriever breeds (Spangler *et al.* 1994).

Tumours of the spleen are less common in cats. A splenic form of mast cell tumour (lymphoreticular MCT – Chapter 4) is the most common tumour of the feline spleen and accounts for 15% of splenic disease in this species (Spangler & Culbertson 1992).

Aetiology

In general the aetiology of splenic tumours is not known. Breed predisposition for haemangiosarcoma and possibly splenic sarcoma in dogs might implicate genetic factors. In cats FeLV is implicated in the aetiology of lymphoma and forms of leukaemia which may affect the spleen (Chapter 15).

Pathology

Tables 17.7 and 17.8 demonstrate the diversity of tumours that may arise in the spleen. Most of these tumours have been considered elsewhere and do not require further discussion.

Haemangiosarcoma is the most important

Table 17.7 Tumours of the canine spleen.

Primary tumours
Haemangioma
Haemangiosarcoma
Sarcoma – various – see text

Secondary or multicentric tumours
Lymphoproliferative and myeloproliferative conditions
   including lymphoma
Haemangiosarcoma
Mast cell tumour
Other malignant tumours with widespread metastases,
   e.g. melanoma

Non-neoplastic causes of splenomegaly or splenic mass
Nodular hyperplasia
Haematoma
Thrombosis and infarction
Congestion
Extramedullary haematopoiesis
Torsion

Table 17.8 Tumours of the feline spleen.

Primary tumours
Mast cell tumour
Haemangiosarcoma
Sarcoma – various

Secondary or multicentric tumours
Lymphoproliferative and myeloproliferative conditions,
   including lymphoma
Haemangiosarcoma
Other malignant tumours with widespread metastases,
   e.g. adenocarcinoma

Non-neoplastic causes of splenomegaly or splenic mass
Nodular hyperplasia
Haematoma
Congestion
Extramedullary haematopoiesis

---

tumour of the canine spleen, but haemangioma and haematoma are also quite common at this site and sometimes it can be difficult to differentiate these conditions clinically and histopathologically, for example when major haemorrhage occurs within a haemangiosarcoma. It may be necessary to examine multiple sections from the lesion before a certain diagnosis can be reached. Haemangioma and haemangiosarcoma may both present as a single mass or as multiple nodules within the spleen. Haemangiosarcoma arising at other sites may also metastasise to the spleen. It is a matter for debate as to whether the heart or the spleen is the most common site for development of haemangiosarcoma in the dog. In some cases with widespread tumour metastases it is difficult to be certain which location is the primary focus or whether the tumour might be multicentric.

The spleen may also be a site for development of primary tumours of mesenchymal origin, 'sarcomas' (Fig. 17.4). Some such tumours are well differentiated and can be classified according to their morphology on haematoxylin and eosin (H&E) sections, for example, liposarcoma. However, many lack such clear differentiation leading to diagnoses of 'undifferentiated sarcoma'. When more detailed immunohistochemical staining is performed on these tumours it appears that they, along with splenic fibrosarcoma and leiomyosarcoma, might share a common origin from smooth muscle or splenic myofibroblasts (Spangler *et al.* 1994).

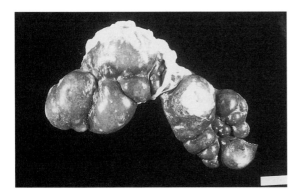

Fig. 17.4 Primary splenic sarcoma from a flat-coated retriever. This tumour was diagnosed as a histiocytic sarcoma.

Tumour behaviour/paraneoplastic syndromes

Haemangiosarcoma is a highly malignant tumour with haematogenous metastasis occurring early in the course of the disease. Rupture of the primary tumour can lead to acute and fatal haemorrhage (see below). Primary or secondary tumours may be associated with DIC. In contrast, haemangioma of the spleen is a slowly growing tumour and can attain large proportions before diagnosis. Metastasis does not occur.

Primary mesenchymal tumours of the spleen can be divided into three categories on the basis of their biological behaviour (Spangler *et al.* 1994):

- Benign, non-invasive tumours (leiomyoma, lipoma) – these do not metastasise and are associated with long patient survival times
- Intermediate tumours (mesenchymoma) – median survival period of 12 months with 50% one year survival
- Malignant tumours (fibrosarcoma, leiomyosarcoma, undifferentiated sarcoma, histiocytic sarcoma) – these are capable of metastasis and are associated with relatively short postoperative survival times (median survival four months, 80–100% mortality after 12 months).

Presentation/signs

For low grade and benign tumours abdominal distension due to the enlarging tumour mass may be the first sign of the problem or the mass may be detected during routine clinical examination. Such tumours can reach large proportions without causing clinical signs. Splenic sarcomas may cause non-specific signs of malaise but are also most often detected on clinical examination, radiography or ultrasound or at the time of exploratory celiotomy.

In contrast the presenting signs of splenic haemangiosarcoma may be dramatic:

- Acute collapse may follow rupture of the primary mass leading to a haemoperitoneum
- Less specific signs of lethargy, weakness, pallor and anorexia may be detected prior to a major abdominal bleed
- Bleeding due to DIC may be a presenting sign in some cases

- Splenic haemangiosarcoma may also be detected as an incidental finding in the absence of overt clinical signs.

Investigations

Bloods

In cases of splenic haemangiosarcoma the haemogram may show a number of changes:

- Anaemia – may be regenerative if due to blood loss, or microangiopathic due to fragmentation of red blood cells during passage through a meshwork of fibrin in the microvascular network of the tumour.
- Acanthocytes (damaged red cells) and schistocytes (red blood cell fragments) – highly indicative of haemangiosarcoma.
- Thrombocytopenia – due to bleeding, sequestration of platelets within the microvascular network of the tumour or DIC.

In cases with DIC, clotting studies will reveal abnormalities in both primary and secondary haemostasis, fibrin degradation products will be elevated and fibrinogen and antithrombin III decreased.

Imaging techniques

Splenomegaly or a splenic mass may be detected on plain radiographs of the abdomen, and these may also show evidence of abdominal fluid in cases with haemorrhage. Ultrasonography can provide useful information about the structure of a splenic mass or masses and their relationship with normal spleen. The vascular nature of haemangiosarcoma may be seen on ultrasound as a mixed or non-homogeneous mass with echolucent areas in contrast to the more homogeneous denser structure of normal spleen.

Radiography of the thorax and ultrasonography of other abdominal organs, especially the liver and kidneys, is indicated to detect metastases.

Biopsy/FNA

Fine needle aspirates may assist in cytological diagnosis in cases of generalised splenomegaly or where splenic lesions appear solid on ultrasonography. It is not advisable to attempt FNA in cases where splenic lesions have a vascular appearance on ultrasound. It is unlikely that the resulting samples would be diagnostic; usually blood is all that is collected from such lesions but, more importantly, the procedure carries a significant risk of causing haemorrhage into the abdomen and possible seeding of tumour cells.

Splenic biopsy may be indicated in cases with diffuse splenomegaly or multinodular splenic disease. Needle biopsy techniques may be used under ultrasound guidance or incisional biopsies collected at celiotomy. The latter allows visualisation of the whole spleen and thus better selection of representative lesions for biopsy.

In cases where there is a distinct mass in the spleen, excisional biopsy by splenectomy is preferable. Not only is this technically easier to perform but also provides the pathologist with sufficient material to achieve the correct diagnosis. This is particularly important for differentiating haemangioma and haemangiosarcoma.

Staging

The clinical staging system for canine haemangiosarcoma is shown in Table 17.5. In both splenic haemangiosarcoma and splenic sarcoma, the extent of the tumour within the spleen is of less importance than whether the tumour has invaded through the splenic capsule. Nodal metastases are uncommon but radiography and ultrasonography are required to evaluate the patient for haematogenous metastases.

Treatment

Surgery

Surgical removal of the tumour by splenectomy is the treatment of choice for splenic haemangiosarcoma and splenic sarcoma. Unfortunately this is not a curative treatment for most splenic sarcomas. In the case of haemangiosarcoma, survival times following splenectomy range from 19 to 143 days (Wood *et al.* 1998) and most dogs die as a result of metastasis. For splenic sarcomas a median survival time of four months has been reported and metastases were a frequent reason for euthanasia in these patients (Spangler *et al.* 1994).

Radiotherapy

Radiotherapy is not indicated in the treatment of splenic tumours.

Chemotherapy

In most cases of splenic haemangiosarcoma micrometastases are present at the time of diagnosis of the primary tumour; these progress rapidly and are the reason for poor survival times following splenectomy. Post-operative chemotherapy is indicated in an attempt to prevent or delay the progression of this micrometastatic disease. Chemotherapy protocols based on doxorubicin with cyclophosphamide and vincristine have been used in this adjuvant setting with median survival times from 141–179 days (Hammer *et al.* 1991; Sorenmo *et al.* 1993). Doxorubicin used as a single agent has been reported to achieve similar survival times (Ogilvie *et al.* 1996).

Post-operative chemotherapy would be a logical treatment for dogs with splenic sarcoma, but less is known about the chemosensitivity of such tumours. Larger scale clinical trials are required to better define the role of chemotherapy in the management of splenic tumours.

Prognosis

As outlined above the prognosis for dogs with splenic haemangiosarcoma is poor. There appears to be little difference in survival for those animals with stage I versus stage II disease, i.e. rupture of the tumour does not appear to affect prognosis (Wood *et al.* 1998). The prognosis for splenic sarcoma is also poor, although there is a wider range of survival times for such tumours. Mitotic index has been shown to be of prognostic importance in this group of tumours: those tumours with a mitotic index <9 showed significantly longer survival than those with a mitotic index >9 (Spangler *et al.* 1994).

MALIGNANT (AND SYSTEMIC) HISTIOCYTOSIS

Malignant histiocytosis is characterised by neoplastic proliferation of cells of histiocytic (monocyte) lineage. Several disorders of histiocytes have been described in animals (see Chapter 4) but of these only canine cutaneous histiocytoma is common. There is still uncertainty about the precise nature of this group of tumours.

Epidemiology

Malignant histiocytosis is a rare tumour first recognised in the Bernese mountain dog and still strongly associated with this breed, although it has also been reported in the golden retriever, rottweiler, dobermann, English springer spaniel and flat-coated retriever (Kerlin & Hendrick 1996). In the Bernese it typically affects older dogs, seven to eight years of age, and is more common in males. Malignant histiocytosis has been documented in cats.

Systemic histiocytosis is another rare histiocytic disorder affecting the Bernese mountain dog but this is a condition of younger animals, with age of onset at three to four years (Paterson *et al.* 1995).

Although the clinical signs and presentation of these two conditions differ, the fact that they are both disorders of histiocytic cells and are both relatively common in the Bernese mountain dog has led to the suggestion that they may be manifestations of a common underlying defect (Moore & Rosin 1986).

Aetiology

There are indications that histiocytosis is an inherited disease in the Bernese mountain dog and it has been suggested that the mode of inheritance is polygenic rather than a simple autosomal recessive or dominant trait (Padgett *et al.* 1995).

Pathology

Malignant histiocytosis is characterised by the development of solid tumour masses in a variety of organs (Fig. 17.5a,b). The most common sites for the tumour are:

- Spleen
- Liver

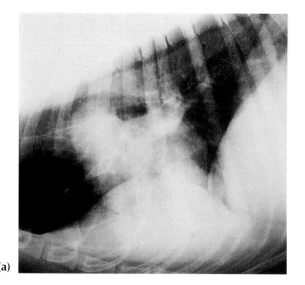

(a)

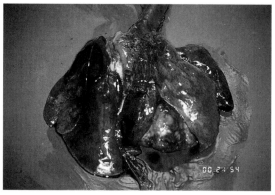

(b)

Fig. 17.5 (a) Lateral thoracic radiograph of a Bernese mountain dog showing a large soft tissue mass in the ventral thorax, displacing the heart dorsally. A soft tissue opacity around the bifurcation of the trachea suggests an enlargement of the tracheobronchial lymph nodes. (Previously published in *Veterinary Record* (1996), (138), 440–44, with permission) **(b)** Gross appearance of the mass at post mortem examination.

• Lymph nodes
• Lungs.

Involvement of the spinal column has also been reported (Ramsey *et al.* 1996). In contrast to systemic histiocytosis, the eyes and skin are rarely involved.

The tumours consist of sheets of large, pleomorphic cells with foamy cytoplasm often showing evidence of erythrophagocytosis. Mitotic activity is high and abnormal mitotic figures are often present. Interspersed between these cells are multinucleate giant cells, and an infiltrate of lymphocytes and neutrophils is often present. Immunostaining for tissue-specific enzymes (especially lysozyme) is necessary to distinguish this anaplastic tumour from poorly differentiated sarcomas or carcinomas.

Tumour behaviour/paraneoplastic syndromes

Malignant histiocytosis is a highly malignant and very aggressive disease that runs a rapid and fatal course. Affected animals usually present with multiple lesions, often involving several organs.

Systemic histiocytosis is a more chronic disease involving the skin, peripheral lymph nodes, eyes and other tissues and is characterised by a fluctuating course.

Presentation/signs

In malignant histiocytosis most tumours are sited internally. In many cases the clinical signs are non-specific, for example:

• Anorexia
• Weight loss
• Lethargy, depression
• Anaemia.

In other cases the signs may reflect the organs involved, for example:

• Cough or dyspnoea may be indicative of a lung mass
• Lameness and paresis, spinal cord involvement.

The clinical signs and presentation of systemic histiocytosis have been discussed in Chapter 4.

Investigations

Bloods

A severe (often regenerative) anaemia is a common finding in dogs with malignant histiocytosis. Bone marrow aspirates may assist in the diagnosis of such cases to demonstrate malignant histiocytic proliferation with erythrophagocytosis.

Biochemical parameters may demonstrate abnormalities related to failure of specific organs.

Imaging techniques

Plain survey radiographs of the thorax and abdomen may demonstrate the presence of a soft tissue mass or masses or enlargement of abdominal organs. Ultrasonographic examination of the liver and spleen may show evidence of lesions within these tissues. Further, more detailed studies may be indicated according to preliminary findings.

Biopsy/FNA

If lesions are accessible for fine needle aspiration, the finding of anaplastic mononuclear cells with vacuolated cytoplasm, multinucleated cells and bizarre mitotic figures may provide cytological evidence of a malignant, anaplastic tumour. However, the diagnosis of malignant histiocytosis will usually depend on histological examination of biopsy material or material collected at post mortem examination.

Staging

There is no clinical staging system described for malignant histiocytosis.

Treatment and prognosis

Although chemotherapy has been attempted no treatment has proved effective in the management of malignant histiocytosis. This is an aggressive and rapidly fatal disease and the prognosis is grave.

Systemic histiocytosis is a chronic progressive disease that fluctuates with periods of improvement and recrudescence. Immunosuppressive therapy does not appear to alter the course of the disease. The disease is rarely fatal but euthanasia is often requested by the owners due to the debilitating nature of the condition.

References

Atwater, S.W., Powers, B.E., Park, R.D. *et al.* (1994) Canine thymoma: 23 cases (1980–1991). *Journal of the American Veterinary Medical Association*, (205), 1007–13.

Aronsohn, M. (1985a) Canine thymoma. *Veterinary Clinics of North America*, 15 (4), 755–67.

Aronsohn, M. (1985b) Cardiac haemangiosarcoma in the dog: a review of 38 cases. *Journal of the American Veterinary Medical Association*, (187), 922–6.

Brown, N.O., Patnaik, A.K., MacEwan, E.G. (1985) Canine haemangiosarcoma. *Journal of the American Veterinary Medical Association*, (186), 56–8.

Closa, J.M., Font, A. & Mascort, J. (1999) Pericardial mesothelioma in a dog: long-term survival after pericardiectomy in combination with chemotherapy. *Journal of Small Animal Practice*, (40), 383–6.

Day, M.J., Lucke, V.M. & Pearson, H. (1995) A review of pathological diagnoses made from 87 canine splenic biopsies. *Journal of Small Animal Practice*, (36), 426–33.

Day, M.J. (1997) Review of thymic pathology in 30 cats and 36 dogs. *Journal of Small Animal Practice*, (38), 393–403.

Frey, A.J. & Bets, C.W. (1977) A retrospective survey of splenectomy in the dog. *Journal of the American Animal Hospital Association*, (13), 730–34.

Glickman, L.T., Domanski, L.M., Maguire, T.G. *et al.* (1983) Mesothelioma in pet dogs associated with exposure of their owners to asbestos. *Environmental Research*, (32), 305.

Gores, B.R., Berg, J., Carpenter, J.L. *et al.* (1994) Surgical treatment of thymoma in cats: 12 cases (1987–1992). *Journal of the American Veterinary Medical Association*, (204), 1782–5.

Hammer, A.S., Couto, C.G., Filppi, J. *et al.* (1991) Efficacy and toxicity of VAC chemotherapy (vincristine, doxorubicin and cyclophosphamide) in dogs with haemangiosarcoma. *Journal of Veterinary Internal Medicine*, (5), 160–66.

Hopkins, A.L. (1993) Canine myasthenia gravis. *Journal of Small Animal Practice*, (33), 477–84.

Kerlin, R.L. & Hendrick, M.J. (1996) Malignant fibrous histiocytoma and malignant histiocytosis in the dog – convergent or divergent phenotypic differentiation? *Veterinary Pathology*, (33), 713–16.

de Madron, E., Helfand, S.C. & Stebbins, K.E. (1987) Use of chemotherapy for the treatment of cardiac haemangiosarcoma in a dog. *Journal of the American Veterinary Medical Association*, (190), 887–91.

Moore, A.S., Kirk, C. & Cardona, A. (1991) Intracavitary cisplatin chemotherapy experience in six dogs. *Journal of Veterinary Internal Medicine*, (5), 227–31.

Moore, P.F. & Rosin, A. (1986) Malignant histiocytosis of Bernese mountain dogs. *Veterinary Pathology*, (23), 1–10.

Morrison, W.B. & Trigo, F.J. (1984) Clinical characterisation of pleural mesothelioma in seven dogs. *Compendium on Continuing Education*, (6), 342–8.

Ogilvie, G.K., Powers, B.E., Mallinckrodt, C.H. *et al.* (1996) Surgery and doxorubicin in dogs with hemangiosarcoma. *Journal of Veterinary Internal Medicine*, (6), 379–84.

Owen, L.N. (1980) TNM Classification of Tumours in Domestic Animals. World Health Organisation, Geneva.

Owen, T.J., Bruyette, D.S. & Layton, C.E. (1996) Chemodectoma in dogs. *Compendium on Continuing Education*, (18), 253–65.

Paterson, S., Boydell, P. & Pike, P. (1995) Systemic histiocytosis in the Bernese mountain dog. *Journal of Small Animal Practice*, (36), 233.

Padgett, G.A., Madewell, B.R., Kellert, E.T. *et al.* (1995) Inheritance of histiocytosis in Bernese mountain dogs. *Journal of Small Animal Practice*, (36), 93–8.

Patnaik, A.K., Lui, S.K., Hurvitz, A.I. *et al.* (1975) Canine chemodectoma (extra-adrenal paragangliomas) – a comparative study. *Journal of Small Animal Practice*, (16), 785–801.

Ramsey, I.K., McKay, J.S., Rudorf, H. & Dobson, J.M. (1996) Malignant histiocytosis in three Bernese mountain dogs. *Veterinary Record*, (138), 440–44.

Rusbridge, C., White, R.N., Elwood, C.M. & Wheeler, S.J. (1996) Treatment of acquired myasthenia gravis associated with thymoma in two dogs. *Journal of Small Animal Practice*, (36), 376–80.

Scott-Moncrieff, J.C., Cook, J.R. & Lantz, G.C. (1990) Acquired myasthenia gravis in a cat with thymoma. *Journal of the American Veterinary Medical Association*, (196), 1291–3.

Sisson, D., Thomas, W.P., Ruehl, W.W. *et al.* (1984) Diagnostic value of pericardial fluid analysis in the dog. *Journal of the American Veterinary Medical Association*, (184), 51–5.

Sorenmo, K.U., Jeglum, K.A. & Helfand, S.C. (1993) Chemotherapy of canine haemangiosarcoma with doxorubicin and cyclophosphamide. *Journal of Veterinary Internal Medicine*, (7), 370–76.

Spangler, W.L. & Culbertson, M.R. (1992) Prevalence and type of splenic diseases in cats: 455 cases (1985–1991). *Journal of the American Veterinary Medical Association*, (201), 773–6.

Spangler, W.L., Culbertson, M.R. & Kass, P.H. (1994) Primary mesenchymal (nonangiomatous/nonlymphomatous) neoplasms occuring in the canine spleen: anatomic classification, immunohistochemistry and mitotic activity correlated with patient survival. *Veterinary Pathology*, (31), 37–47.

Tilley, L.P., Band, B., Patnaik, A.K. & Liu, S.K. (1981) Cardiovascular tumours in the cat. *Journal of the American Animal Hospital Association*, (17), 1009–21.

Turrell, J.M. (1987) Principles of radiation therapy. II Clinical Applications. In: *Veterinary Cancer Medicine*, (eds G.H. Theilen & B.R. Madewell), pp. 148–56. Lea & Febiger, Philadelphia.

Wood, C.A., Moore, A.S, Gliatto, J.M. *et al.* (1998) Prognosis for dogs with Stage I or II splenic haemangiosarcoma treated by splenectomy alone: 32 cases (1991–1993). *Journal of the American Animal Hospital Association*, (34), 417–21.

Appendices

- I   General reading list
- II   Actions, indications and toxicity of cytotoxic agents used in veterinary practice
- III Body weight:surface area conversions
- IV   Protocols for administration of doxorubicin and cisplatin
- V   Glossary of drugs and dosages included in text

I GENERAL READING LIST

Allwood, M. & Wright, P. (eds) (1993) *The Cytotoxics Handbook*, 2nd edn. Radcliffe Medical Press, Oxford.

Brown, N.O. (ed.) (1985) *Clinical Veterinary Oncology*. The Veterinary Clinics of North America series, 15 (3). W.B. Saunders, Philadelphia.

Brown, N.O. (ed.) (1985) *Canine Haematopoietic Tumours*. The Veterinary Clinics of North America series, 15 (4). W.B. Saunders, Philadelphia.

Chabner, B.A. & Collins, J.M. (eds) (1990) *Cancer Chemotherapy*. J.B. Lippincott, Philadelphia.

Dobson, J.M. & Gorman, N.T. (1993) *Cancer Chemotherapy in Small Animal Practice*. Library of Veterinary Practice Series, Blackwell Science Ltd, Oxford.

Feldman, E.C. & Nelson, R.W. (1996) *Canine & Feline Endocrinology and Reproduction*, 2nd edn. W.B. Saunders Company, Philadelphia.

Goldschmidt, M.H. & Shofer, F.S. (1992) *Skin Tumours of the Dog and Cat*. Pergamon Press, Oxford.

Goute C.G. (ed.) (1990) *Clinical Management of the Cancer Patient*. The Veterinary Clinics of North America series, 20 (4). W.B. Saunders, Philadelphia.

Hahn, K. & Richarson, R.C. (ed.) (1995) *Cancer Chemotherapy. A Veterinary Handbook*. Williams & Wilkins, Pennsylvania.

Morrison, W.B. (1998) *Cancer in Dogs and Cats. Medical & Surgical Management*. Williams & Wilkins, Pennsylvania.

Moulton, J.E. (ed.) (1990) *Tumours in Domestic Animals*, 3rd edn. University of California Press.

Ogilvie, G.K. & Moore, A.S. (1995) *Managing the Veterinary Cancer Patient (A Practice Manual)*. Veterinary Learning Systems Co., Inc., Trenton, New Jersey.

Pavletic, M.M. (1999) *Atlas of Small Animal Reconstructive Surgery*, 2nd edn. W.B. Saunders Company, Philadelphia.

Rijnberk, A. (ed.) (1996) *Clinical Endocrinology of Dogs and Cats*, Kluwer Academic Publishers, Dordrecht, Boston, London.

Slatter, D. (1993) *Textbook of Small Animal Surgery*, 2nd edn. W.B. Saunders Company, Philadelphia.

Theilen, G.H. & Madewell, B.R. (1987) *Veterinary Cancer Medicine*, 2nd edn. Lea & Febiger, Philadelphia.

White, R.A.S. (ed.) (1991) *BSAVA Manual of Small Animal Oncology*. British Small Animal Veterinary Association Publications, Cheltenham.

Withrow, S.J. & MacEwen, E.G. (1996) *Small Animal Clinical Oncology*, 2nd edn. J.B. Lippincott Company, Philadelphia.

II   ACTIONS, INDICATIONS AND TOXICITY OF CYTOTOXIC AGENTS USED IN VETERINARY PRACTICE

1. ALKYLATING AGENTS

Action: Substitute alkyl radicals (R-CH2-CH3) for hydrogen atoms in the DNA molecule. Alkylation of nucleotide bases causes breaks, cross-linkages and abnormal base pairing in DNA, all of which interfere with replication of DNA and transcription of RNA. These actions are not cell cycle specific.

Toxicity: All agents may cause: Myelosuppression

Gastrointestinal toxicity, anorexia, vomiting, diarrhoea.

May also affect gametogenesis and cause alopecia or thinning of coat in some breeds of dog.

	Individual agents/dose	Indications	Specific toxicity
Nitrogen mustard derivatives	*Cyclophosphamide* *Endoxana*™ (*Cytoxan – US*) 50 mg/m² po every other day, or daily for first 4 days of each week or 250–300 mg/m² po or iv every 3 weeks (do not exceed 250 mg/m² in dogs)	Lymphoma and leukaemia Multiple myeloma (sarcomas/carcinomas in combination protocols) Immunosuppression	Urologic – haemorrhagic cystitis
	Chlorambucil *Leukeran*™ 2–10 mg/m² po daily or every other day	Chronic lymphocytic leukaemia Multiple myeloma Lymphoma (maintenance) (Polycythaemia vera) (Immunosuppression)	Myelosuppression – mild
	Melphalan *Alkeran*™ 1–5 mg/m² po daily or every other day	Multiple myeloma Lymphoma (Carcinomas and sarcomas in combination protocols)	Myelosuppression – may be delayed in onset
Ethenamine derivatives	*Thiotepa* (triethylenethiophosphoramide) see specific protocols	Malignant effusions by instillation into body cavities Carcinoma of bladder by instillation	Myelosuppression – can follow local instillation
Alkyl suphonates	*Busulphan* *Myleran*™ 2–6 mg/m² po daily	Chronic granulocytic leukaemia Polycythaemia vera	Pulmonary fibrosis Endocrinological disorders Ocular – lens changes All rare
Triazine derivatives In addition to alkylating actions, also inhibits DNA and protein synthesis	*Dacarbazine* *DTIC-Dome*™ 100 mg/m² iv every 7 days or 200–250 mg/m² daily on days 1–5 repeating every 21–28 days	Lymphoma	Irritant – perivascular reactions (Hepatotoxicity)
Nitrosureas Lipophilic agents, pass into cerebrospinal fluid	*Carmustine* *BiCNU*™ 50 mg/m² iv every 3–6 weeks	Brain tumours – malignant glioma	Myelosuppression: cumulative and delayed due to stem cell toxicity (Pulmonary fibrosis)
	Lomustine *CCNU*™ 60–90 mg/m² po every 3–6 weeks	Brain tumours – as above (?Mast cell tumours)	Myelosuppression as above Neurological reactions

II Continued.

2. ANTI-METABOLITES

Action: These agents are structural analogues of metabolites required for purine and/or pyrimidine synthesis. They interfere with DNA and RNA synthesis by enzyme inhibition or by causing synthesis of non-functional molecules. Antimetabolites are cell cycle specific, acting during the S phase of the cell cycle.

Toxicity: All agents may cause: Myelosuppression
Gastrointestinal toxicity (anorexia, vomiting, diarrhoea).
Some agents may cause renal or neurological toxicity as noted

	Individual agents/dose	Specific indications	Specific toxicity
Antifolates	*Methotrexate* *Maxtrex*™ 1–3 mg/m² po daily (see specific protocols)	Lymphoma and leukaemia TVT (Sertoli cell tumour) (Soft tissue sarcoma and osteosarcoma)	Renal tubular necrosis
Pyrimidine analogues	*5-Fluorouracil* 150–200 mg/m² iv every 7 days (*Efudix*™ – topical preparation)	Carcinomas – especially mammary Topical – basal and squamous cell carcinoma of the skin	Neurological toxicity – cerebellar ataxia and seizures *Do not use in cats*
	Cytarabine/Cytosine arabinoside 100 mg/m² iv or sc daily for 2–4 days or 75 mg/m² by infusion over 24 hours	Lymphoma and leukaemia Especially in acute leukaemias	
Purine analogues	*6-Mercaptopurine* *Puri-nethol*™ 50 mg/m² po daily or every other day	Lymphoma and leukaemia	
	6-Thioguanine *Lanvis*™ 50 mg/m² po daily or every other day	Lymphoma and leukaemia	
	Azathioprine *Azamune*™, *Berkaprine*™, *Imuran*™ 1–2 mg/kg po every 24–48 hours	Immunosuppression	(Hepatic toxicity reported in humans) Use with care in cats

(continued on p. 282.)

II Continued.

3. ANTI-TUMOUR ANTIBIOTICS

Action: These compounds, which are derived from soil fungi; form stable complexes with DNA, thus inhibiting DNA synthesis and transcription. These actions are not cell cycle specific. This group contains some of the most potent and broad spectrum anti-cancer agents indentified to date.

Toxicity: Myelosuppression is the major, dose-limiting toxicity (except bleomycin)
Gastro-intestinal toxicity – dose related
Also cause a diverse range of selective toxicities as detailed below.

Individual agents/dose	Specific indications	Specific toxicity
Doxorubicin (formerly *Adriamycin*) Dogs 30 mg/m^2 iv every 21 days or 10 mg/m^2 iv every 7 days Cats 20 mg/m^2 po every 3–6 weeks	Lymphoma and leukaemia Soft tissue and osteogenic sarcoma (Carcinomas)	Hypersensitivity Vesicant – perivascular reaction Cardiac toxicity (acute and chronic/cumulative) Nephrotoxic in cats Alopecia
Epirubicin (*Pharmorubicin*^{TM}) 30 mg/m^2 iv every 21 days	As above	Hypersensitivity Vesicant – perivascular reaction Cardiac toxicity (acute and chronic/cumulative – less than doxorubicin) Alopecia
Mitozantrone (*Novantrone*^{TM}) 3–5 mg/m^2 iv every 21 days	Lymphoma and leukaemia ?Soft tissue sarcoma ?Carcinomas	Irritant – perivascular reaction Cardiac toxicity (less than doxorubicin) Seizures reported in cats
Actinomycin D (dactinomycin) 0.75 mg/m^2 iv every 21 days	Lymphoproliferative disorders	Alopecia Vesicant – perivascular reaction

4. VINCA ALKALOIDS

Action: Vinca alkaloids bind specifically to microtubular proteins (tubulin) and inhibit the formation of the mitotic spindle, thus blocking mitosis and causing a metaphase arrest. These actions are cell cycle specific, acting during the M phase.

Toxicity: see below

Individual agents/dose	Indications	Specific toxicity
Vincristine (*Oncovin*^{TM}) 0.5–0.75 mg/m^2 iv every 7 days	Lymphoma and leukaemia ?Mast cell tumours TVT (Thrombocytopenia)	Vesicant – perivascular reaction Peripheral and autonomic neuropathies Alopecia – mild
Vinblastine (*Velbe*^{TM}, *Velban*^{TM}) 2.0–2.5 mg/m^2 iv every 7 days	Lymphoma and leukaemia (Mammary and testicular carcinomas)	Myelosuppression Vesicant – perivascular reaction Neurological Gastro-intestinal

II Continued.

5. MISCELLANEOUS
PLATINUM CO-ORDINATION COMPOUNDS

Action: Inhibit protein synthesis by the formation of both inter and intra cross links in the strands of DNA. The N7 atom of guanine is particularly reactive and platinum cross-links between adjacent guanine bases on the same DNA strand are most readily demonstrated. These agents also act with other nucleophiles such as the sulphydryl groups of proteins and these reactions may produce some of the toxic effects.

Toxicity: Severe toxicity has limited veterinary use of these drugs.
Gastro-intestinal toxicity is common with acute and severe vomiting mediated by direct actions on the chemoreceptor trigger zone. Nephrotoxicity is the main concern.

Individual agents/dose	Indications	Specific toxicity
Cisplatin (*Platinol*™) $50-70\,mg/m^2$ iv every 4 weeks	Osteogenic sarcoma Carcinomas	Nephrotoxicity – acute proximal tubular necrosis Gastrointestinal tract – vomiting (Vesicant) (Myelosuppression) *Do not use in cats*
Carboplatin (*Paraplatin*™) $300\,mg/m^2$ iv every 3–4 weeks	Osteogenic sarcoma Carcinomas	Myelosuppression Nephrotoxic – less than cisplatin Nausea and vomiting – less than cisplatin Irritant – perivascular reaction
L-asparaginase – cristantaspase (*Erwinase*™) *Action*: An enzyme which hydrolyses asparagine. Most normal mammalian tissues synthesise sufficient asparagine for protein synthesis. Lymphoid tumours do not have this ability and are therefore susceptible to the actions of asparaginase.	Lymphoproliferative disease (?mast cell tumours) Dose rate: $10000-40000\,IU/m^2$ im every 7 days	Hypersensitivity reactions Gastrointestinal Haemorrhagic pancreatitis has been reported in the dog
Hydroxyurea *Action*: Inhibits DNA synthesis. Acts by inhibiting the enzyme ribonucleoside diphosphate reductase. This enzyme acts at a critical and rate limiting step in the biosynthesis of DNA. This action is cell cycle specific (S phase).	Polycythaemia vera Chronic granulocytic leukaemia Dose rate: $50\,mg/m^2$ daily to effect or $80\,mg/kg$ every 3 days	Myelosuppression
Mitotane *Action*: o,p'DDD is a derivative of the chlorinated hydrocarbon insecticides. It causes destruction of the zona fasiculata and reticularis of the adrenal cortex, through actions on cytochrome P_{450} dependent enzymes in adrenocortical cells.	Hyperadrenocorticism $50\,mg/kg$ daily to effect then weekly	Nausea, vomiting Hypoadrenocorticism

III   BODY WEIGHT: SURFACE AREA CONVERSIONS

Table for conversion of body weight to surface area (dogs).			
kg	M^2	kg	M^2
0.5	0.06	26.0	0.88
1.0	0.10	27.0	0.90
2.0	0.15	28.0	0.92
3.0	0.20	29.0	0.94
4.0	0.25	30.0	0.96
5.0	0.29	31.0	0.99
6.0	0.33	32.0	1.01
7.0	0.36	33.0	1.03
8.0	0.40	34.0	1.05
9.0	0.43	35.0	1.07
10.0	0.46	36.0	1.09
11.0	0.49	37.0	1.11
12.0	0.52	38.0	1.13
13.0	0.55	39.0	1.15
14.0	0.58	40.0	1.17
15.0	0.60	41.0	1.19
16.0	0.63	42.0	1.21
17.0	0.66	43.0	1.23
18.0	0.69	44.0	1.25
19.0	0.71	45.0	1.26
20.0	0.74	46.0	1.28
21.0	0.76	47.0	1.30
22.0	0.78	48.0	1.32
23.0	0.81	49.0	1.34
24.0	0.83	50.0	1.36
25.0	0.85		

Table for conversion of body weight to surface area (cats).			
kg	M^2	kg	M^2
2.0	0.159	3.6	0.235
2.2	0.169	3.8	0.244
2.4	0.179	4.0	0.252
2.6	0.189	4.2	0.260
2.8	0.199	4.4	0.269
3.0	0.208	4.6	0.277
3.2	0.217	4.8	0.285
3.4	0.226	5.0	0.292

IV PROTOCOLS FOR ADMINISTRATION OF DOXORUBICIN AND CISPLATIN

Doxorubicin administration

(1) Calculate required dose of drug according to body weight:surface area conversion. Usual dose = 30 mg/m^2.
(2) Reconstitute doxorubicin according to manufacturer's instructions with water for injection or with saline, ideally in biological safety cabinet. Load drug into syringe for administration. *NB*: Gloves, face mask and protective clothing should be used.
(3) Place an intravenous catheter into the cephalic vein and tape firmly in place, making sure it is patent and flushes easily with saline. Connect 500 ml 0.9% saline via giving set and luer locking three-way tap.
(4) Pre-medicate with anti-histamine, e.g. chlorpheniramine.
(5) Set saline to fast drip rate and administer the doxorubicin into the side port of the giving set over a 20–30 minute period, monitoring heart rate and rhythm, integrity of vein and observing for any adverse reactions. Discontinue the infusion if any problems occur.
(6) Flush through the catheter and distal end of the giving set with saline prior to disconnecting. Dispose of the bag, giving set, catheter and all other contaminated materials as cytotoxic waste, i.e. double bag and destroy by high temperature incineration.
(7) Continue to monitor the patient for the next 30–60 minutes for any delayed reaction.

NB: Gloves and face protection should be worn at all times and great care should be taken not to spill any doxorubicin or contaminate work surfaces
In the event of extravasation of doxorubicin or epirubicin the following action is recommended:
Infiltrate the area with 2–5 ml 2.1% sodium bicarbonate, leave for 2 min and aspirate off. Paint DMSO topically to the extravasated area, 2-hourly. Apply hydrocortisone cream and cold compresses.

Cisplatin administration

(for actual protocols see Chapter 6, Table 6.4)
(1) Check haematology and renal function (BUN/creatinine).
(2) Calculate required dose of drug according to body weight:surface area conversion – usual dose = 70 mg/m^2.
(3) Place an intravenous catheter into the cephalic vein and tape firmly in place, making sure it is patent and flushes easily with saline.
(4) Calculate required volume of saline per hour and drip rate necessary to administer it. Connect up bag of 0.9% saline, and administer subsequent bags as needed. Monitor urine production – allow plenty of opportunities to urinate.
(5) If using mannitol, add required volume to a 500 ml bag of saline (empty some saline out of bag first to allow for extra volume) and change drip to this bag, approximately 30 minutes before cisplatin is due.
(6) Add required dose of cisplatin to a 500 ml bag of saline (empty some saline out of bag first). *NB*: Face mask, gloves, eye protection and over-clothing should be used.
(7) Pre-medicate with anti-emetic, e.g. metoclopramide (1 mg/kg im) and then connect cisplatin bag. Infuse slowly over 15–30 minutes.
(8) Disconnect cisplatin bag and dispose of carefully as cytotoxic waste. Reconnect 0.9% saline and complete infusion protocol.

NB: All urine should be regarded as contaminated for 24 hours after administration and protective clothing and gloves should be worn to handle the patient during this period.
In the event of extravasation of cisplatin the following action is recommended:
Infiltrate the area with 2–5 ml of 3% sodium thiosulphate, aspirate off. Give 1500 units hyaluronidase around the area and apply heat and compression.

In the event of extravasation of vincristine or vinblastine the following action is recommended:
Infiltrate the area with 1500 units of hyaluronidase and apply heat and compression.

V   GLOSSARY OF DRUGS AND DOSAGES INCLUDED IN TEXT

* Signifies human medicinal product not licensed for veterinary use.

Alendronate (Fosamax™) POM*

Forms: Oral 10 mg tablet.
Dose: Dogs: 10 mg q 24 hours po.

Bismuth subsalicylate (PeptoBismol™) GSL*

Actions: Cytoprotectant and anti-inflammatory actions on GIT
Indications: Prevention/treatment of doxorubicin induced enterocolitis.
Form: Oral suspension.
Dose: 3–15 ml po q 6–8 hours.

Bisphosphonates

Action: Bisphosphonates are adsorbed onto hydroxyapatite crystals, slowing their rate of formation and dissolution.
Indications: Used for symptomatic treatment of hypercalcaemia, when other therapies are not effective. (Possible palliative role in treatment of bone tumours.)

Bromocriptine (Bromocriptine, Parodel™) POM*

Action: Dopamine agonist which inhibits release of prolactin and growth hormone by the pituitary gland.
Indications: Has been used in the management of pituitary-dependent hyperadrenocorticism (PDH) in dogs, although not very effective. Possible use for counteracting excess growth hormone in acromegaly in cats, again not very effective.
Forms: Oral: 1 mg, 2.5 mg tablets, 5 mg, 10 mg capsules.
Dose: PDH in dogs: 0.05 mg/kg po every 12 hours.

Butorphanol (Torbugesic™, Torbutrol™) POM

Action: Mixed agonist/antagonist opioid with medium duration of action.

Indications: Potent antitussive. Suppression of mild to moderate pain.
Forms: Injectable 10 mg/ml solution, oral 1 mg, 5 mg, 10 mg tablets.
Dose: For analgesia: Dogs: 0.3–0.4 mg/kg iv, im, sc, q 6–8 hours
                          Cats: 0.05–0.6 mg/kg im, sc q 6–8 hours.

Cabergoline (Galastop™) POM

Action: Ergoline derivative with potent and selective inhibitory effect on prolactin secretion.
Indications: Treatment of pseudopregnancy in bitches and termination of lactation.
Forms: Oral: aqueous solution, 50 µg/ml.
Dose: Bitches for pseudopregnancy: 5 µg/kg po every 24 hours for 4–6 days.

Calcium carbonate (Canovel™ calcium tablets) GSL

Indications: Calcium supplementation, also used as intestinal phosphate binder to reduce phosphate absorption in patients with renal failure and as an antacid.
Forms: Oral: 420 mg calcium carbonate tablet.
Dose: Dogs and cats: 20–100 mg/kg po q 8 hours.

Carbimazole (Neo-Mercazole™) POM*

Action: Carbimazole is metabolised to the active drug methimazole which intereferes with the synthesis of thyroid hormones.
Indications: To control thyroid hormone levels in cats with hyperthyroidism.
Forms: Oral: 5 mg tablet.
Dose: 5 mg/cat po every 8 hours.

Chlorpheniramine (Piriton™) P*

Action: Antihistamine H_1 antagonist.
Indications: Used in the management/prevention of allergies and anaphylactic reactions.
Forms: Injectable 10 mg/ml solution
              Oral: 4 gm tablet, 2 mg/5 ml oral syrup.
Dose: Dogs: Small – medium 2.5–5 mg im q 12 hours (or as premedication)

Medium – large 5–10 mg im q 12
hours (or as premedication)
(Cats: 2–4 mg/cat po q 8–12 hours).
Note: Maximum recommended dose is 0.5 mg/kg
q 12 hours in both cats and dogs.

Cimetidine (Tagamet™) POM*

Action: Histamine (H$_2$) receptor antagonist.
Indications: Prevention   and   management   of
gastric and duodenal ulceration.
Forms: Injectable: 100 mg/ml solution.
Intravenous infusion: 4 mg/ml in NaCl.
Oral: 200 mg,   400 mg,   800 mg   tablets,
40 mg/ml syrup.
Dose: Dogs: 5–10 mg/kg iv, im, po q 6–8 hours.
Cats: 2.5–5 mg/kg iv, im, po q 8–12 hours.
Note: Retards oxidative hepatic drug metabolism
by binding to P450. This may increase the plasma
levels of some drugs and could exacerbate side-
effects such as leucopenia.

Clodronate (Bonefos™, Loron™) POM*

Forms: Injectable 30 mg/ml, 60 mg/ml, oral 400 mg
capsule.
Dose: Dogs: 5–14 mg/kg q 24 hours iv. or 10–30
mg/kg q 8–12 hours po.

Cyproheptadine (Periactin™) P*

Action: Antihistamine and serotonin antagonist.
Indications: Various indications described including symptomatic relief in cases of allergic skin
disease. Used in oncological patients as an
appetite stimulant.
Forms: Oral: 4 mg tablet.
Dose: For appetite stimulation: cats and dogs:
0.1–0.5 mg/kg po q 8–12 hours.
Deoxycortone acetate/pivalate

Deoxycortone acetate/pivalate

Action: Steroid secreted by the adrenal cortex
which has primarily mineralocorticoid activity
and no significant glucocortioid action.
Indications: Treatment of adrenal insufficiency.
Forms: Solution for injection.
Dose: Dogs: starting dose of 2.2 mg/kg by deep im
injection every 4 weeks.

Desmopressin (DDAVP) POM*

Action: Analogue of vasopressin.
Indications: Diagnosis and treatment of central
diabetes insipidus.
Forms: Intranasal drops: 100 mg/ml solution
(for topical use).
Injectable: 4 mg/ml solution.
Dose: For treatment of diabetes insipidus
Cats: 5 mg/cat topically onto the
conjunctiva every 8–24 hours
Dogs: 5–40 mg/dog topically onto the
conjunctiva every 8–24 hours.

Diazoxide (Eudemine™) POM*

Actions: Benzothiazide   diuretic   which   also
inhibits insulin secretion by blocking calcium
mobilisation.
Indications: In   the   management   of   hypoglycaemia associated with insulinoma.
Forms: Oral 50 mg tablet.
Dose: Dogs: hypoglycaemia: 3.3 mg/kg po every 8
hours, increasing to 20 mg/kg po every 8 hours.

Dihydrotachysterol

Action: Vitamin D analogue, influences calcium
and   phosphorus   metabolism.   Raises   serum
calcium within 1–7 days.
Indications: Hypocalcaemia.
Forms: Oral: 0.25 mg/ml aqueous liquid.
Dose: 0.01–0.03 mg/kg po every 24 hours initially
then   0.01–0.02 mg/kg   every   24–48 hours   for
maintenance.

Dimethylsulphoxide (DMSO) POM*

Actions: Various pharmacological actions including free radical scavenging, membrane stabilisation, analgesia and anti-inflammatory actions.
Indications: Various but including topical use in
the management of cyclophosphamide induced
haemorrhagic cystitis.
Forms: 50%, 90% liquid.
Dose: For topical application to urinary bladder.
10 ml of 50% solution, diluted in equal volume
of sterile water, instilled into bladder for 20
minutes. Repeat at weekly intervals if necessary.
Notes: Solution is very hygroscopic and should be

kept in tightly closed container. DMSO is rapidly absorbed through intact skin; handle with care and wear gloves. Do not mix with potentially toxic compounds as DMSO may promote their systemic absorption.

Edrophonium chloride (Edrophonium, Camsilon™) POM*

Actions: Rapid and short-acting anticholinesterase drug.
Indications: In the diagnosis of myasthenia gravis.
Forms: Injectable: 10 mg/ml solution.
Dose: Dogs: 0.11–0.22 mg/kg iv
Cats: 2.5 mg/cat iv
Improvement should be noted within 30 seconds and wane within 5 minutes.
Note: Atropine should be available (0.05 mg/kg) to control cholinergic side-effects.

Etidronate (Didronel™) POM*

Forms: Injectable 50 mg/ml, 60 mg/ml, oral 200 mg tablet.
Dose: Dogs: 7.5 mg/kg q 24 hours iv for 3 days or 20 mg/kg q 24 hours po. (?Efficacy of oral route.)

G-CSF: Filgrastim (Neupogen) POM, Lenograstim (Granocyte) POM*

Actions: Human recombinant granulocyte colony stimulating factors (rHuG-CSF), stimulates granulocyte production.
Indications: Management of chemotherapy-induced neutropenia, neutrophil counts rise within 24 hours of treatment.
Forms: Filgrastim: Injectable: 300 μg/ml (30 million units per ml) solution.
Lenograstim: Injectable 263 μg powder in vial for reconstitution.
Dose: Filgrastim: Cats, dogs: 5–20 μg/kg sc q 12–24 hours for 1–2 weeks.
Lenograstim: Cats, dogs; insufficient information.

Fludrocortisone acetate (Florinef™) POM*

Actions: Mineralocorticoid with weak glucocorticoid activity.
Indications: Treatment of hypoadrenocorticism.

Forms: Oral: 0.1 mg tablet.
Dose: Dogs and cats start at 0.01 mg/kg po every 24 hours. Monitor sodium and potassium levels and adjust dose accordingly.

Frusemide (Diuride™, Frusecare™, Lasix™) POM

Actions: 'Loop diuretic', inhibits reabsorption of chloride and sodium in the ascending loop of Henle and thus promotes naturesis and reduces water reabsorption.
Indications: Diuresis, e.g. hypercalcuric nephropathy.
Forms: Injectable: 50 mg/ml solution
Oral: 20 mg, 40 mg, 1 g tablets.
Dose: Standard dose 2 mg/kg po q 8–12 hours. For hypercalcaemic nephropathy may give up to 5 mg/kg bolus iv then begin 5 mg/kg/hour infusion. Maintain hydration and electrolyte balance with normal saline and added KCl. Monitor urine output and calcium.
Note: Ensure patient is hydrated before therapy.

Isotretinoin (Roaccutane™)* (Hospital only)

Acitretin (Neotigason™)* (Hospital only)

Action: Vitamin A derivatives used in treatment of severe acne in human patients.
Indications: Possible therapeutic benefit in treatment of epitheliotrophic lymphoma.
Forms: 5 mg, 25 mg capsules.
Dose: Isotretinoin: 1.7–3.7 mg/kg po daily
Acitretin: 0.7–1.0 mg/kg po daily.
Note: These agents are teratogenic and will only be supplied on a named patient basis.

Ketoconazole (Nizoral™) POM*

Actions: Broad spectrum imidazole antifungal agent. Also inhibits cytochrome P450 dependent enzymes which results in decreased synthesis of adrenal and gonadal steroids.
Indications: In addition to antifungal properties, has been used in the treatment of hyperadrenocorticism (HAC) in dogs.
Forms: Oral: 200 mg tablet, 100 ml, 5 ml oral suspension.
Dose: Dogs: for HAC 5 mg/kg po every 12 hours

for 7 days increasing to 10 mg/kg q 12 hours if no adverse effects seen.

Lithium carbonate (Camcolit) POM*

Actions: Stimulates bone marrow stem cells.
Indications: May be of value in the treatment of cytotoxic drug-induced myelosuppression, aplastic anaemia, cyclic haematopoiesis.
Forms: Oral: 250 mg, 400 mg tablets.
Dose: Dogs: 10 mg/kg po q 12 hours.
Note: Avoid concurrent use with diuretics, NSAIDs, ACE inhibitors and calcium channel blockers.

Medroxyprogesterone acetate (Promone-E™, Perlutex™) POM

Actions: Long acting progestogen.
Indications: Various including control of oestrus in queen and bitch, management of prostatic hypertrophy, treatment of feline miliary dermatitis.
Forms: Injectable: 25 mg/ml, 50 mg/ml suspension
Oral: 5 mg tablet.
Dose: Depends on indication. For prostatic hypertrophy in dogs 50–100 mg/dog sc every 3–6 months.

Megoestrol acetate (Ovarid™) POM

Actions: Oral progestagen.
Indications: Prevention and postponement of oestrus in the bitch and queen and management of pseudopregnancy. ?Treatment of oestrogen-dependent mammary tumours.
Forms: Oral: 5 mg, 20 mg tablets.
Dose: Depends on indication.

Metoclopramide (Emequell™, Maxalon*) POM

Actions: Anti-emetic and upper GI tract stimulant. Inhibits vomiting by blocking dopamine at the chemoreceptor trigger zone, also inhibits the vomiting reflex peripherally by: increasing oesophageal sphincter pressure, gastric tone and contractions and peristaltic activity in the upper small intestine and by relaxing the pyloric sphincter.
Indications: Treatment/prevention of vomiting.

Forms: Injectable: 5 mg/ml solution
Oral: 10 mg tablet (Emequell), 1 mg/ml syrup (Maxalon).
Dose: Cats and dogs: 0.5–1 mg/kg im, sc po q 6–8 hours, or 1–2 mg/kg as a slow iv infusion over 24 hours.
Note: May cause sedation, extrapyramidal effects and changes in behaviour especially if administered iv. Also reduces renal blood flow which may exacerbate pre-existing renal disease (see cisplatin administration).

Metyrapone (Metopirone) POM*

Action: Reduces cortisol synthesis by competitive inhibition of 11b-hydroxylation, thereby blocking the conversion of 11-deoxycortisol to cortisol.
Indication: In humans may be used as a test of anterior pituitary function. May have a role in the medical management of hyperadrenocorticism in cats (see text).
Forms: Oral: 250 mg capsules.
Dose: Cats: 65 mg/kg every 8–12 hours.

Note: Potential side-effects include, depression, tremors, ataxia, hypocortisolaemia.

Octreotide (Sandostatin™) POM*

Action: Somatostatin analogue.
Indications: To decrease growth hormone levels in acromegaly. Also inhibits secretion of insulin by normal and neoplastic cells and thus may be useful in the management of insulinoma.
Forms: Injectable: 50, 200, 500 ug/ml solution.
Dose: 1 μg/kg sc q 8 hours. Information on the use of this drug in cats and dogs is limited.

Omeprazole (Losec™) POM*

Actions: Proton pump inhibitor, potent inhibitor of gastric acid secretion.
Indications: Treatment of gastric hyperacidity and ulceration, especially associated with gastrin producing tumours (gastrinoma) and mast cell tumours.
Forms: Oral 10 mg, 20 mg, 40 mg capsules.
Dose: Dogs: 0.5–1.5 mg/kg po every 24 hours.

Ondansetron (Zofran™) POM*

Actions: $5HT_3$ antagonist.
Indications: Prevention and treatment of radiation or chemotherapy induced emesis.

Forms: Injection 2 mg/ml
Oral: 4 mg, 8 mg tablets (very expensive), syrup 4 mg/5 ml (Suppositories: 16 mg).
Dose: 0.1 mg/kg iv immediately before chemotherapy and every 6 hours thereafter.

Pamidronate (Aredia™) POM*

Forms: Injectable 50 mg/ml, 60 mg/vial, powder for reconstitution.
Dose: Dogs: 0.9–1.3 mg/kg infusion over 24 hours, once.
Notes: Adverse effects may include: nausea, vomiting, hypocalaemia, hypophosphataemia, hypomagnesaemia and hypersensitivity reactions.

Phenoxybenzamine (Dibenyline) POM*

Actions: Alpha adrenergic blocker.
Indications: In the treatment of hypertension in animals with phaeochromocytoma prior to surgery (in conjunction with a beta blocker). Also used for treatment of reflex dyssynergia.
Forms: Oral 10 mg capsule.
Dose: Dogs: hypertension associated with phaeochromocytoma: 0.2–1.5 mg/kg po every 12 hours, starting at a low dosage and increasing until the hypertension is controlled.
Note: Should be used in conjunction with a beta blocker for treatment of phaeochromocytoma to avoid possible hypertensive crisis.

Piroxicam POM*

Actions: NSAID which inhibits cyclo-oxygenase-1. Anti-inflammatory, antipyretic and analgesic effects.
Indications: In addition to standard NSAID effects, piroxicam has been used for palliative treatment of transitional cell carcinoma of the canine urinary bladder.
Forms: Oral 10 mg, 20 mg capsules.
Dose: Dogs: 0.3 mg/kg po q 24 hours.
Note: Possible gastro-intestinal and renal toxicity.

Propantheline bromide (Pro-Banthine) POM*

Actions: Anti-muscarinic, anti-cholinergic agent.
Indications: Various including, peripherally acting anti-emetic and antispasmodic.

Forms: Oral: 15 mg tablet.
Dose: GI indications: 0.25 mg/kg po q 8–12 hours.

Propranolol (Inderal, Propranolol) POM*

Actions: Beta adrenoceptor antagonist, antagonises chronotropic and inotropic effects of beta 1 adrenoceptors on the heart and blocks vasodilatory actions of beta 2 adrenoceptors.
Indications: In the treatment of cardiac arrhythmias and tachycardia, hypertension, and to reduce some of the cardiac effects of hyperthyroidism prior to surgery.
Forms: Oral 10 mg, 40 mg, 80 mg, 160 mg tablets.
Dose: Cats: 2.5–5 mg/cat po every 8 hours.

Pyridostigmine (Mestinon) POM*

Actions: Long acting anticholinesterase agent.
Indications: Used in the treatment of myasthenia gravis.
Forms: Oral 60 mg tablets.
Dose: Dogs: 0.2–5 mg/kg po every 8–12 hours.
Note: May cause cholinergic effects necessitating dose reduction.

Ranitidine (Zantac™) POM*

Action: Histamine (H_2) receptor antagonist.
Indications: Prevention and management of gastric and duodenal ulceration.
Forms: Injectable: 25 mg/ml solution.
Oral: 150 mg, 300 mg tablets, 12.5 mg/ml syrup.
Dose: Dogs: Ranitidine: 2 mg/kg slow iv sc po q 8–12 hours.
Cats: Ranitidine: 2 mg/kg/day constant iv infusion, 2.5 mg/kg slow iv q 12 hours, 3.5 mg/kg po q 12 hours.
Note: Retards oxidative hepatic drug metabolism by binding to P450. This may increase the plasma levels of some drugs and could exacerbate side-effects such as leucopenia.

Sucralfate (Antepsin™) POM*

Actions: Complex of aluminium hydroxide and sulphated sucrose, binds to proteinaceous exudate in GI tract thus protecting against further erosion. Also stimulates mucosal defences and repair mechanisms.

Indications: Oesophageal, gastric and duodenal ulceration.
Forms: Oral: 1 g tablet, 0.2 g/ml suspension.
Dose: Cats: 250 mg/cat po q 8–12 hours.
  Dogs: <20 kg, 500 mg/dog po q 6–8 hours, >20 kg 1–2 g/dog po q 6–8 hours.
Note: Sucralfate may decrease bioavailability of H_2 antagonists and interfere with absorption of fluoroquinolones.

Tamoxifen (Tamoxifen, Nolvadex™) POM*

Action: Tamoxifen is an oestrogen receptor antagonist.
Indications: Adjuvant, hormonal treatment for breast cancer in post-menopausal women at high risk of metastatic disease following surgical management of primary tumour. Efficacy of this drug in bitches is unproven (see Chapter 12).
Forms: 10 mg, 20 mg and 40 mg tablets.
Dose: Women: 20 mg daily
  Therapeutic dose not established in the bitch.

Tetracosactrin (ACTH) (Synacthen) POM*

Action: Analogue of adrenocorticotrophic hormone (ACTH).
Indications: Used to stimulate cortisol production for the diagnosis of hyperadrenocorticism.
Forms: Injectable: 0.25 mg/ml solution.
Dose: Cats and dogs < 5 kg body weight, 0.125 mg iv. Dogs > 5 kg body weight 0.25 mg iv.

For further details on ACTH stimulation test and interpretation of results see texts on endocrinology.

Thyroxine (L-thyroxine, soloxine) POM

Action: Levothyroxine is a synthetic form of thyroxine.
Indications: Hypothyroidism
Forms: Oral: 0.05 mg, 0.1 mg, 0.2 mg, 0.3 mg, 0.5 mg, 0.8 mg tablets.
Dose: Cats and dogs, 0.02–0.04 mg/kg/day po. Monitor serum T4 levels.

Index